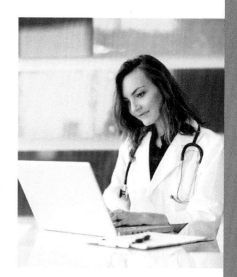

Sarcoidosis

Editors

ROBERT P. BAUGHMAN
DANIEL A. CULVER

CLINICS IN CHEST MEDICINE

www.chestmed.theclinics.com

December 2015 • Volume 36 • Number 4

ELSEVIER

1600 John F. Kennedy Boulevard • Suite 1800 • Philadelphia, Pennsylvania, 19103-2899

http://www.theclinics.com

CLINICS IN CHEST MEDICINE Volume 36, Number 4
December 2015 ISSN 0272-5231, ISBN-13: 978-0-323-40240-8

Editor: Patrick Manley
Developmental Editor: Casey Jackson

Clinics in Chest Medicine (ISSN 0272-5231) is published quarterly by Elsevier Inc., 360 Park Avenue South, New York, NY 10010-1710. Months of issue are March, June, September, and December. Periodicals postage paid at New York, NY and additional mailing offices. Subscription prices are $345.00 per year (domestic individuals), $556.00 per year (domestic institutions), $165.00 per year (domestic students/residents), $380.00 per year (Canadian individuals), $690.00 per year (Canadian institutions), $470.00 per year (international individuals), $690.00 per year (international institutions), and $230.00 per year (international and Canadian students/residents). International air speed delivery is included in all Clinics subscription prices. All prices are subject to change without notice. **POSTMASTER:** Send address changes to Clinics in Chest Medicine, Elsevier Health Sciences Division, Subscription Customer Service, 3251 Riverport Lane, Maryland Heights, MO 63043. **Customer Service: Telephone: 1-800-654-2452** (U.S. and Canada); **1-314-447-8871** (outside U.S. and Canada). **Fax: 1-314-447-8029. E-mail: journalscustomerservice-usa@elsevier.com (for print support); journalsonlinesupport-usa@elsevier.com (for online support).**

Reprints. For copies of 100 or more of articles in this publication, please contact the Commercial Reprints Department, Elsevier Inc., 360 Park Avenue South, New York, NY 10010-1710. Tel.: 212-633-3874; Fax: 212-633-3820; E-mail: reprints@elsevier.com.

Clinics in Chest Medicine is covered in *MEDLINE/PubMed (Index Medicus), Current Contents/Clinical Medicine, EMBASE/Excerpta Medica, Science Citation Index,* and *ISI/BIOMED.*

Contributors

EDITORS

ROBERT P. BAUGHMAN, MD
Professor, Department of Medicine, University of Cincinnati Medical Center, Cincinnati, Ohio

DANIEL A. CULVER, DO
Department of Pulmonary Medicine, Respiratory Institute; Department of Pathobiology, Lerner Research Institute, Cleveland Clinic, Cleveland, Ohio

AUTHORS

ROBERT P. BAUGHMAN, MD
Department of Medicine, University of Cincinnati, Cincinnati, Ohio

ROB S.B. BEANLANDS, MD
Division of Cardiology, University of Ottawa Heart Institute, Ottawa, Ontario, Canada

JEFFREY S. BERMAN, MD
Professor of Medicine and Director, Sarcoidosis Center, Boston University Medical Center, Boston, Massachusetts

JEAN-FRANÇOIS BERNAUDIN, MD, PhD
Assistance Publique Hôpitaux de Paris, Pathology Department, Tenon Universitary Hospital, Paris, France

DAVID BIRNIE, MD, MB ChB
Division of Cardiology, University of Ottawa Heart Institute, Ottawa, Ontario, Canada

NANCY CASANOVA, MD
Department of Medicine, Arizona Respiratory Center, University of Arizona Health Sciences Center, University of Arizona, Tucson, Arizona

LINDSAY J. CELADA, PhD
Department of Pathology, Microbiology and Immunology, Vanderbilt University School of Medicine, Nashville, Tennessee

SANTABHANU CHAKRABARTI, MBBS, MD
Division of Cardiology, Department of Medicine, University of British Columbia, Vancouver, British Columbia, Canada

DANIEL A. CULVER, DO
Department of Pulmonary Medicine, Respiratory Institute; Department of Pathobiology, Lerner Research Institute, Cleveland Clinic, Cleveland, Ohio

JOLANDA DE VRIES, MSc, PhD
ILD Care Foundation Research Team, Bennekom, The Netherlands; Department of Medical Psychology, St. Elisabeth Hospital Tilburg, Tilburg, The Netherlands; Department of Medical and Clinical Psychology, Tilburg University, Tilburg, The Netherlands

WONDER P. DRAKE, PhD
Department of Pathology, Microbiology and Immunology; Division of Infectious Diseases, Department of Medicine, Vanderbilt School of Medicine, Nashville, Tennessee

MARJOLEIN DRENT, MD, PhD
Professor of Interstitial Lung Diseases, Departments of Pharmacology and Toxicology, Faculty of Health, Medicine and Life Science, Maastricht University, Maastricht, The Netherlands; ILD Center of Excellence, St. Antonius Hospital, Nieuwegein, The Netherlands; ILD Care Foundation Research Team, Bennekom, The Netherlands

BORIS DUCHEMANN, MD
Assistance Publique Hôpitaux de Paris, Pulmonary Department, Avicenne Universitary Hospital, Bobigny, France

PETER J. ENGEL, MD
Ohio Heart and Cardiovascular Center, Christ Hospital, Cincinnati, Ohio

TASHA E. FINGERLIN, PhD
Center for Genes, Environment and Health, National Jewish Health, Denver, Colorado; Department of Biostatistics and Informatics, University of Colorado, Aurora, Colorado

OLIVIA FREYNET, MD
Assistance Publique Hôpitaux de Paris, Pulmonary Department, Avicenne Universitary Hospital, Bobigny, France

JOE G.N. GARCIA, MD
Senior Vice President for Health Sciences, Department of Medicine, Arizona Respiratory Center, University of Arizona Health Sciences Center, University of Arizona, Tucson, Arizona

PRAVEEN GOVENDER, MB BCh
Assistant Professor of Medicine and Associate Director, Sarcoidosis Center, Boston University Medical Center, Boston, Massachusetts

JAN C. GRUTTERS, MD, PhD
ILD Center of Excellence, St. Antonius Hospital, Utrecht, Nieuwegein, The Netherlands; Division of Heart and Lungs, University Medical Center, Utrecht, The Netherlands

LORNE J. GULA, MD, MSc
Division of Cardiology, London Health Sciences Centre, London, Ontario, Canada

ANDREW C.T. HA, MD
Department of Medicine, Peter Munk Cardiac Centre, University Health Network, University of Toronto, Toronto, Ontario, Canada

NABEEL HAMZEH, MD
Division of Environmental Occupational Health and Sciences, National Jewish Health, Denver, Colorado; Division of Pulmonary and Critical Care Sciences, Department of Medicine, School of Medicine, University of Colorado, Aurora, Colorado

CHARLENE HAWKINS, PhD
Division of Infectious Diseases, Department of Medicine, Vanderbilt University Medical School, Nashville, Tennessee

ELSKE HOITSMA, MD, PhD
ILD Care Foundation Research Team, Bennekom, The Netherlands; Department of Neurology, Alrijne Hospital, Leiden, The Netherlands

JOE JACOB, MD
Department of Radiology, Royal Brompton Hospital, London, United Kingdom

FLORENCE JENY, MD
EA2363, University Paris 13, COMUE Sorbonne-Paris-Cité; Assistance Publique Hôpitaux de Paris, Pulmonary Department, Avicenne Universitary Hospital, Bobigny, France

MARC A. JUDSON, MD
Professor, Division of Pulmonary and Critical Care Medicine, Department of Medicine, Albany Medical College, Albany, New York

MARIANNE KAMBOUCHNER, MD
Assistance Publique Hôpitaux de Paris, Pathology Department, Avicenne Universitary Hospital, Bobigny, France

RUTH G. KEIJSERS, MD, PhD
Department of Nuclear Medicine, St. Antonius Hospital, Utrecht, Nieuwegein, The Netherlands

KENNETH S. KNOX, MD
Department of Medicine, Arizona Respiratory Center, University of Arizona Health Sciences Center; Pulmonary Division, Department of Medicine, Arizona Health Sciences Center, University of Arizona, Tucson, Arizona

VASILEIOS KOURANOS, MD, MSc
Interstitial Lung Disease Unit, Royal Brompton Hospital, London, United Kingdom

JOACHIM MÜLLER-QUERNHEIM, MD
Full Professor of Medicine and Head of Department of Pneumology, University Medical Center, Freiburg, Germany

LISA A. MAIER, MD, MSPH
Division of Environmental Occupational Health and Sciences, National Jewish Health, Denver, Colorado; Division of Pulmonary and Critical Care Sciences, Department of Medicine, School of Medicine, University of Colorado, Aurora, Colorado

STEVEN NATHAN, MD
Advanced Lung Disease, INOVA Medical Care,
Falls Church, Virginia

PABLO NERY, MD
Division of Cardiology, University of Ottawa
Heart Institute, Ottawa, Ontario, Canada

HILARIO NUNES, MD, PhD
EA2363, University Paris 13, COMUE
Sorbonne-Paris-Cité; Assistance Publique
Hôpitaux de Paris, Pulmonary Department,
Avicenne Universitary Hospital, Bobigny,
France

SIRICHAI PASADHIKA, MD
Vitreoretinal and Uveitis Service, Legacy
Devers Eye Institute, Portland, Oregon

CAROLE PLANÈS, MD, PhD
EA2363, Université Paris 13, COMUE
Sorbonne-Paris-Cité; Assistance Publique
Hôpitaux de Paris, Physiology Department,
Avicenne Universitary Hospital, Bobigny,
France

MISHA ROSENBACH, MD
Department of Dermatology, University of
Pennsylvania, Philadelphia, Pennsylvania

JAMES T. ROSENBAUM, MD
Chief of Ophthalmology, Legacy Devers Eye
Institute, Portland, Oregon

BARNEY J. STERN, MD
Professor of Neurology; Interim Chair,
Department of Neurology, University of
Maryland School of Medicine, Baltimore,
Maryland

BERT STROOKAPPE, MSc
ILD Care Foundation Research Team,
Bennekom, The Netherlands; Department of
Physical Therapy, Gelderse Vallei Hospital
(ZGV) Ede, The Netherlands

JINNY O. TAVEE, MD
Director, Neuromuscular Fellowship Program;
Assistant Professor of Neurology,
Neuromuscular Center, Cleveland Clinic Lerner
College of Medicine, Cleveland Clinic
Foundation, Cleveland, Ohio

DOMINIQUE VALEYRE, MD
EA2363, University Paris 13, COMUE
Sorbonne-Paris-Cité; Assistance Publique
Hôpitaux de Paris, Pulmonary Department,
Avicenne Universitary Hospital, Bobigny,
France

MARCEL VELTKAMP, MD, PhD
ILD Center of Excellence, St. Antonius
Hospital, Utrecht, Nieuwegein, The
Netherlands

KAROLYN A. WANAT, MD
Departments of Dermatology and Pathology,
University of Iowa, Iowa City, Iowa

ATHOL U. WELLS, MD, PhD
Consultant Physician, Interstitial Lung Disease
Unit, Royal Brompton Hospital, London, United
Kingdom

MARLIES S. WIJSENBEEK, MD, PhD
Department of Pulmonary Medicine,
Erasmus Medical Center, University Medical
Center Rotterdam, Rotterdam, Netherlands

TONG ZHOU, PhD
Department of Medicine, Arizona Respiratory
Center, University of Arizona Health Sciences
Center, University of Arizona, Tucson, Arizona

GERNOT ZISSEL, PhD
Department of Pneumology, Center for
Medicine, Medical Center, University of
Freiburg, Freiburg, Germany

Contents

> Current hypotheses on the pathogenesis of sarcoidosis assume that it is induced by a nondegradable antigen inducing immune reactions, which are mediated by a panel of immune cells of the innate and adoptive immune system. This immune reaction leads to an accumulation of immune cells that is mainly alveolar macrophages, T cells, and neutrophils in the lung. As the antigen persists and cannot be eliminated, the ongoing immune reaction results in granuloma formation and remodeling of the lung. The current review aims to elucidate the different roles of the cellular players in the immunopathogenesis of sarcoidosis.

> Sarcoidosis is a granulomatous disease of unknown etiology, most commonly involving the lung, skin, lymph node, and eyes. Molecular and immunologic studies continue to strengthen the association of sarcoidosis with infectious antigens. Independent studies report the presence of microbial nucleic acids and proteins within sarcoidosis specimens. Complementary immunologic studies also support the role of infectious agents in sarcoidosis pathogenesis. Case reports and clinical trials have emerged regarding the efficacy of antimicrobials. They support increasing efforts to identify novel therapeutics, such as antimicrobials, that will have an impact on the observed increase in sarcoidosis morbidity and mortality.

> Sarcoidosis is a disease with highly variable presentation and progression. Although it is hypothesized that disease phenotype is related to genetic variation, how much of this variability is driven by genetic factors is not known. The HLA region is the most strongly and consistently associated genetic risk factor for sarcoidosis, supporting the notion that sarcoidosis is an exposure-mediated immunologic disease. Most of the genetic etiology of sarcoidosis remains unknown in terms of the specific variants that increase risk in various populations, their biologic functions, and how they interact with environmental exposures.

> Sarcoidosis is a diagnosis of exclusion; there exists neither a pathognomonic clinical feature nor a perfect diagnostic test. Missed diagnosis and overdiagnosis are common. A careful history and physical examination look for "footprints" of sarcoidosis or features suggesting alternative diagnoses. Some presentations are classic and do not require tissue confirmation. A tissue biopsy should be performed if doubt exists.

Sampling intrathoracic disease by transbronchial or ultrasound-guided biopsy of mediastinal lymph nodes provide high diagnostic yield with low complication rates. Even with tissue confirmation, diagnosis is never secure and follow-up is required to be fully confident of the diagnosis.

Chest imaging has a central role in the diagnosis and monitoring of sarcoidosis. For staging of pulmonary disease on chest radiograph. Scadding stages are still widely used. High-resolution CT (HRCT), however, is more accurate in visualizing the various manifestations of pulmonary sarcoidosis as well its complications. A generally accepted HRCT scoring system is lacking. Fluorodeoxyglucose F 18 positron emission tomography can visualize disease activity better than conventional makers in a significant proportion of patients. In patients with extensive changes on HRCT but no parenchymal fluorodeoxyglucose F 18 uptake, prudence with regard to initiation or intensification of immunosuppressive treatment is warranted.

This article briefly reviews conventional biomarkers used clinically to (1) support a diagnosis and (2) monitor disease progression in patients with sarcoidosis. Potential new biomarkers identified by genome-wide screening and the approaches to discover these biomarkers are described.

Sarcoidosis is a systemic disease, with lung involvement in almost all cases. Abnormal chest radiography is usually a key step for considering diagnosis. Lung impact is investigated through imaging, pulmonary function, and, when required, 6-minute walk test, cardiopulmonary exercise testing, or right heart catheterization. There is usually a reduction of lung volumes, and forced vital capacity is the most accurate parameter to reflect the impact of pulmonary sarcoidosis with or without pulmonary infiltration at imaging. Various evolution patterns have been described. Increased risk of death is associated with advanced pulmonary fibrosis or cor pulmonale, particularly in African-American patients.

Neurosarcoidosis is known as the great mimicker and may appear similar to lymphoma, multiple sclerosis, and other diseases affecting the nervous system. Although definitive diagnosis requires histologic confirmation of the affected neural tissue, characteristic clinical manifestations, gadolinium-enhanced MRI patterns and specific cerebrospinal fluid findings can help support the diagnosis in the absence of neural biopsy. An understanding of the common clinical presentations and diagnostic findings is central to the evaluation and management of neurosarcoidosis.

Cardiac Sarcoidosis   657

David Birnie, Andrew C.T. Ha, Lorne J. Gula, Santabhanu Chakrabarti, Rob S.B. Beanlands, and
Pablo Nery

> Studies suggest clinically manifest cardiac involvement occurs in 5% of patients
> with pulmonary/systemic sarcoidosis. The principal manifestations of cardiac
> sarcoidosis (CS) are conduction abnormalities, ventricular arrhythmias, and heart
> failure. Data indicate that a 20% to 25% of patients with pulmonary/systemic
> sarcoidosis have asymptomatic (clinically silent) cardiac involvement. An interna-
> tional guideline for the diagnosis and management of CS recommends that patients
> be screened for cardiac involvement. Most studies suggest a benign prognosis for
> patients with clinically silent CS. Immunosuppression therapy is advocated for clin-
> ically manifest CS. Device therapy, with implantable cardioverter defibrillators, is
> recommended for some patients.

Ocular Sarcoidosis   669

Sirichai Pasadhika and James T. Rosenbaum

> Sarcoidosis is one of the leading causes of inflammatory eye disease. Ocular
> sarcoidosis can involve any part of the eye and its adnexal tissues and may cause
> uveitis, episcleritis/scleritis, eyelid abnormalities, conjunctival granuloma, optic neu-
> ropathy, lacrimal gland enlargement, and orbital inflammation. Glaucoma and cata-
> ract can be complications from inflammation itself or adverse effects from therapy.
> Ophthalmic manifestations can be isolated or associated with other organ involve-
> ment. Patients with ocular sarcoidosis can present with a wide range of clinical pre-
> sentations and severity. Multidisciplinary approaches are required to achieve the
> best treatment outcomes for both ocular and systemic manifestations.

Cutaneous Sarcoidosis   685

Karolyn A. Wanat and Misha Rosenbach

> The skin is the second most common organ affected in sarcoidosis, which can affect
> patients of all ages and races, with African-American women having the highest
> rates of sarcoidosis in the United States. The cutaneous manifestations are protean
> and can reflect involvement of sarcoidal granulomas within the lesion or represent
> reactive non-specific inflammation, as seen with erythema nodosum. Systemic
> work-up is necessary in any patient with cutaneous involvement of sarcoidal granu-
> lomas, and treatment depends on other organ involvement and severity of clinical
> disease. Skin-directed therapies are first line for mild disease, and immunomodula-
> tors or immunosuppressants may be necessary.

Pulmonary Hypertension in Sarcoidosis   703

Robert P. Baughman, Peter J. Engel, and Steven Nathan

> Pulmonary hypertension is a complication of sarcoidosis leading to dyspnea and
> associated with increased morbidity and mortality. Sarcoidosis-associated pulmo-
> nary hypertension (SAPH) can be due to several factors, including vascular involve-
> ment by the granulomatous inflammation, compression of the pulmonary arteries by
> adenopathy, fibrotic changes within the lung, and left ventricular diastolic dysfunc-
> tion. Several case series have suggested that some patients with SAPH benefit from
> specific therapy for pulmonary hypertension. A randomized, placebo-controlled trial
> found 16 weeks' bosentan therapy to be associated with significant improvement in
> pulmonary artery pressure. Future studies may better define who would respond to
> treatment of pulmonary hypertension.

PROGRAM OBJECTIVE

The goal of the *Clinics in Chest Medicine* is to provide practitioners with state-of-the-art information that is clinically useful, concise, well referenced, and comprehensive.

TARGET AUDIENCE

All practicing physicians and healthcare professionals who provide patient care utilizing findings from *Chest Medicine Clinics of North America*.

LEARNING OBJECTIVES

Upon completion of this activity, participants will be able to:
1. Review the genetics and players in the immunopathogenesis of sarcoidosis.
2. Discuss the manifestations of cardiac, cutaneous, nervous, and ocular sarcoidosis.
3. Recognize the treatments for and side effects of sarcoidosis, and evaluate factors in patients' quality of life.

ACCREDITATION

The Elsevier Office of Continuing Medical Education (EOCME) is accredited by the Accreditation Council for Continuing Medical Education (ACCME) to provide continuing medical education for physicians.

The EOCME designates this enduring material for a maximum of 15 *AMA PRA Category 1 Credit*(s)™. Physicians should claim only the credit commensurate with the extent of their participation in the activity.

All other health care professionals requesting continuing education credit for this enduring material will be issued a certificate of participation.

DISCLOSURE OF CONFLICTS OF INTEREST

The EOCME assesses conflict of interest with its instructors, faculty, planners, and other individuals who are in a position to control the content of CME activities. All relevant conflicts of interest that are identified are thoroughly vetted by EOCME for fair balance, scientific objectivity, and patient care recommendations. EOCME is committed to providing its learners with CME activities that promote improvements or quality in healthcare and not a specific proprietary business or a commercial interest.

The planning committee, staff, authors and editors listed below have identified no financial relationships or relationships to products or devices they or their spouse/life partner have with commercial interest related to the content of this CME activity:
Rob S.B. Beanlands, MD; Jeffrey S. Berman, MD; Jean-François Bernaudin, MD, PhD; David Birnie, MD, MB ChB; Nancy Casanova, MD; Lindsay J. Celada, PhD; Santabhanu Chakrabarti, MBBS, MD; Jolanda De Vries, MSc, PhD; Wonder P. Drake, MD; Marjolein Drent, MD, PhD; Boris Duchemann, MD; Peter J. Engel, MD; Tasha E. Fingerlin, PhD; Anjali Fortna; Olivia Freynet, MD; Joe G.N. Garcia, MD; Praveen Govender, MB BCh; Jan C. Grutters, MD, PhD; Lorne J. Gula, MD, MSc; Andrew C.T. Ha, MD; Charlene Hawkins, PhD; Elske Hoitsma, MD, PhD; Joe Jacob, MD; Florence Jeny, MD; Marianne Kambouchner, MD; R.G. Keijsers, MD, PhD; Kenneth S. Knox, MD; Vasileios Kouranos, MD, MSc; Patrick Manley; Joachim Müller-Quernheim, MD; Palani Murugesan; Pablo Nery, MD; Hilario Nunes, MD, PhD; Sirichai Pasadhika, MD; Carole Planès, MD, PhD; Misha Rosenbach, MD; Erin Scheckenbach; Bert Stookappe, MSc; Dominique Valeyre, MD; Marcel Veltkamp, MD, PhD; Karolyn A. Wanat, MD; Athol U. Wells, MD, PhD; Marlies Wijsenbeek, MD, PhD; Tong Zhou, PhD; Gernot Zissel, PhD.

The planning committee, staff, authors and editors listed below have identified financial relationships or relationships to products or devices they or their spouse/life partner have with commercial interest related to the content of this CME activity:
Robert P. Baughman, MD is on the speakers' bureau for Mallinckrodt; Bayer AG; and Genentech, Inc., is a consultant/advisor for Celgene Corporation; Mallinckrodt; Gilead; Actelion Pharmaceuticals; Johnson and Johnson Services, Inc.; and Genentech, Inc., has research support from Celgene Corporation; Mallinckrodt; Bayer AG; Gilead; Actelion Pharmaceuticals; Johnson and Johnson Services, Inc.; and Genentech, Inc. His spouse/partner has research support from Celgene Corporation; Mallinckrodt; Gilead; Actelion Pharmaceuticals; Johnson and Johnson Services, Inc.; and Genentech, Inc., has research support from Celgene Corporation; Mallinckrodt; Gilead; Actelion Pharmaceuticals; and Genentech, Inc.
Daniel A. Culver, DO is a consultant/advisor for, with research support from, Mallinckrodt.
Nabeel Hamzeh, MD is on the speakers' bureau for Mallinckrodt, receives research support from Mallinckrodt; National Institutes of Health; and Prothena Corporation plc, and his spouse/partner receives research support from National Institutes of Health.
Marc A. Judson, MD is a consultant/advisor for Mallinckrodt; Celgene Corporation; and Mitsubishi Tanabe Pharma Corporation.
Lisa A. Maier, MD, MSPH is a consultant/advisor for Novartis Pharmaceuticals Corporation and Foundation for Sarcoidosis Research, and has research support from National Institutes of Health and Janssen Global Services, LLC.
Steven Nathan, MD is on the speakers' bureau for, is a consultant/advisor for, and receives research support from, Gilead; United Therapeutics Corporation; and Bayer AG.
James T. Rosenbaum, MD is a consultant/advisor for AbbVie Inc; Xoma; Santen Pharmaceutical Co., Ltd.; sanofi-aventis U.S. LLC.; UCB, Inc.; Medimmune, LLC; UptoDate, Inc.; Eyevensys; Cavtherx; Topivert LTD; and TheraKine.
Barney J. Stern, MD receives royalties/patents from UptoDate, Inc.

Jinny O. Tavee, MD is a consultant/advisor for Araim Pharmaceuticals, Inc., and receives research support from Mallinckrodt and Araim Pharmaceuticals, Inc.

UNAPPROVED/OFF-LABEL USE DISCLOSURE

The EOCME requires CME faculty to disclose to the participants:

1. When products or procedures being discussed are off-label, unlabelled, experimental, and/or investigational (not US Food and Drug Administration [FDA] approved); and
2. Any limitations on the information presented, such as data that are preliminary or that represent ongoing research, interim analyses, and/or unsupported opinions. Faculty may discuss information about pharmaceutical agents that is outside of FDA-approved labelling. This information is intended solely for CME and is not intended to promote off-label use of these medications. If you have any questions, contact the medical affairs department of the manufacturer for the most recent pre-scribing information.

TO ENROLL

To enroll in the *Chest Medicine Clinics* Continuing Medical Education program, call customer service at 1-800-654-2452 or sign up online at http://www.theclinics.com/home/cme. The CME program is available to subscribers for an additional annual fee of USD $225.

METHOD OF PARTICIPATION

In order to claim credit, participants must complete the following:

1. Complete enrolment as indicated above.
2. Read the activity.
3. Complete the CME Test and Evaluation. Participants must achieve a score of 70% on the test. All CME Tests and Evaluations must be completed online.

CME INQUIRIES/SPECIAL NEEDS

For all CME inquiries or special needs, please contact elsevierCME@elsevier.com.

CLINICS IN CHEST MEDICINE

RELATED INTEREST

Medical Clinics of North America, Vol. 99, No. 5 (September 2015)
Comprehensive Care of the Patient with Chronic Illness
Douglas S. Paauw, *Editor*

THE CLINICS ARE AVAILABLE ONLINE!
Access your subscription at:
www.theclinics.com

CLINICS IN CHEST MEDICINE

Preface
Sarcoidosis

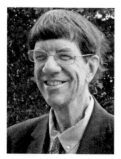
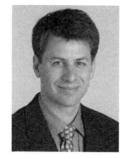

Robert P. Baughman, MD   Daniel A. Culver, DO

Editors

Sarcoidosis remains a disease of unknown etiology with a variable presentation and clinical outcome. Despite these limitations, researchers have gained valuable insights into the disease over the past five years. As editors of this issue, we asked a group of experts in this area to provide timely reviews about various aspects of the disease. We believe the authors have done a tremendous job.

We start off with Drs Zissel and Müller-Quernheim regarding the immunologic response of the disease, including the formation of the granuloma. This is followed by Dr Celada and colleagues, who give a detailed discussion of the various potential causes of sarcoidosis. This is followed by Dr Fingerlin and colleagues at National Jewish, who provide a review of what we know about the genetics of the disease.

The next portion begins with the approach to diagnosis of Drs Govender and Berman. This is followed by an article on imaging led by Drs Keijsers, Veltkamp, and Grutters. In the final article in this section, Dr Casanova and colleagues give details about how novel biomarkers in sarcoidosis may be identified using genome-based approaches.

The next set of articles contains articles on individual organs affected by sarcoidosis, including lungs (Dr Valeyre and colleagues), neurologic (Drs Tavee and Stern), cardiac (Drs Birnie and colleagues), eye (Drs Pasadhika and Rosebaum),

and skin (Drs Wanat and Rosenbach). This is followed by discussion of pulmonary hypertension (Dr Baughman, Engel, and Nathan) and severe sarcoidosis (Drs Kouranos, Jacob, and Wells). Dr Drent and colleagues discuss the consequences of sarcoidosis, while Dr Judson explains the quality-of-life assessment measures. Finally, Drs Wijsenbeek and Culver discuss general treatment strategies. Overall, this issue summarizes many aspects of sarcoidosis. We hope that you learn as much as we have about this disease.

We also want to thank Dr Richard Matthay for the opportunity to put this together and Casey Jackson for her help in compiling this issue.

Robert P. Baughman, MD
Department of Medicine
University of Cincinnati Medical Center
1001 Holmes, Eden Avenue
Cincinnati, OH 45267, USA

Daniel A. Culver, DO
Cleveland Clinic Foundation
9500 Euclid Avenue
Cleveland, OH 44195, USA

E-mail addresses:
bob.baughman@uc.edu (R.P. Baughman)
CULVERD@ccf.org (D.A. Culver)

Clin Chest Med 36 (2015) xv
http://dx.doi.org/10.1016/j.ccm.2015.09.001
0272-5231/15/$ – see front matter © 2015 Published by Elsevier Inc.

Cellular Players in the Immunopathogenesis of Sarcoidosis

Gernot Zissel, PhD, Joachim Müller-Quernheim, MD*

KEYWORDS

- Saracoidosis • Alveolar macrophage • T cells • TH1 • TH17 • Treg • Cytokines • TNF

KEY POINTS

- Granuloma induction is a coordinated immunologic response requiring the orchestrated action of different cell types.
- The coordination between these cells is regulated by cytokines with tumor necrosis factor as a mediator of high importance.
- The set of immune cells involved and the intensity of the immune reaction induced may determine acute and chronic disease.
- Granuloma induction is elicited by an environmental factor based on and shaped by the genetic background of patients.
- Although several probable sarcoidosis antigens have been identified in the recent past, a single causative, granuloma-inducing agent in sarcoidosis is still lacking.

INTRODUCTION

Every year the knowledge on mediators, receptors, and, during the last years, on genes possibly involved in sarcoidosis is growing. Nevertheless, its cause, its large variability, and the regulatory network involved remains enigmatic. This enigma indicates that, although we know some key players, our view on this disease is merely based on concepts or models than on secure knowledge of the underlying processes and pathways. The main reasons are twofold: the lack of a causal agent and the lack of a reliable animal model in sarcoidosis.

In general, the formation of granuloma requires the presence of activated T cells and macrophages embedded in a specific cytokine milieu. T cells are specifically activated by recognizing antigens with their antigen-specific T-cell receptor (TCR) presented by antigen-presenting cells (APCs). TCRs are highly specific, and the T-cell pool in sarcoidosis discloses signs of TCR enrichment; therefore, the search for a sarcoidosis antigen concentrates on a specific antigen-activating T cells. Although there was some recent progress in identifying T-cell–stimulating peptides in sarcoidosis, their origin is still elusive.

Although the T cells seem to be key players, it is generally accepted that the pathogenesis of sarcoidosis is mediated by a panel of immune reactions mediated by both the innate and the adoptive immune system. This activation is controlled by a plethora of cytokines found to be released in increased amounts by diverse immune cells and by increased expression of activation markers on the cell surface, which might also be released or shed and can be found in body fluids. This rather mechanistic view of the immune processes is shaped by regulatory and cell biological processes and defects as demonstrated by new data from genetic studies.

Department of Pneumology, Center for Medicine, Medical Center - University of Freiburg, Hugstetter Street 55, Freiburg 79106, Germany
* Corresponding author.
E-mail address: joachim.mueller-quernheim@uniklinik-freiburg.de

Clin Chest Med 36 (2015) 549–560
http://dx.doi.org/10.1016/j.ccm.2015.08.016
0272-5231/15/$ – see front matter © 2015 Elsevier Inc. All rights reserved.

From this, the immunopathogenesis of sarcoidosis is driven by a network of cells and processes of the innate and adoptive immune system and their products, which are discussed in the following article.

THE INNATE IMMUNE SYSTEM
Receptors of the Innate Immune System

Throughout the evolution, organisms had to face a potentially hostile environment and defend themselves from invading microorganisms using specialized cells equipped with structures to detect, kill, and eliminate invading microorganisms from the body. These cells are called macrophages, which can be found in all vertebrates and even in invertebrates like the fruit fly Drosophila. Cells of the innate immune system detect invading microorganisms using a set of membrane-bound or intracellular receptors called pattern recognition receptors (PRRs), including Toll-like receptors (TLRs), nucleotide-binding oligomerization domain (NOD)-like, and retinoic acid inducible gene (RIG)-I like receptors.

Microorganisms exhibit a wide range of invariable molecular patterns, which unambiguously differentiate these cells from cells of the infected host. These structures are called pathogen-associated molecular patterns (PAMPs) and summarize molecules like lipopolysaccharide (LPS), nonmethylated DNA, and others.

TLRs also recognize endogenous ligands. Because these ligands are released in association with tissue injury or trauma, the name damage-associated molecular patterns (DAMPs) or alarmins is suggested. DAMPs are rapidly released by damaged but not by apoptotic cells and may also be released by some living cells (reviewed in[1]).

In sarcoidosis, the plasma level of the S100 acute-phase molecules S100A8 (migration inhibitory factor-related protein [MRP]8, calprotectin)[2,3] and S100A9 (MRP14, calgranulin B)[4] are found to be increased and S100+ cells are involved in early phases of granuloma induction.[5] Both molecules bind to TLR4 and receptor for advanced glycation endproducts (RAGE) and are able to initiate an immune response including nuclear factor kappa B (NFκB) activation and induction of cytokine release.[6,7] Defensins are also increased in sarcoidosis[8] and might also activate the innate immune system via TLR4.[9] Peptides released by neutrophils are rich in defensins and induce tumor necrosis factor (TNF) release in alveolar macrophages from patients with active sarcoidosis but not from controls.[10] Recently it was demonstrated that serum amyloid A is found in sarcoidosis granuloma and activates NFκB via TLR2.[11]

TLR2 also influences adaptive immunity, as the blockade of TLR2 by specific antibodies downregulates T-cell recognition of the mycobacterial antigens like ESAT-6 (early secreted antigenic target 6) and the mycobacterial catalase G (mKatG).[12] It has been shown that recognition of ESAT-6 by TLR2 inhibits MyD88 activation and subsequent interleukin 12 (IL-12) release.[13]

Binding of a ligand to its specific receptor may be modulated by gene modifications. For TLR9, TLR4, or TLR2, it was reported that single nucleotide polymorphisms (SNPs) caused either diminished receptor function leading to reduced mediator production[14,15] or in contrast resulted in increased release of proinflammatory mediators.[16] Thus, TLR polymorphisms might either result in missing detection of an invading pathogen, which would normally be recognized and eradicated by the innate immune system. In this case, the microorganism escapes immune surveillance and persists in the host. In contrast, polymorphisms leading to overstimulation of the immune system the altered TLR might induce an inadequately strong immune response to a normally harmless microbe or a commensal. Thus, polymorphisms in PRRs might be linked to initiation and progress of the disease.[17–23] These differences in activated receptor expression may account for the different reactions to TLR stimulation observed in sarcoidosis.[24]

Neutrophil Granulocytes

An important player of the innate immune system is the neutrophil granulocyte (NG). NGs are attracted by chemokines like CXCL8 (Interleukin-8 [IL-8]), CXCL5 (epithelial-derived neutrophil-activating peptide 78 [ENA-78]), and others. These mediators are released by monocytes and macrophages but also after adequate stimulation by other cells, for example, alveolar epithelial cells type II.[25] Neutrophils are equipped with a variety of PRRs to detect invading microbes and, therefore, they are very effective in phagocytizing and killing these organisms. However, they also release a wide panel of proteases and reactive oxygen intermediates (ROIs), which damage the lung tissue; therefore, excessive activation of neutrophils may be harmful to the lung.

Although neutrophil accumulation inducing chemokines like IL-8 are increased in sarcoidosis, especially in patients with progressing disease or chest radiograph type II,[26–28] the percentage of neutrophils in the bronchoalveolar lavage is rather low. Interestingly, several studies found a positive correlation of CXCL8 or CXCL5 and the number or percentage of neutrophils in bronchoalveolar lavage (BAL) in idiopathic pulmonary fibrosis (IPF) but not in sarcoidosis.[27,28] Nevertheless, it was found that the increase in the percentage of neutrophils in BAL is associated with progressing disease and a significantly increased risk for the necessity for steroid therapy.[29,30]

Superoxide dismutase (SOD) from neutrophils catalyzes the generation of ROIs, which is probably responsible for tissue damage in the lung interstitium. Indeed, the proportion of carbonylated proteins in the lung is significantly higher in sarcoidosis compared with control lungs.[31] In the presence of a free radical like ROI, fatty acids (mostly arachidonic acid) are degraded into isoprostanes. These isoprostanes are markers for oxidative stress in exhaled breath condensate[32] but also exert proinflammatory activities.[33,34]

Alveolar Macrophages

There is a body of evidence indicating a fundamental role of pulmonary macrophages in the pathogenesis of sarcoidosis; for example, as multinucleated giant cells derive from (alveolar) macrophages, their number is increased in the lungs of patients with sarcoidosis and produce spontaneously mediators like TNF. Particularly TNF is thought to be the most important granuloma-promoting factor in sarcoidosis. The trigger of this increased TNF release is unknown; however, in a recent publication, Chen and colleagues[11] reported that serum amyloid A induces TNF release via TLR2 and NFκB activation. And again, these investigators found that serum amyloid A is mostly located within cells in the granuloma, which are also important in TNF production. The role of alveolar macrophages might be dual; at one side they are phagocytic cells removing debris, particles, and microorganisms without being activated and, therefore, without initiating an inflammatory response. However, once activated via PRRs by PAMPS or DAMPS, alveolar macrophages initiate a strong inflammatory response and might also mediate the transmission from the innate to the adaptive immune response by serving as costimulatory and APCs.

When the innate immune system fails to contain an infection or an antigenic structure, these microorganisms or structures have to face the second line of immune defense: the adaptive immune system. The adaptive immune system is compiled by various cell types like T cells, B cells, and APCs; their action is orchestrated by the cytokine network.

THE ADAPTIVE IMMUNE SYSTEM
Antigen-Presenting Cells

Dendritic cells
Unfortunately, there are only few data available regarding the role of dendritic cells (DCs) in the immunopathogenesis of sarcoidosis. Based on their phenotype, DCs are divided in 2 subtypes, the plasmacytoid and the myeloid dendritic cells. Plasmacytoid DCs belong to the innate immune system. They express a variety of TLRs and play an important role in immunity and secrete high amounts of interferon α (IFNα) after TLR-mediated stimulation. However, in sarcoidosis, no difference in the number of plasmacytoid DCs in BAL fluid compared with control subjects could be found.[35]

According to general views on T-cell/DC interactions, the lymphoid tissue is the preferred place where mature myeloid DCs activate naive T cells. Therefore, the lymphadenopathy associated with sarcoidosis may reflect an ongoing accumulation of APCs in hilar lymph nodes. In sarcoidosis, however, it seems that the lymph node is not the primary site of antigen recognition, as it was demonstrated that the DCs in the local lymph node are less activated than the cells in the alveoli.[36] In BAL, there are different reports available. Although most of them report no differences in the percentage of DC within the total cells recovered,[35,37] increased as well as equal absolute numbers of DCs are reported. However, the proportion of immature DCs was higher in sarcoidosis as indicated by an decreased expression of CD1a,[35] whereas others report a large heterogeneity of these DCs in sarcoidosis.[37] Reduced CD1a expression is of interest because CD1a⁻ cells are poor APCs.[38] In the peripheral blood, only a tendency to decrease the numbers of DCs was observed.[39] Although these cells did not demonstrate differences in the expression of costimulatory molecules, these cells disclose diminished stimulatory capacity compared with DCs from controls, which might be the cause for the relative anergy found in skin testing for recall antigens in patients with sarcoidosis. In recent articles, however, no differences in the mixed lymphocyte reaction stimulating capacity in peripheral myeloid dendritic cells (mDCs) could be detected.[37,40] Rather, the investigators found a diminished immunologic response of the sarcoidosis peripheral mononuclear lymphocytes to allogeneic stimuli.[40] Therefore, the definite role of DCs in sarcoidosis remains open.

Alveolar macrophages
A pivotal step in the generation of specific T-cell responses is the activation of T cells by the recognition of an antigen, a process that depends on the APC. T cells recognize antigen by their TCR only when the antigen is presented within the antigen-binding groove of a major histocompatibility complex (MHC) class II molecule. Therefore, antigen

must be ingested by the APC, inserted into the MHC molecule, and transported to its surface to be presented to T cells. For full T-cell activation, APCs have to deliver additional costimulatory signals. Thus, phagocytes acting as APCs are an important bridge between the innate and the adaptive immune system.

In sarcoidosis, an increased expression of costimulatory and adhesion molecules on alveolar macrophages from patients with sarcoidosis has been observed.[41] This altered phenotype enables these cells to act as highly efficient APCs causing proliferation of T cells, which is in contrast to control alveolar macrophages suppressing T-cell proliferation.

Vice a versa, in patients with sarcoidosis, the gene coding for butyrophilin-like 2 (BTNL2), a molecule inhibiting T-cell activation[42] and induction of regulatory T cells (Tregs),[43] contains an SNP resulting in a truncated molecule. Although there is now a dispute whether or not this SNP is in linkage disequilibrium with certain HLA molecules and might, therefore, be secondary to another disease marker, carriers of this SNP are unable to generate an intact protein. This truncated molecule is not able to insert in the cell membrane and, therefore, leads to a reduced control of T-cell activation. This SNP is significantly associated with familial and sporadic sarcoidosis in Caucasians[44,45] and to a lower extend in African Americans.[46] At least in Caucasian patients, this association could be verified in a meta-analysis.[47]

The increased expression of the molecules named earlier reflects a proinflammatory activation state of the alveolar macrophages in sarcoidosis. Macrophages can be activated in different ways. Activation of macrophages by LPS, IFNγ, or both is called classic activation. In analogy to the prototypic T-cell activation, this activation pattern is also called M1. M1 macrophages release increased amounts of proinflammatory cytokines and disclose increased expression of CD16, CD32, CD64, and costimulatory molecules. Therefore, these macrophages foster inflammatory reactions. In contrast, stimulation of macrophages with IL-4, IL-10, IL-13, or immune complexes is called alternative activation or M2 and results in the release of mediators like CCL17, CCL18, CCL22, IL-1Ra, and others.

The M1 activation seems to be fostered by the lack of expression or function of the peroxisome proliferator-activated receptor-γ (PPARγ), a nuclear receptor originally described to regulate fatty acid storage and glucose metabolism. However, it is known that PPARγ also negatively regulates the function of several immune cells, most prominently in alveolar macrophages and DC. In sarcoidosis it has been shown that PPARγ expression and function is diminished[48,49] possibly due to a polymorphism in the Peroxisome proliferator-activated receptor gamma (PPARγ) gene, which is enriched in sarcoidosis.[50] The lack of PPARγ also increases the reactivity of macrophages to granulogenic stimuli like carbon nanotubes as they induce more granuloma and M1-associated cytokines in mice lacking PPARγ compared with control mice.[51,52] Indeed, drugs targeting PPARγ have been shown to induce a shift from M1 to M2 activation pattern in macrophages.[53] Again, a loss in PPARγ expression and function renders the macrophages irresponsive to inhibiting signals. Thus, loss of function or expression of PPARγ might be a predisposing factor for granuloma induction.

T Cells

T helper 1 versus T helper 2 cells

T-cell activation is mandatory for the development of any granulomatous response. This notion is supported by the observation that T-cell depleted mice are incapable of granuloma formation.[54] Activation of T cells elicits a diverse world of T-cell subsets named T helper (TH) 1 or TH2 or by their main product, for example, TH17.[55]

TH1 cells develop in the presence of IL-12 released by macrophages and DCs. Their leading product is IFNγ, but they also release lymphotoxin, TNF, and other mediators. TH1 cells are also characterized by the expression of the transcription factor T-box expressed in T cells (T-bet). The main polarizing cytokine of TH2 cells is IL-4, which is also the main product of this subset. IL-4 is necessary for B-cell development and activation and downregulates the release of proinflammatory cytokines by macrophages and induces an alternative activation of these cells.[56] The characterizing transcription factor is GATA3. TH17 cells express the transcription factor RORγt (Retinoic acid-Related Orphan Receptor γ-T [T, thymus, where it is mostly found]); their main products are the cytokines of the IL-17-family, mainly IL-17A and IL-17F, but other mediators are also released. TH17 cells are induced by the coordinated action of IL-1, IL-6, transforming growth factor β (TGFβ), and IL-23.[57]

Most of the findings with regard to T-cell response in sarcoidosis is characteristic of a regular T-cell mediated response to antigen and is highly suggestive of the presence of one or more persistent, poorly degradable antigens. This activation induces proliferation of the T cells and increased T-cell numbers as seen in the lungs of patients with sarcoidosis.

Another possibility is a preferential homing of activated T cells to the lung. T cells activated in peripheral lymph nodes differentiate into 2 different subsets, either TH1 or TH2 cells. Initially these subsets were functionally defined as TH1 cells foster cellular immunity and TH2 cells humoral immunity. However, these subsets also express different sets of chemokine receptors; therefore, their accumulation is regulated by different chemokines. The receptors CXCR3, CCR5, and CXCR6 are preferentially expressed on TH1 cells, whereas the expression of CCR3, CCR4, and CCR8 is merely restricted to TH2 cells.[58] Activated T cells in sarcoidosis lungs release IFNγ and IL-2 and express the chemokine receptors CXCR3 and CXCR6[59]; therefore, these cells may be characterized as TH1 cells. This classification is corroborated by the demonstration of increased expression of the transcription factor T-bet, underlining the TH1 characteristics of the T cells in sarcoidosis lungs.[60] Chemokines attracting TH1 cells like CXCL9, CXCL10, and CXCL16 are also found to be released by alveolar macrophages and alveolar epithelial cells type II.[26,59,61,62] In addition, the concentration of the chemokines found in BAL fluid or BAL cell culture supernatants is significantly related to the degree of alveolitis and the course of the disease.[63] Thus, besides a local activation of memory cells, it is conceivable that cells activated at extrapulmonary sites enter the blood stream and are attracted into the lung by the pulmonary chemokine milieu. The important role of TH1 cells in granuloma induction has been shown using a nonpeptide inhibitor of CXCR3 and CCR5. This inhibitor not only decreases the accumulation of TH1 cells but also ameliorates the granuloma formation in a model of pulmonary granulomatosis in mice.[64]

In contrast, the marker cytokines of TH2 cells, IL-4, IL-5, IL-10, and IL-13, cannot be found elevated in sarcoidosis body fluids or cell culture supernatants of sarcoidosis T cells. Both lineages derive from naive TH0 cells, which are able to release the whole panel of cytokines and differentiate in either TH1 or TH2 cells after antigen stimulation depending on antigen concentration, the affinity of the antigen to the MHC class II molecules, and its nature. Bäumer and colleagues[65] could demonstrate that T-cell clones derived from peripheral blood, BAL cells, and lung parenchyma of patients with sarcoidosis disclose the entire spectrum of cytokine patterns after nonspecific activation. TH2-like cells could be demonstrated in all 3 body compartments, including BAL. From this, one may assume that, although TH2 cells are present, they are not activated or even suppressed, which may contribute to the immunopathogenesis by maintaining a cytokine imbalance in the lung.

Regulatory T cells

In most cases, sarcoidosis comes to a spontaneous resolution, which suggests that the eliciting antigen is eliminated and the inflammatory response is terminated. A successful immune response needs to be downregulated, and T cells with regulatory capacity like Tregs constitute a tool of the immune system for this purpose. Tregs are identified by their bright expression of the IL-2R and the transcription factor FoxP3 (Forkhead-Box-Protein 3). There are conflicting results on the presence and function of Tregs in sarcoidosis. In one study, high numbers of Tregs are observed in blood, lung, and lymph nodes of patients with Löfgren disease.[66] In contrast, in patients with chronic active disease, Tregs are reduced in the lung.[67] However, the same group reported later increased numbers of Tregs in the local lymph nodes compared with BAL and peripheral blood in a mixed group of patients with and without Löfgren syndrome. A new article reports extremely high levels of FoxP3$^+$CD127$^-$ Tregs (75%) in the BAL of patients with sarcoidosis and significantly lower levels in controls.[68] The authors' own results describe diminished percentages of Tregs in chronic sarcoidosis but normal values in nonactive sarcoidosis and in patients with spontaneous remission.[69] Reduced BAL Treg numbers result in a diminished control of pulmonary T-effector cell response in sarcoidosis. Tregs dampen the proliferation and cytokine release of effector T cells, which facilitates a remission of disease. In sarcoidosis, however, studies suggest that Tregs are dysfunctional, again with conflicting results. In one report, peripheral blood Tregs do not suppress T-effector cell IFNγ and TNF release, whereas others found impaired Tregs only in the lung.[68] In consequence, at least the reduced regulatory capacity of Tregs in the sarcoidosis lung leads to the fact that sarcoidosis Tregs do not suppress granuloma formation, whereas Tregs from nonsarcoidosis patients do.[70] This diminished efficacy of Treg in sarcoidosis might be related to the increased presence of TNF in these patients. It was shown that TNF decreases the inhibitory capacity of Tregs, which is accompanied by a downregulation of FoxP3 expression.[71] Indeed, the authors could demonstrate that an experimental therapy with vasoactive intestinal peptide of patients suffering from sarcoidosis increases the number of Tregs in BAL and restores their suppressive capacity.[69] It has been shown that both IL-2 as well as TGFβ must be present for the efficient induction of Tregs.[72] Both mediators are present in high levels in patients with active disease,[73–75] the clinical course with the highest frequency of spontaneous remission. Thus, the increased levels of TGFβ and

IL-2 might counterbalance the increased TNF levels; therefore, normal numbers of Tregs with proper function are found.[69]

T helper 17 cells in sarcoidosis

TH17 cells mediate the recruitment of neutrophils and macrophages to the infected tissue, hence, increasing bacterial clearing. Suppression of IL-17 or TH17 cells diminishes immunity against extracellular bacteria and favors persistence of infection. There is an important interrelation of TH1, Treg, and TH17 cells. TH17 cells are induced by a TCR trigger in the presence of TGFβ, IL-6, and IL-23. Each of these mediators exerts a distinct role in TH17 development. IL-6 and IL-23 seem to be indispensable in TH17 generation, but also IL-1 and IL-21 seem to be engaged in this process. IL-23 is a cytokine belonging to the IL-12 family, thus it shares the subunit p40 with all other cytokines of this family. IL-23 is a heterodimer of p40 and the subunit p19 whereas the TH1-driving cytokine IL-12 uses the subunits P40 and p35. Thus, the similarity of the driving mediators demonstrates the close proximity of TH1 and TH17 commitment.[76]

The role of TGFβ in TH17 commitment is less clear. In mice, it seems that TGFβ is also a prerequisite for Th17 generation. In man, it seems that a low dose of TGFβ is required to suppress processes interfering with TH17 generation but has no direct role in TH17 generation. However, a high dose of TGFβ induces Treg, dampening all immune responses. In contrast, activation of TH17 cells suppresses TH1 activation, whereas the TH1 product IFNγ inhibits TH17 commitment and IL-17 release. In addition, this view is complicated by the finding that IFNγ treated APCs foster TH17 commitment; but the release of Il-17 is still diminished by this mediator.[77–79]

Although current literature fosters the idea that the main role of TH17 cells is the coordination of immune defense against extracellular bacteria, there is evidence that IL-17 is also involved in the immune defense against intracellular bacteria, such as Listeria monocytogenes or Francisella tularensis. In mycobacterial infection, a low dose of antigen induces the release of IL-17 by γδ T cells, which is most interestingly independent from TCR activation of these cells but requires IL-23 release by infected DCs. In the model of granuloma induction by Schistosoma mansoni eggs, it was demonstrated that IL-17 plays also a role in granuloma formation, as blockade of IL-17 inhibits granuloma generation.[80]

There are now an increasing number of publications on TH17 cells or IL-17 release in sarcoidosis available. However, at first glance, the situation is far from being clear. In most of the publications, T cells from peripheral blood are analyzed. In a few articles, BAL T cells and tissue were also examined for the presence of TH17 cells or IL-17 release or expression. Most investigators found an increase in TH17 cells in peripheral blood mononuclear cells (PBMNC) as well as in BAL.[81–84] These investigators used flow cytometry to detect IL-17+CD4+ T cells either alone or together with other markers. In all of these investigations, the cells were stimulated in an unspecific manner in order to see a maximum of cytokine production for proper analysis in flow cytometry. In this case, all cells are activated, irrespective of any possible antigen specificity. The situation is a bit more complicated as soon as the cells are activated by a potential antigen. An investigation from Japan used for T-cell stimulation viable Propionibacterium acnes and Bacillus Calmette-Guérin (BCG) as well as ESAT-6. After stimulation with P acnes, they found a significant increase in IL-17 mRNA expression only in healthy controls but not in patients with sarcoidosis. In contrast, no difference was found when the cells were stimulated with BCG.[85] These conflicting results may be attributed to the complicated activation of TH17 cells as mentioned earlier. High levels of IFNγ, which is present in sarcoidosis, may prime the APC to foster the development of TH17 cells but simultaneously inhibits the activation of these cells and diminishes IL-17 release. However, meanwhile others found increased percentages of TH17 in sarcoidosis compared with controls using a mycobacterial antigen like ESAT-6 or mKatG as stimuli.[86,87] These data would indeed point to an involvement of TH17 cells in the pathogenesis of sarcoidosis. A potential role of these cells might be the generation or maintaining of granuloma formation, as Facco and colleagues[81] not only found increased percentages of TH17 cells mainly in patients suffering from active disease but they also found alveolar macrophages producing IL-17 in patients with active disease but not in patients with inactive disease or controls. They also found a substantial expression of IL-17 in the granuloma itself, again expressed by macrophages (giant cells) and by T cells within the granuloma.

GRANULOMA FORMATION VERSUS FIBROSIS IN SARCOIDOSIS: A CONSEQUENCE OF DIFFERENTIAL IMMUNE RESPONSES

General Considerations

As outlined earlier, the immune responses in sarcoidosis are manifold and might reflect the diverse phenotypes of sarcoidosis. It is intriguing that acute sarcoidosis (Löfgren syndrome) is associated with an intense activation of TH1 cells and M1 macrophages as characterized by exaggerated IFNγ and TNF release. Although acute sarcoidosis is frequently accompanied by fever, arthralgia, and uveitis, it is in most cases a self-limiting disease. This point demonstrates that intense immune responses in sarcoidosis are not deleterious per se. Investigations in nonacute forms of sarcoidosis demonstrate that certain immune activation patterns can be associated with different clinical forms of sarcoidosis. As outlined earlier, the mediator release is a biological landmark indicating the different activation states of the immune system; the exaggerated mediator release activates immune cells in diverse ways, that is shifting the balance of T-helper and T-effector cells, inducing Tregs, or differential activation of M1 or M2 macrophages. Thus, differences in immune responses in sarcoidosis define the clinical course of the disease.

The most prominent immune response structures in sarcoidosis are the granulomas. Granulomas are highly organized structures and created by macrophages, epithelioid cells, giant cells, T cells, and fibroblasts. It is generally accepted that initiation of granuloma formation requires T-cell activation. In contrast, diminished T-cell response inhibits granuloma formation. This point is nicely shown by Taflin and colleagues[70] who demonstrated that functional Tregs diminish in vitro granuloma formation. In addition, TNF released by alveolar macrophages is also required for the induction and maintenance of granuloma, as patients with sarcoidosis with macrophage aggregates in their lung parenchyma, which may be regarded as granulomas in status nascendi, disclosed higher levels of TNF release as patients with differentiated granulomas.[88] In addition, from the absent therapeutic effects of the TNF-receptor 2-fusion protein etanercept, which blocks merely soluble TNF and only to a lower extend membrane-bound TNF[89]; we conclude that in addition to free, soluble TNF membrane-bound TNF is necessary for granuloma formation and maintenance. Consequently, TNF antibodies like infliximab or adalimumab blocking both forms of TNF are more efficient in sarcoidosis therapy.[90]

However, fatal sarcoidosis is not associated with exaggerated granuloma formation but with the progress of the disease to fibrotic remodeling of the lung affecting 5% to 15% of the patients.[91,92] Fibrotic sarcoidosis is fatal; it affects younger patients as, for example, idiopathic pulmonary fibrosis and leads to an early death.[93] In general, fibrotic sarcoidosis or type IV disease is regarded to be an end-stage disease with an inflammatory burnout of the lung. However, in a small study using explanted lungs of patients with sarcoidosis type IV, such an end-stage lung was seen only in 3 out of 7 cases.[94] In 4 cases, the investigators found chronic interstitial pneumonitis indicating that there are still on-going inflammatory processes. Most interestingly, the investigators found fibroblast foci resembling the pattern in usual interstitial pneumonia. The authors' own results demonstrate that at least the macrophages are still activated and release increased amounts of chemokines like CCL18.[56,95] Thus, sarcoidosis type IV is also a condition with ongoing remodeling processes and macrophage activity.

Granuloma Induction

From the nature of the immune responses discussed earlier, the authors are now able to draft a scenario of granuloma induction in sarcoidosis. The starting point is the detection of an antigen by T cells and the activation of macrophages by PAMPS or DAMPS. The stimulus persists as the granuloma-inducing agent is either resistant to degradation or is repeatedly delivered. The potential antigens ranking from infectious or environmental agents to autoantigens meet all these requirements. They either derive from bacteria known to be at least partially protease resistant[12,96] or they may be delivered as autoantigens.[97,98] These antigens are presented to CD4 T cells in context of MHC II or to CD8 T cells by cross-presentation in context of MHC I in conditions of increased accessory function of the alveolar macrophages,[99] reduced counter-regulation due to the lack of membrane-anchored BTNL2,[42,44] and a decrease in Tregs[67,69] or their functional impairment.[66,68] These conditions allow efficient T-cell activation leading to an exaggerated immune response against these antigens, which under normal conditions might not initiate an immune activation. T cells activated in these conditions proliferate and release chemokines attracting additional inflammatory cells and activate macrophages by IFNγ to release chemokines attracting additional T cells. In consequence, these activated T cells resemble physiologically activated T cells with no differences to T cells activated in other immune responses.

In addition, the granuloma-inducing agent also activates alveolar macrophages to release chemokines attracting T cells and neutrophils. It is known that the mycobacterial antigen ESAT-6 activates TLR2-dependent immune responses,[12,13] and TLR2 might also be the receptor for other mycobacterial products. *Propionibacterium*-induced granuloma formation depends on TLR9 activation,[100] but products of *Propionibacterium* also trigger TLR2.[23] It is also possible that the T-cell activation is independent from the activation of alveolar macrophages or more precisely that the T-cell activation by an antigen is independent of the macrophage stimulus. For example, it is conceivable that in a condition in which T cells are activated by autoantigens,[98] alveolar macrophages might be activated by alarmins like acute phase proteins, for example, serum amyloid A.[101]

Activated T cells surrounding the outer border of the granuloma as well as activated cells within the granuloma release IFNγ amplifying alveolar macrophage activation and possibly release IL-17 adding to granuloma formation and maintenance. As the intensity of T-cell activation is different in acute and chronic sarcoidosis, high numbers of T cells release larger quantities of mediators like IFNγ in acute disease, which is lower or even missing in chronic sarcoidosis. Alveolar macrophages release, for example, TNF, IL-17, macrophage colony-stimulating factor (M-CSF), and granulocyte-macrophage colony-stimulating factor (GM-CSF) necessary for the induction and maintenance of a functionally intact granuloma and IL-12 and IL-18 fostering the differentiation of TH1 T cells.[102] Under the influence of M-CSF and GM-CSF, the macrophages conflate to multinucleated giant cells. Epithelial cells enclose the inner circle of the granuloma to contain the possibly harmful and nondegradable agent. At least in the skin sarcoidosis granuloma are surrounded by DCs[103] monitoring the environment for escaping antigen and subsequently activating T cells.

Successful immune responses result either in a total removal of the eliciting agent followed by a *reconstitutio ad integrum* and a downregulation of the immune processes involved, for example, by TGFβ delivered by various cell types, for example, Tregs or alveolar macrophages.[75] This effect may be seen mostly in acute sarcoidosis leading to spontaneous remission. In contrast, incomplete removal of the eliciting agent results in the maintenance of the granuloma or even ongoing granuloma formation to contain the causative agent. The latter may result in phases of inflammatory responses and repeated granuloma formation with subsequent clinical deterioration as often seen in chronic sarcoidosis.

Development of Fibrosis

In comparison with acute sarcoidosis, chronic sarcoidosis is characterized by diminished T-cell activation as demonstrated by lower cytokine release.[73] The resulting paucity in IFNγ targets both the alveolar macrophages, as IFNγ is an important activator of alveolar macrophages and the fibroblast itself, as IFNγ inhibits matrix production by fibroblasts.[104] Nevertheless, alveolar macrophages in chronic sarcoidosis still release proinflammatory cytokines[105] as well as increased amounts of the profibrotic chemokine CCL18,[56,95] a chemokine characterizing M2 macrophages. Thus, engagement of the innate PRRs induce macrophage activation, which might be boosted by chemokines like CCL2 released by alveolar epithelial cells type II.[106] This scenario is corroborated by the fact that CCL2 is also increased in patients with persistent and recurrent disease.[107] Nevertheless, this scenario is rather unlikely, as the limited activation of alveolar macrophages would not result in sufficient granuloma formation. In addition, the involvement of T cells in sarcoidosis granuloma is mandatory.[108] Thus, it is more likely that after granuloma formation T-cell activation is downregulated or, more likely, shifts from a TH1- to a TH2-dominated phenotype. Downregulation of T-cell activation but persistent macrophage activation again might result in a shift from classic to alternative activation as described earlier. Interestingly, Ten Berge and colleagues[82] found IL-17/IL-4 double-positive T cells in peripheral blood more so in the BAL of patients with sarcoidosis, which may also contribute to a shift from a proinflammatory TH1 to a profibrotic TH2 environment. Tregs, although possibly functionally limited in chronic sarcoidosis, are still present and release TGFβ, which is also able to induce a shift from M1 to M2.[109]

PERSPECTIVES

The knowledge of cellular players in sarcoidosis is not only a question of academic interest. Despite all definite progress achieved in the field of a possible sarcoidosis antigen, a causative agent in sarcoidosis is still lacking. Thus, new therapeutic strategies aim to target cellular key players or more precisely their mediators. As outlined earlier, not all of these mediators might be found in every subtype or every stage of the disease. Thus, for a successful therapy targeting a specific mediator in sarcoidosis, we need to know whether this mediator is present and active in the respective disease stage, which requires knowledge about the cytokine network in the different disease stages. Thus, the integration of genomic, metabolomic, and proteomic data by means of bioinformatics and systems biology in order to elucidate pathways and patterns involved in sarcoidosis is urgently needed. In aggregate, a future successful treatment of sarcoidosis will require a personalized approach targeting the cytokines and receptors of the pathologic pathways activated in a specific stage of the disease.

REFERENCES

1. Bianchi ME. DAMPs, PAMPs and alarmins: all we need to know about danger. J Leukoc Biol 2007; 81(1):1–5.

2. Pechkovsky DV, Zalutskaya OM, Ivanov GI, et al. Calprotectin (MRP8/14 protein complex) release during mycobacterial infection in vitro and in vivo. FEMS Immunol Med Microbiol 2000;29(1):27–33.

3. Korthagen NM, Nagtegaal MM, van Moorsel CH, et al. MRP14 is elevated in the bronchoalveolar lavage fluid of fibrosing interstitial lung diseases. Clin Exp Immunol 2010;161(2):342–7.

4. Bargagli E, Olivieri C, Prasse A, et al. (S100A9) levels in bronchoalveolar lavage fluid of patients with interstitial lung diseases. Inflammation 2008; 31(5):351–4.

5. Veress B, Malmskold K. The distribution of S100 and lysozyme immunoreactive cells in the various phases of granuloma development in sarcoidosis. Sarcoidosis 1987;4(1):33–7.

6. Riva M, Källberg E, Bjork P, et al. Induction of NFkappaB responses by the S100A9 protein is TLR4-dependent. Immunology 2012;137(2): 172–82.

7. Yonekawa K, Neidhart M, Altwegg LA, et al. Myeloid related proteins activate Toll-like receptor 4 in human acute coronary syndromes. Atherosclerosis 2011;218(2):486–92.

8. Ashitani J, Matsumoto N, Nakazato M. Elevated alpha-defensin levels in plasma of patients with pulmonary sarcoidosis. Respirology 2007;12(3): 339–45.

9. Biragyn A, Ruffini PA, Leifer CA, et al. Toll-like receptor 4-dependent activation of dendritic cells by beta-defensin 2. Science 2002;298(5595): 1025–9.

10. Paone G, Lucantoni G, Leone A, et al. Human neutrophil peptides stimulate tumor necrosis factor-alpha release by alveolar macrophages from patients with sarcoidosis. Chest 2009;135(2): 586–7.

11. Chen ES, Song Z, Willett MH, et al. Serum amyloid A regulates granulomatous inflammation in sarcoidosis through Toll-like receptor-2. Am J Respir Crit Care Med 2010;181(4):360–70.

12. Oswald-Richter KA, Culver DA, Hawkins C, et al. Cellular responses to mycobacterial antigens are present in bronchoalveolar lavage fluid used in the diagnosis of sarcoidosis. Infect Immun 2009; 77(9):3740–8.

13. Pathak SK, Basu S, Basu KK, et al. Direct extracellular interaction between the early secreted antigen ESAT-6 of Mycobacterium tuberculosis and TLR2 inhibits TLR signaling in macrophages. Nat Immunol 2007;8(6):610–8.

14. Kubarenko AV, Ranjan S, Rautanen A, et al. A naturally occurring variant in human TLR9, P99L, is associated with loss of CpG oligonucleotide responsiveness. J Biol Chem 2010;285(47): 36486–94.

15. Figueroa L, Xiong Y, Song C, et al. The Asp299Gly polymorphism alters TLR4 signaling by interfering with recruitment of MyD88 and TRIF. J Immunol 2012;188(9):4506–15.

16. Broen JC, Bossini-Castillo L, van Bon L, et al. A rare polymorphism in the gene for Toll-like receptor 2 is associated with systemic sclerosis phenotype and increases the production of inflammatory mediators. Arthritis Rheum 2012; 64(1):264–71.

17. Asukata Y, Ota M, Meguro A, et al. Lack of association between toll-like receptor 4 gene polymorphisms and sarcoidosis-related uveitis in Japan. Mol Vis 2009;15:2673–82.

18. Pabst S, Bradler O, Gillissen A, et al. Toll-like receptor-9 polymorphisms in sarcoidosis and chronic obstructive pulmonary disease. Adv Exp Med Biol 2013;756:239–45.

19. Schürmann M, Kwiatkowski R, Albrecht M, et al. Study of Toll-like receptor gene loci in sarcoidosis. Clin Exp Immunol 2008;152(3):423–31.

20. Veltkamp M, Grutters JC, van Moorsel CH, et al. Toll-like receptor (TLR) 4 polymorphism Asp299Gly is not associated with disease course in Dutch sarcoidosis patients. Clin Exp Immunol 2006; 145(2):215–8.

21. Veltkamp M, van Moorsel CH, Rijkers GT, et al. Genetic variation in the Toll-like receptor gene cluster (TLR10-TLR1-TLR6) influences disease course in sarcoidosis. Tissue Antigens 2012; 79(1):25–32.

22. Veltkamp M, Van Moorsel CH, Rijkers GT, et al. Toll-like receptor (TLR)-9 genetics and function in sarcoidosis. Clin Exp Immunol 2010;162(1):68–74.

23. Veltkamp M, Wijnen PA, van Moorsel CH, et al. Linkage between Toll-like receptor (TLR) 2 promotor and intron polymorphisms: functional effects and relevance to sarcoidosis. Clin Exp Immunol 2007;149(3):453–62.

24. Wiken M, Grunewald J, Eklund A, et al. Higher monocyte expression of TLR2 and TLR4, and enhanced pro-inflammatory synergy of TLR2 with NOD2 stimulation in sarcoidosis. J Clin Immunol 2009;29(1):78–89.

25. Pechkovsky DV, Zissel G, Ziegenhagen MW, et al. Effect of proinflammatory cytokines on interleukin-8 mRNA expression and protein production by isolated human alveolar epithelial cells type II in primary culture. Eur Cytokine Netw 2000;11(4): 618–25.

26. Sugiyama K, Mukae H, Ishii H, et al. Elevated levels of interferon gamma-inducible protein-10 and epithelial neutrophil-activating peptide-78 in patients with pulmonary sarcoidosis. Respirology 2006;11(6):708–14.

27. Cui A, Anhenn O, Theegarten D, et al. Angiogenic and angiostatic chemokines in idiopathic pulmonary fibrosis and granulomatous lung disease. Respiration 2010;80(5):372–8.

28. Vasakova M, Sterclova M, Kolesar L, et al. Bronchoalveolar lavage fluid cellular characteristics, functional parameters and cytokine and chemokine levels in interstitial lung diseases. Scand J Immunol 2009;69(3):268–74.

29. Tutor-Ureta P, Citores MJ, Castejon R, et al. Prognostic value of neutrophils and NK cells in bronchoalveolar lavage of sarcoidosis. Cytometry B Clin Cytom 2006;70(6):416–22.

30. Ziegenhagen MW, Rothe ME, Schlaak M, et al. Bronchoalveolar and serological parameters reflecting the severity of sarcoidosis. Eur Respir J 2003;21(3):407–13.

31. Rottoli P, Magi B, Cianti R, et al. Carbonylated proteins in bronchoalveolar lavage of patients with sarcoidosis, pulmonary fibrosis associated with systemic sclerosis and idiopathic pulmonary fibrosis. Proteomics 2005;5(10):2612–8.

32. Piotrowski WJ, Kurmanowska Z, Antczak A, et al. Exhaled 8-isoprostane in sarcoidosis: relation to superoxide anion production by bronchoalveolar lavage cells. Inflamm Res 2010; 59(12):1027–32.

33. Milne GL, Yin H, Hardy KD, et al. Isoprostane generation and function. Chem Rev 2011;111(10): 5973–96.

34. Janssen LJ, Catalli A, Helli P. The pulmonary biology of isoprostanes. Antioxid Redox Signal 2005;7(1–2):244–55.

35. Lommatzsch M, Bratke K, Bier A, et al. Airway dendritic cell phenotypes in inflammatory diseases of the human lung. Eur Respir J 2007;30(5):878–86.

36. Munro CS, Campbell DA, Du Bois RM, et al. Dendritic cells in cutaneous, lymph node and pulmonary lesions of sarcoidosis. Scand J Immunol 1987;25(5):461–7.

37. Ten Berge B, Kleinjan A, Muskens F, et al. Evidence for local dendritic cell activation in pulmonary sarcoidosis. Respir Res 2012;13:33.

38. van Haarst JM, Verhoeven GT, de Wit HJ, et al. CD1a+ and CD1a- accessory cells from human bronchoalveolar lavage differ in allostimulatory potential and cytokine production. Am J Respir Cell Mol Biol 1996;15(6):752–9.

39. Mathew S, Bauer KL, Fischoeder A, et al. The anergic state in sarcoidosis is associated with diminished dendritic cell function. J Immunol 2008; 181(1):746–55.

40. Kulakova N, Urban B, McMichael AJ, et al. Functional analysis of dendritic cell-T cell interaction in sarcoidosis. Clin Exp Immunol 2009; 159(1):82–6.

41. Zissel G, Prasse A, Muller-Quernheim J. Sarcoidosis–immunopathogenetic concepts. Semin Respir Crit Care Med 2007;28(1):3–14.

42. Nguyen T, Liu XK, Zhang Y, et al. BTNL2, a butyrophilin-like molecule that functions to inhibit T cell activation. J Immunol 2006;176(12):7354–60.

43. Swanson RM, Gavin MA, Escobar SS, et al. Butyrophilin-like 2 modulates B7 costimulation to induce Foxp3 expression and regulatory T cell development in mature T cells. J Immunol 2013;190(5): 2027–35.

44. Valentonyte R, Hampe J, Huse K, et al. Sarcoidosis is associated with a truncating splice site mutation in BTNL2. Nat Genet 2005;37(4):357–64.

45. Li Y, Wollnik B, Pabst S, et al. BTNL2 gene variant and sarcoidosis. Thorax 2006;61(3):273–4.

46. Rybicki BA, Walewski JL, Maliarik MJ, et al. The BTNL2 gene and sarcoidosis susceptibility in African Americans and whites. Am J Hum Genet 2005;77(3):491–9.

47. Lin Y, Wei J, Fan L, et al. BTNL2 gene polymorphism and sarcoidosis susceptibility: a meta-analysis. PLoS One 2015;10(4):e0122639.

48. Barna BP, Culver DA, Abraham S, et al. Depressed peroxisome proliferator-activated receptor gamma (PPargamma) is indicative of severe pulmonary sarcoidosis: possible involvement of interferon gamma (IFN-gamma). Sarcoidosis Vasc Diffuse Lung Dis 2006;23(2):93–100.

49. Culver DA, Barna BP, Raychaudhuri B, et al. Peroxisome proliferator-activated receptor gamma activity is deficient in alveolar macrophages in pulmonary sarcoidosis. Am J Respir Cell Mol Biol 2004;30(1):1–5.

50. Maver A, Medica I, Salobir B, et al. Peroxisome proliferator-activated receptor gamma/Pro12Ala polymorphism and peroxisome proliferator-activated receptor gamma coactivator-1 alpha/Gly482Ser polymorphism in patients with sarcoidosis. Sarcoidosis Vasc Diffuse Lung Dis 2008; 25(1):29–35.

51. Huizar I, Malur A, Patel J, et al. The role of PPAR-gamma in carbon nanotube-elicited granulomatous lung inflammation. Respir Res 2013;14:7.

52. Barna BP, Huizar I, Malur A, et al. Carbon nanotube-induced pulmonary granulomatous disease: twist1 and alveolar macrophage M1 activation. Int J Mol Sci 2013;14(12):23858–71.

53. Hasegawa-Moriyama M, Ohnou T, Godai K, et al. Peroxisome proliferator-activated receptor-gamma agonist rosiglitazone attenuates postincisional pain by regulating macrophage polarization. Biochem Biophys Res Commun 2012;426(1):76–82.

54. Hänsch HC, Smith DA, Mielke ME, et al. Mechanisms of granuloma formation in murine Mycobacterium avium infection: the contribution of CD4+ T cells. Int Immunol 1996;8(8):1299–310.

55. Sallusto F, Lanzavecchia A. Heterogeneity of CD4+ memory T cells: functional modules for tailored immunity. Eur J Immunol 2009;39(8):2076–82.

56. Pechkovsky DV, Prasse A, Kollert F, et al. Alternatively activated alveolar macrophages in pulmonary fibrosis-mediator production and intracellular signal transduction. Clin Immunol 2010; 137(1):89–101.

57. Bi Y, Yang R. Direct and indirect regulatory mechanisms in TH17 cell differentiation and functions. Scand J Immunol 2012;75(6):543–52.

58. Zhu J, Paul WE. CD4 T cells: fates, functions, and faults. Blood 2008;112(5):1557–69.

59. Agostini C, Cabrelle A, Calabrese F, et al. Role for CXCR6 and its ligand CXCL16 in the pathogenesis of T-cell alveolitis in sarcoidosis. Am J Respir Crit Care Med 2005;172(10):1290–8.

60. Kriegova E, Fillerova R, Tomankova T, et al. T-helper cell type-1 transcription factor T-bet is upregulated in pulmonary sarcoidosis. Eur Respir J 2011;38(5): 1136–44.

61. Takeuchi M, Oh IK, Suzuki J, et al. Elevated serum levels of CXCL9/monokine induced by interferon-gamma and CXCL10/interferon-gamma-inducible protein-10 in ocular sarcoidosis. Invest Ophthalmol Vis Sci 2006;47(3):1063–8.

62. Morgan AJ, Guillen C, Symon FA, et al. Expression of CXCR6 and its ligand CXCL16 in the lung in health and disease. Clin Exp Allergy 2005;35(12): 1572–80.

63. Capelli A, Di Stefano A, Lusuardi M, et al. Increased macrophage inflammatory protein-1alpha and macrophage inflammatory protein-1beta levels in bronchoalveolar lavage fluid of patients affected by different stages of pulmonary sarcoidosis. Am J Respir Crit Care Med 2002; 165(2):236–41.

64. Kishi J, Nishioka Y, Kuwahara T, et al. Blockade of Th1 chemokine receptors ameliorates pulmonary granulomatosis in mice. Eur Respir J 2011;38(2): 415–24.

65. Bäumer I, Zissel G, Schlaak M, et al. Th1/Th2 cell distribution in pulmonary sarcoidosis. Am J Respir Cell Mol Biol 1997;16(2):171–7.

66. Miyara M, Amoura Z, Parizot C, et al. The immune paradox of sarcoidosis and regulatory T cells. J Exp Med 2006;203(2):359–70.

67. Idali F, Wahlstrom J, Muller-Suur C, et al. Analysis of regulatory T cell associated forkhead box P3 expression in the lungs of patients with sarcoidosis. Clin Exp Immunol 2008;152(1):127–37.

68. Rappl G, Pabst S, Riemann D, et al. Regulatory T cells with reduced repressor capacities are extensively amplified in pulmonary sarcoid lesions and sustain granuloma formation. Clin Immunol 2011;140(1):71–83.

69. Prasse A, Zissel G, Lutzen N, et al. Inhaled vasoactive intestinal peptide exerts immuno-regulatory effects in sarcoidosis. Am J Respir Crit Care Med 2010;182(4):540–8.

70. Taflin C, Miyara M, Nochy D, et al. FoxP3+ regulatory T cells suppress early stages of granuloma formation but have little impact on sarcoidosis lesions. Am J Pathol 2009;174(2):497–508.

71. Valencia X, Stephens G, Goldbach-Mansky R, et al. TNF downmodulates the function of human CD4+CD25hi T-regulatory cells. Blood 2006; 108(1):253–61.

72. Davidson TS, DiPaolo RJ, Andersson J, et al. Cutting edge: IL-2 is essential for TGF-beta-mediated induction of Foxp3+ T regulatory cells. J Immunol 2007;178(7):4022–6.

73. Mollers M, Aries SP, Dromann D, et al. Intracellular cytokine repertoire in different T cell subsets from patients with sarcoidosis. Thorax 2001;56(6): 487–93.

74. Müller-Quernheim J, Pfeiffer S, Männel D, et al. Lung restricted activation of the alveolar macrophage/monocyte system in pulmonary sarcoidosis. Am Rev Respir Dis 1992;145:187–92.

75. Zissel G, Homolka J, Schlaak J, et al. Anti-inflammatory cytokine release by alveolar macrophages in pulmonary sarcoidosis. Am J Respir Crit Care Med 1996;154(3 Pt 1):713–9.

76. Ringkowski S, Thomas PS, Herbert C. Interleukin-12 family cytokines and sarcoidosis. Front Pharmacol 2014;5:233.

77. Schmitt N, Ueno H. Regulation of human helper T cell subset differentiation by cytokines. Curr Opin Immunol 2015;34:130–6.

78. McAleer JP, Kolls JK. Directing traffic: IL-17 and IL-22 coordinate pulmonary immune defense. Immunol Rev 2014;260(1):129–44.

79. Song X, Gao H, Qian Y. Th17 differentiation and their pro-inflammation function. Adv Exp Med Biol 2014;841:99–151.

80. Chen D, Xie H, Luo X, et al. Roles of Th17 cells in pulmonary granulomas induced by Schistosoma japonicum in C57BL/6 mice. Cell Immunol 2013; 285(1–2):149–57.

81. Facco M, Cabrelle A, Teramo A, et al. Sarcoidosis is a Th1/Th17 multisystem disorder. Thorax 2011; 66(2):144–50.

82. Ten Berge B, Paats MS, Bergen IM, et al. Increased IL-17A expression in granulomas and in circulating memory T cells in sarcoidosis. Rheumatology (Oxford) 2012;51(1):37–46.

83. Huang H, Lu Z, Jiang C, et al. Imbalance between Th17 and regulatory T-cells in sarcoidosis. Int J Mol Sci 2013;14(11):21463–73.

84. Tondell A, Moen T, Borset M, et al. Bronchoalveolar lavage fluid IFN-gamma+ Th17 cells and regulatory T cells in pulmonary sarcoidosis. Mediators Inflamm 2014;2014:438070.

85. Furusawa H, Suzuki Y, Miyazaki Y, et al. Th1 and Th17 immune responses to viable Propionibacterium acnes in patients with sarcoidosis. Respir Investig 2012;50(3):104–9.

86. Richmond BW, Ploetze K, Isom J, et al. Sarcoidosis Th17 cells are ESAT-6 antigen specific but demonstrate reduced IFN-gamma expression. J Clin Immunol 2013;33(2):446–55.

87. Ostadkarampour M, Eklund A, Moller D, et al. Higher levels of interleukin IL-17 and antigen-specific IL-17 responses in pulmonary sarcoidosis patients with Lofgren's syndrome. Clin Exp Immunol 2014;178(2):342–52.

88. Fehrenbach H, Zissel G, Goldmann T, et al. Alveolar macrophages are the main source for tumour necrosis factor-alpha in patients with sarcoidosis. Eur Respir J 2003;21(3):421–8.

89. Scallon B, Cai A, Solowski N, et al. Binding and functional comparisons of two types of tumor necrosis factor antagonists. J Pharmacol Exp Ther 2002;301(2):418–26.

90. Crommelin HA, Vorselaars AD, van Moorsel CH, et al. Anti-TNF therapeutics for the treatment of sarcoidosis. Immunotherapy 2014;6(10):1127–43.

91. Baughman RP, Teirstein AS, Judson MA, et al. Clinical characteristics of patients in a case control study of sarcoidosis. Am J Respir Crit Care Med 2001;164(10 Pt 1):1885–9.

92. Chappell AG, Cheung WY, Hutchings HA. Sarcoidosis: a long-term follow up study. Sarcoidosis Vasc Diffuse Lung Dis 2000;17(2):167–73.

93. Nardi A, Brillet PY, Letoumelin P, et al. Stage IV sarcoidosis: comparison of survival with the general population and causes of death. Eur Respir J 2011;38(6):1368–73.

94. Shigemitsu H, Oblad JM, Sharma OP, et al. Chronic interstitial pneumonitis in end-stage sarcoidosis. Eur Respir J 2010;35(3):695–7.

95. Prasse A, Pechkovsky DV, Toews GB, et al. A vicious circle of alveolar macrophages and fibroblasts perpetuates pulmonary fibrosis via CCL18. Am J Respir Crit Care Med 2006;173(7):781–92.

96. Chen ES, Wahlstrom J, Song Z, et al. T cell responses to mycobacterial catalase-peroxidase profile a pathogenic antigen in systemic sarcoidosis. J Immunol 2008;181(12):8784–96.

97. Wahlstrom J, Dengjel J, Persson B, et al. Identification of HLA-DR-bound peptides presented by human bronchoalveolar lavage cells in sarcoidosis. J Clin Invest 2007;117(11):3576–82.

98. Wahlstrom J, Dengjel J, Winqvist O, et al. Autoimmune T cell responses to antigenic peptides presented by bronchoalveolar lavage cell HLA-DR molecules in sarcoidosis. Clin Immunol 2009;133(3):353–63.

99. Zissel G, Ernst M, Schlaak M, et al. Accessory function of alveolar macrophages from patients with sarcoidosis and other granulomatous and non-granulomatous lung diseases. J Investig Med 1997;45(2):75–86.

100. Kalis C, Gumenscheimer M, Freudenberg N, et al. Requirement for TLR9 in the immunomodulatory activity of Propionibacterium acnes. J Immunol 2005;174(7):4295–300.

101. Alessandrini F, Beck-Speier I, Krappmann D, et al. Role of oxidative stress in ultrafine particle-induced exacerbation of allergic lung inflammation. Am J Respir Crit Care Med 2009;179(11):984–91.

102. Shigehara K, Shijubo N, Ohmichi M, et al. IL-12 and IL-18 are increased and stimulate IFN-gamma production in sarcoid lungs. J Immunol 2001;166(1):642–9.

103. Ota M, Amakawa R, Uehira K, et al. Involvement of dendritic cells in sarcoidosis. Thorax 2004;59(5):408–13.

104. Eickelberg O, Pansky A, Koehler E, et al. Molecular mechanisms of TGF-(beta) antagonism by interferon (gamma) and cyclosporine A in lung fibroblasts. FASEB J 2001;15(3):797–806.

105. Strausz J, Männel DN, Pfeifer S, et al. Spontaneous monokine release by alveolar macrophages in chronic sarcoidosis. Int Arch Allergy Appl Immunol 1991;96:68–75.

106. Pechkovsky DV, Goldmann T, Ludwig C, et al. CCR2 and CXCR3 agonistic chemokines are differently expressed and regulated in human alveolar epithelial cells type II. Respir Res 2005;6(1):75.

107. Petrek M, Kolek V, Szotkowska J, et al. CC and C chemokine expression in pulmonary sarcoidosis. Eur Respir J 2002;20(5):1206–12.

108. Bergeron A, Bonay M, Kambouchner M, et al. Cytokine patterns in tuberculous and sarcoid granulomas: correlations with histopathologic features of the granulomatous response. J Immunol 1997;159(6):3034–43.

109. Liu G, Ma H, Qiu L, et al. Phenotypic and functional switch of macrophages induced by regulatory CD4+CD25+ T cells in mice. Immunol Cell Biol 2011;89(1):130–42.

The Etiologic Role of Infectious Antigens in Sarcoidosis Pathogenesis

Lindsay J. Celada, PhD[a], Charlene Hawkins, PhD[b],
Wonder P. Drake, PhD[a,b,*]

KEYWORDS

- Sarcoidosis • Antimicrobials • Infectious antigens

KEY POINTS

- There is a growing body of literature supporting the role of infectious antigens, in particular mycobacteria and propionibacteria, in sarcoidosis pathogenesis.
- Immunologic studies reveal that mycobacterial virulence factors are the targets of the immune response in sarcoidosis diagnostic bronchoalveolar lavage (BAL).
- Recently, case reports and clinical trials have emerged reporting the efficacy of antimicrobial therapy on cutaneous and pulmonary sarcoidosis. Although the studies are not conclusive, they demonstrate efficacy on endpoints associated with sarcoidosis morbidity and mortality, such as forced vital capacity (FVC).

SARCOIDOSIS EPIDEMIOLOGY SUGGESTS EXPOSURE TO MICROBIAL BIOAEROSOLS

Sarcoidosis is a granulomatous disease of unknown etiology, most commonly involving the lung, skin, lymph node, and eyes.[1] Granulomatous inflammation can be initiated by infectious agents, such as fungi or *Mycobacterium tuberculosis* (MTB), or by noninfectious agents, such as beryllium (chronic beryllium disease). Analysis of sarcoidosis epidemiology suggests that infectious agents have a role in sarcoidosis pathogenesis. Investigators in A Case Control Etiologic Study of Sarcoidosis observed positive associations between sarcoidosis risk and certain occupations, such as agricultural employment, exposure to insecticides, and moldy environments.[2] Another study noted that the hospitalization admissions for African Americans with sarcoidosis in South Carolina increased with proximity to the Atlantic Ocean.[3] A unifying factor in environmental and geographic reports is the possibility of exposure to microbial bioaerosols. Natural waters; water distribution systems; biofilm in pipes; peat and potting soil; water droplets; equipment, such as bronchoscopes and catheters; and moldy buildings are natural habitats for environmental opportunistic mycobacteria.[4] Aerosolization of environmental opportunistic mycobacteria has been associated with the development of other granulomatous diseases of mycobacterial origin, such as hypersensitivity pneumonitis.[5]

This work was supported by National Institutes of Health grants (T32 HL069765 to L.J. Celada; T32 HL094296 to C. Hawkins; and R01 HL117074, U01 112694 to W.P. Drake). Drs L.J. Celada and C. Hawkins have no conflicts of interest to disclose. Dr W.P. Drake serves as a scientific advisor for Celgene.

[a] Department of Pathology, Microbiology and Immunology, Vanderbilt University School of Medicine, 1161 21st Avenue South, A2200 Medical Center North, Nashville, TN 37232, USA; [b] Division of Infectious Diseases, Department of Medicine, Vanderbilt University Medical School, 1161 21st Avenue South, A2200 Medical Center North, Nashville, TN 37232, USA
* Corresponding author. Division of Infectious Diseases, Vanderbilt University Medical School, 21st Avenue South, Medical Center North, Room A-3314, Nashville, TN 37232-2363.
E-mail address: Wonder.Drake@vanderbilt.edu

Clin Chest Med 36 (2015) 561–568
http://dx.doi.org/10.1016/j.ccm.2015.08.001
0272-5231/15/$ – see front matter © 2015 Elsevier Inc. All rights reserved.

MOLECULAR AND IMMUNOLOGIC INVESTIGATIONS REVEAL MICROBIAL PROTEINS AND DNA

The inability to identify microorganisms by histologic staining or to culture microorganisms from pathologic tissues continues to be one of the strongest arguments against a potential role for infectious agents in sarcoidosis pathogenesis. As molecular analysis continues to grow in sensitivity and specificity, current culture and staining methods are known to identify less than 2% of current microbial communities present within the human biological specimens.[6,7] Advanced molecular techniques, such as deep sequencing technologies, also have demonstrated successful identification of novel microorganisms in pathologic tissues not easily identified by traditional methods.[8,9] Molecular analysis of pathologic tissue for microbial nucleic acids and proteins serves as an alternative means of identifying a putative infectious agent. Polymerase chain reaction (PCR) was used to identify the etiologic agents of Whipple disease (*Tropheryma whippelii*)[10] as well as the novel coronavirus as the agent of severe acute respiratory syndrome.[11]

A growing scientific interest involves defining the microbial community within distinct diseases, that is, microbiome analysis. Microbiome analysis was performed on the upper and lower airway of subjects with interstitial lung diseases, including idiopathic interstitial pneumonia (IIP), non-IIP, and sarcoidosis as well as *Pneumocystis jiroveci* pneumonia and healthy controls. The microbiota in lower airways of a majority of patients (30; 90%) primarily consisted of *Prevotellaceae*, *Streptococcaceae*, and *Acidaminococcaceae*; α and β diversity measurements revealed no significant differences in airway microbiota composition between the 5 different groups of patients. It was concluded that IIP, non-IIP, and sarcoidosis are not associated with disordered airway microbiota and a pathogenic role of commensals in the disease process is therefore unlikely.[12] A more targeted molecular approach for microbial pathogens in sarcoidosis granulomas most strongly supports that propionibacteria and/or mycobacteria have a role in sarcoidosis pathogenesis. Japanese researchers report molecular evidence of *Propionibacterium acnes* DNA in sarcoidosis specimens, although the DNA could also be isolated from control specimens.[13] The distinction lies in the quantitative differences in *P acnes* DNA between sarcoidosis and controls. The number of genomes of *P acnes* in BAL cells was correlated with the serum angiotensin-converting enzyme level and the percentage of macrophages in BAL fluid from patients with sarcoidosis. No

significant difference was detected between *P granulosum* and controls.[14] A murine model of sarcoidosis pathogenesis was successfully developed using heat-killed propionibacteria by intratracheal challenge. This model demonstrated the contribution of Toll-like receptor (TLR)-1, TLR-2, and TLR-9 to the development of the polarized, T_H1 immune response.[15] Another study further confirmed the role of TLR-2 in *P acnes*–specific sarcoidosis immune responses by demonstrating that *P acnes*–induced granulomatous pulmonary inflammation was markedly attenuated in TLR-2($-/-$) mice compared with wild-type C57BL/6 animals.[16] A recent meta-analysis involving 9 case-control studies of *P acnes* associated with sarcoidosis revealed a significantly elevated sarcoidosis risk (odds ratio 19.58; 95% CI, 13.06–29.36).[17]

Investigations from independent laboratories worldwide have also reported molecular evidence supporting a significant association between mycobacteria and sarcoidosis. One study reported evidence of mycobacterial 16S ribosomal RNA (rRNA) or RNA polymerase B in 60% of the sarcoidosis granulomas and in none of the controls ($P<.00002$, chi-square).[18] Sequence analysis of the 16S rRNA and *rpoB* amplicons revealed the presence of a novel *Mycobacterium*, genetically most similar to MTB complex (99% positional identity). Using matrix-assisted laser desorption/ionization time-of-flight mass spectrometry, Song and colleagues[19] found MTB katG peptides in 75% of sarcoidosis specimens compared with 14% of control specimens ($P = .0006$), in situ hybridization localized MTB katG, and 16S rRNA DNA to the inside of sarcoidosis granulomas. Analysis of Polish sarcoidosis lymph nodes revealed MTB complex heat shock protein (HSP) 70, HSP 65, and HSP 16.[20] Molecular analysis of American sarcoidosis granulomas also revealed the presence of nucleic acids of the mycobacterial virulence factor, superoxide dismutase A (sodA), in 70% of the sarcoidosis specimens compared with 12% of controls ($P = .001$). Sequence analysis of the amplicons demonstrated close positional identity with MTB complex, yet genetically distinct.[21] DNA of mycobacterial HSPs has been detected in cutaneous lesions of Chinese sarcoidosis patients but absent from control specimens. Sequence analysis was consistent with MTB, *M chelonae*, and *M gordonae*.[22] Another study reported the ability of real-time PCR analysis to quantitatively differentiate sarcoidosis from tuberculosis using receiver operating characteristic curves.[23] Real-time PCR analysis from these independent laboratories demonstrates that if viable mycobacteria are present within the sarcoidosis granulomas, they are present below the sensitivity of the acid-fast bacilli histologic stain.[21,23] Future molecular efforts should delineate if the identified nucleic acids or proteins reflect actively replicating organisms or persistent proteins.

IMMUNE RESPONSES AGAINST MYCOBACTERIAL VIRULENCE FACTORS ARE PRESENT IN SYSTEMIC AND ACTIVE SARCOIDOSIS INVOLVEMENT

An equally important modality to delineate if infectious agents have a role in idiopathic disease is to assess for immune responses against microbial proteins. The presence of humoral and cellular responses against microbial antigens is an insightful method for assessing exposure to infectious agents. Increased lymphocyte proliferation induced by *P acnes* has been reported in patients with active sarcoidosis; however, these responses did not correlate with clinical, roentgenographic, physiologic, and BAL findings in regard to disease severity.[24,25] Sarcoidosis T_H1 and T_H17 immune responses against viable *P acnes* that were significantly different from healthy controls were recently reported.[26]

Immune responses against mycobacteria have also been reported. Along with the detection of peptide fragments consistent with katG protein within sarcoidosis granulomas, the existence of humoral immune responses against mycobacterial katG proteins was demonstrated in sarcoidosis patients. Song and colleagues[16] noted IgG antibodies to recombinant MTB katG in sera from 48% of sarcoidosis patients compared with 0% in sera from purified protein derivative–negative controls (P = .0059). Sarcoidosis is characterized by polarized CD4$^+$ T cells with a T_H1 immunophenotype. The identification of T_H1 CD4$^+$ cellular immune responses against mycobacterial ESAT-6 and katG peptides in sarcoidosis peripheral blood mononuclear cells (PBMCs) suggested that the sarcoidosis immune response may be against mycobacterial virulence factors.[27] Distinctions in cellular recognition patterns against virulence factors, such as antigen 85A (Ag85A), can differentiate mycobacterial species. For example, patients infected with MTB recognize distinct Ag85A peptides from those infected with *M leprae*.[28] Further investigation of the sarcoidosis immune response pattern against Ag85A confirmed that the pattern detected was distinct from those in patients infected with MTB or *M leprae*.[29] Another report demonstrated systemic CD4$^+$ T_H1 immune responses against multiple mycobacterial virulence factors in sarcoidosis patients. These responses were not only against multiple secreted proteins but also against multiple epitopes within a given protein.[30] These findings are more analogous with what is observed in patients with active bacterial infection.

A dual molecular and immunologic analysis of sarcoidosis specimens for the mycobacterial virulence factor, sodA, demonstrated nucleic acids sequences closest to MTB, yet distinct. Translation of those sequences into peptides to stimulate sarcoidosis PBMC resulted in reproduction of the sarcoidosis T_H1 immunophenotype.[21] Mycobacterial proteins, such as soda, are virulence factors that confer pathogenicity to *Mycobacterium* species.[31] It has been demonstrated that the protein secretion system SecA2 is required for the optimal secretion of sodA and katG. Both of these proteins are synthesized without Sec signal sequences and function to detoxify reactive oxygen intermediates generated by the host macrophage. SecA2 is part of a specialized secretion system that contributes to the virulence of pathogenic mycobacteria by countering the oxidative attack of the host and confers their ability to survive within the host macrophage.[32,33]

In addition, CD4$^+$ and CD8$^+$ T-cell immune responses against MTB katG have been detected in sarcoidosis BAL. Comparison of immune responses to mycobacterial katG whole protein between American and Swedish sarcoidosis subjects revealed no differences despite distinctions in patient phenotypic, genetic, and prognostic characteristics. It was also demonstrated that although T_H1 immune responses were present systemically, katG-reactive CD4$^+$ 1 cells preferentially accumulated in the lung, indicating a compartmentalized response.[34] Patients with or without Löfgren syndrome had similar frequencies of katG-specific interferon-gamma–expressing peripheral T cells. This study also demonstrated that circulating katG-reactive T cells were found in chronic active sarcoidosis but not in patients with inactive disease.[34] The loss of immune responses to mycobacterial virulence factors after resolution of tuberculosis has also been observed.[35] Another report demonstrated that immune responses against these mycobacterial virulence factors are present in sarcoidosis diagnostic BAL and that induction of innate immunity by TLR-2 contributes to the polarized T_H1 immune response. Recognition was significantly absent from BAL fluid cells of patients with other lung diseases, including infectious granulomatous diseases.[36] The detection of immune responses against ESAT-6, katG, and sodA confirms exposure of sarcoidosis patients to a pathogenic mycobacterial species. These proteins are typically secreted during the stage of active mycobacterial replication, compared with expression of other proteins that are expressed when mycobacteria are in the latent state.[37,38] The immunologic analysis performed to date provides a mechanism for more in-depth analysis of sarcoidosis pathogenesis. These proteins can be used to delineate immunologic pathways that contribute to sarcoidosis resolution or disease progression.

NONINFECTIOUS ETIOLOGIES OF SARCOIDOSIS

It has been reported that the amyloid precursor protein serum amyloid A (SAA) is strikingly abundant in sarcoidosis tissues, predominantly in a nonfibrillar form, and localized to epithelioid granulomas. SAA has been detected in numerous pulmonary infections, such as tuberculosis, nontuberculous mycobacteria infection, and leprosy.[39–42] By comparison, quantitative immunohistochemistry showed that the extent and distribution of SAA in sarcoidosis is significantly lower in other diseases of granulomatous inflammation.[43] Chen and Moller[44] elaborate a concept of chronic stimulation of the innate immune system by disaggregated host protein SAA within granulomas after a microbial infection that induces a hyperimmune T_H1 immune response to microbial antigens in the absence of ongoing infection. SAA levels are reduced in pulmonary tuberculosis subjects after the initiation of antimicrobial therapy.[40] In addition, antibodies against autoantigens, such as zinc finger protein 688 and mitochondrial ribosomal protein L43, have been identified in sarcoidosis BAL and serum. High interindividual heterogeneity was noted.[45] Using pulmonary CD4+ T cells from 16 HLA-DRB1*0301+ patients, HLA-DR molecules were affinity purified and bound peptides acid eluted. The peptidies were separated by reversed-phase high-performance liquid chromatography and analyzed by liquid chromatography–mass spectrometry, resulting in the identification of autoantigens, such as vimentin, and ATP synthase.[46] These data support that immune responses against self-antigens are present in local and systemic sites of sarcoidosis subjects.

MICROBIAL INDUCTION OF SARCOIDOSIS CD4+ T-CELL DYSFUNCTION

Investigation of sarcoidosis immune function on T-cell receptor (TCR) stimulation reveals significant distinctions from healthy controls. The presence of chronic immune stimulation due to persistent microbial antigens has been reported to reduce T-cell function. Sarcoidosis T lymphocytes have also been characterized by reduced cytokine expression and proliferative capacity as well as up-regulation of the inhibitory receptor, programmed death-1 (PD-1), all immunologic phenomena associated with elevated antigenic burdens.

As defined by Wherry and colleagues,[47] T-cell exhaustion occurs as a result of chronic antigen stimulation that, over the duration of antigen exposure, results in a gradual reduction in the cell's ability to optimally respond to TCR stimulation. As such, although healthy T cells produce high levels of cytokine and exhibit high levels of proliferation and low levels of apoptosis in response to antigen, exhausted T cells gradually lose these normal functions until they can no longer respond to antigen and instead undergo apoptosis on TCR activation. PD-1 up-regulation on T cells plays a significant role in acquisition of the exhaustion phenotype. As an inhibitory coreceptor, signaling between PD-1 and its ligands, PDL1 and PDL2, functions to modulate tolerance to self antigens and limit the robustness of the adaptive immune response to foreign antigens. Exhausted T cells express high levels of PD-1 that correlates well with the systematic loss of cellular function. Recent findings that PD-1 is up-regulated on dysfunctional sarcoidosis T cells as well as the T cells of other granulomatous diseases characterized by microbial antigens, such as MTB[48–50] and schistosomiasis,[51] suggest that this phenotype could result from persistent antigen exposure (**Fig. 1, Table 1**).

Up-regulation of the PD-1 receptor and reduced proliferative capacity in sarcoidosis BAL and peripheral CD4+ T cells were recently reported.[52] Restoration of sarcoidosis CD4+ T-cell proliferative capacity to healthy control levels was apparent after PD-1 pathway blockade.[52] Various mechanisms by which PD-1 interferes with T-cell proliferation have been well described. PD-1 has been reported to inhibit CD4+ T-cell proliferation by blocking cell cycle progression through the suppression of Skp2 transcription.[53,54] Skp2 is the substrate recognition component of the ubiquitin ligase complex SCF^{Skp2} that binds to and degrades $p27^{kip1}$, a cyclin-dependent kinase (CDK) inhibitor, thereby allowing continuation of the cell cycle. PD-1 cell cycle impediment and, therefore, proliferation hindrance have been shown to be the result of PI3K/Akt and ERK pathway inactivation.[53,54] PD-1 inhibition of T-cell proliferation has been correlated with increased p27 availability and repression of Cdc25A, a CDK-activating phosphatase.[53,54] PD-1 engagement has also been demonstrated to attenuate TCR signaling by preventing ZAP70 and PKCθ activation.[55]

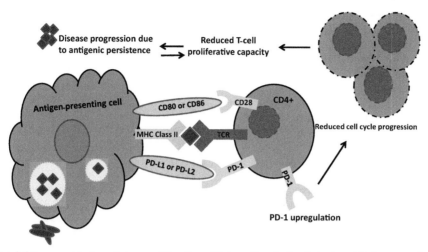

Fig. 1. PD-1 inhibits sarcoidosis cellular proliferation. High antigenic loads induce PD-1 up-regulation, which alters cell cycle progression. Cell cycle progression is necessary for normal CD4$^+$ T-cell proliferation to clear microbial or autoantigens, thus leading to clinical resolution. Persistent antigen further PD-1 up-regulation and loss of cellular function.

The reported up-regulation of PD-1 is particularly important because it has been associated with the emergence of human lymphotropic viruses, such as Epstein-Barr virus and cytomegalovirus.[56–58] These same viruses have been associated with sarcoidosis pathogenesis.[59,60]

CLINICAL TRIALS OF ANTIMICROBIAL THERAPY IN SARCOIDOSIS

After the publication of molecular and immunologic support for a role of microorganisms in sarcoidosis pathogenesis, such as fungi, propionibacteria, and mycobacteria, there has been an increasing number of case reports and clinical trials regarding efficacy with antimicrobial therapy. Numerous prior reports of the tetracyclines, in particular, doxycycline and minocycline, have been published in subjects with cutaneous sarcoidosis.[61–63] Although minocycline has antimicrobial effects against *P acnes*, its mechanism of action is thought immunomodulatory.[64] A recent report of the efficacy of clarithromycin, which has efficacy against propionibacteria and mycobacteria, was reported in a Japanese woman with systemic sarcoidosis.[65] Conclusive delineation of the mechanism of action is pending.

Fungal antigens are also reported to contribute to sarcoidosis pathogenesis.[66] Clinical and radiographic improvement after administration of antifungal therapy, such as posaconazole (300 mg/d) or ketoconazole (200 mg/d) with or without corticosteroids, has been reported in Slovenian sarcoidosis patients. The investigators conducted an open-labelled, patient-preference trial of steroids (methylprednisolone 0.4 mg/kg, antifungal agents (posaconazole 300 mg/d or ketoconazole 200 mg/d), or steroids/antifungal agents. The most significant clinical radiographic improvement was detected in the antifungal group; they also reported a reduction in disease recurrence among those on antifungal therapy. Study limitations include the lack of randomization as well as not being conducted in a double-blind fashion.

Two clinical trials regarding the efficacy of antimycobacterial therapy in sarcoidosis pathogenesis have been reported. A double blind, placebo-controlled investigation of an antimycobacterial regimen consisting of concomitant levofloxacin, ethambutol, azithromycin and rifampin (CLEAR) compared with placebo was conducted in subjects with cutaneous sarcoidosis. In the intention-to-treat analysis, the CLEAR-treated group had a mean (SD) decrease in lesion diameter of −8.4 (14.0) mm compared with an increase of 0.07 (3.2) mm in the placebo-treated group

Table 1
Evidence for etiologic agents in sarcoidosis pathogenesis

Etiology	Evidence
Mycobacteria	M, I, E[18–22,27,29,30]
Propionibacteria	M, I[13–15,24–26]
Fungal antigens	M[66]
Autoantigens	M, I[45,46]

Abbreviations: E, epidemiologic; I, immunologic; M, molecular.

(P = .05). The CLEAR group had a significant reduction in granuloma burden and experienced a mean (SD) decline of −2.9 (2.5) mm in lesion severity compared with a decline of −0.6 (2.1) mm in the placebo group (P = .02). The observed clinical reductions were present at the 180-day follow-up period. Transcriptome analysis of sarcoidosis CD4[+] T cells revealed reversal of pathways associated with disease severity and enhanced T-cell function after TCR stimulation.[67]

In addition, an open-label investigation of this same regimen was conducted in pulmonary sarcoidosis subjects; 15 chronic, pulmonary sarcoidosis patients with FVCs between 45% and 80% of predicted were enrolled. The primary efficacy endpoint was change in absolute FVC from baseline to completion of therapy. Secondary endpoints were change in functional capacity measured by Six Minute Walk Distance (6MWD) and quality-of-life assessment measured by St. George's Respiratory Questionnaire (SGRQ). Of 15 patients enrolled, 11 completed 4 weeks of therapy, and 8 completed 8 weeks of therapy. The CLEAR regimen was associated with an FVC increase of 0.23 L at 4 weeks and 0.42 L at 8 weeks (P = .0098 and 0.016, respectively). The 6MWD increased by 87 m from baseline to 8 weeks (P = .0078). The mean score of the validated SGRQ was improved at 8 weeks over baseline (P = .023).[68]

These early trials are promising. Future investigation of the mechanisms by which the antimicrobials work—as antimicrobials, immune modulators, or both—is warranted.

SUMMARY

Recent molecular, genetic, and immunologic studies from independent laboratories support an association with sarcoidosis and microbial antigens, particularly mycobacteria or propionibacteria. The findings among American sarcoidosis subjects are most strongly associated with mycobacteria and, among Japanese sarcoidosis subjects, propionibacteria. Because epidemiologic studies indicate that both sarcoidosis morbidity and mortality is increasing,[69] the impetus on current sarcoidosis researchers is to translate their strong basic research investigations into innovative therapeutics that will have an impact on sarcoidosis pathogenesis and hopefully lead to a cure. The progress to date strongly supports advances toward this goal.

REFERENCES

1. Baughman RP. Sarcoidosis. Clin Dermatol 2007; 25(3):231.

2. Newman LS, Rose CS, Bresnitz EA, et al. A case control etiologic study of sarcoidosis: environmental and occupational risk factors. Am J Respir Crit Care Med 2004;170(12):1324–30.

3. Kajdasz DK, Judson MA, Mohr LC Jr, et al. Geographic variation in sarcoidosis in South Carolina: its relation to socioeconomic status and health care indicators. Am J Epidemiol 1999;150(3):271–8.

4. Falkinham JO III. Nontuberculous mycobacteria in the environment. Clin Chest Med 2002;23(3): 529–51.

5. Hanak V, Kalra S, Aksamit TR, et al. Hot tub lung: presenting features and clinical course of 21 patients. Respir Med 2006;100(4):610–5.

6. DiGiulio DB, Romero R, Amogan HP, et al. Microbial prevalence, diversity and abundance in amniotic fluid during preterm labor: a molecular and culture-based investigation. PLoS One 2008;3(8):e3056.

7. Bik EM, Eckburg PB, Gill SR, et al. Molecular analysis of the bacterial microbiota in the human stomach. Proc Natl Acad Sci U S A 2006;103(3):732–7.

8. Whitley R. The new age of molecular diagnostics for microbial agents. N Engl J Med 2008;358(10): 988–9.

9. Palacios G, Druce J, Du L, et al. A new arenavirus in a cluster of fatal transplant-associated diseases. N Engl J Med 2008;358(10):991–8.

10. Relman DA, Schmidt TM, MacDermott RP, et al. Identification of the uncultured bacillus of Whipple's disease. N Engl J Med 1992;327(5):293–301.

11. Ksiazek TG, Erdman D, Goldsmith CS, et al. A novel coronavirus associated with severe acute respiratory syndrome. N Engl J Med 2003;348(20): 1953–66.

12. Garzoni C, Brugger SD, Qi W, et al. Microbial communities in the respiratory tract of patients with interstitial lung disease. Thorax 2013;68(12):1150–6.

13. Ishige I, Eishi Y, Takemura T, et al. Propionibacterium acnes is the most common bacterium commensal in peripheral lung tissue and mediastinal lymph nodes from subjects without sarcoidosis. Sarcoidosis Vasc Diffuse Lung Dis 2005;22(1):33–42.

14. Ichikawa H, Kataoka M, Hiramatsu J, et al. Quantitative analysis of propionibacterial DNA in bronchoalveolar lavage cells from patients with sarcoidosis. Sarcoidosis Vasc Diffuse Lung Dis 2008;25(1):15–20.

15. McCaskill JG, Chason KD, Hua X, et al. Pulmonary immune responses to Propionibacterium acnes in C57BL/6 and BALB/c mice. Am J Respir Cell Mol Biol 2006;35(3):347–56.

16. Song Z, Marzilli L, Greenlee BM, et al. Mycobacterial catalase-peroxidase is a tissue antigen and target of the adaptive immune response in systemic sarcoidosis. J Exp Med 2005;201:755–67.

17. Zhou Y, Hu Y, Li H. Role of propionibacterium acnes in sarcoidosis: a meta-analysis. Sarcoidosis Vasc Diffuse Lung Dis 2013;30(4):262–7.

18. Drake WP, Pei Z, Pride DT, et al. Molecular analysis of sarcoidosis tissues for mycobacterium species DNA. Emerg Infect Dis 2002;8(11):1334–41.

19. Song Z, Marzilli L, Greenlee BM, et al. Mycobacterial catalase-peroxidase is a tissue antigen and target of the adaptive immune response in systemic sarcoidosis. J Exp Med 2005;201(5):755–67.

20. Dubaniewicz A, Dubaniewicz-Wybieralska M, Sternau A, et al. Mycobacterium tuberculosis complex and mycobacterial heat shock proteins in lymph node tissue from patients with pulmonary sarcoidosis. J Clin Microbiol 2006;44(9):3448–51.

21. Allen SS, Evans W, Carlisle J, et al. Superoxide dismutase A antigens derived from molecular analysis of sarcoidosis granulomas elicit systemic Th-1 immune responses. Respir Res 2008;9:36.

22. Ding XL, Cai L, Zhang JZ. Detection and identification of mycobacterial gene in skin lesions and lymph nodes in patients with sarcoidosis. Zhongguo Yi Xue Ke Xue Yuan Xue Bao 2009;31(1):20–3 [in Chinese].

23. Zhou Y, Li HP, Li QH, et al. Differentiation of sarcoidosis from tuberculosis using real-time PCR assay for the detection and quantification of Mycobacterium tuberculosis. Sarcoidosis Vasc Diffuse Lung Dis 2008;25(2):93–9.

24. Nakata Y, Ejiri T, Kishi T, et al. Alveolar lymphocyte proliferation induced by Propionibacterium acnes in sarcoidosis patients. Acta Med Okayama 1986; 40(5):257–64.

25. Nakata Y, Ejiri T, Kishi T, et al. Alveolar lymphocyte proliferation in sarcoidosis patients induced by Propionibacterium acnes. Nihon Kyobu Shikkan Gakkai Zasshi 1985;23(4):413–9 [in Japanese].

26. Furusawa H, Suzuki Y, Miyazaki Y, et al. Th1 and Th17 immune responses to viable Propionibacterium acnes in patients with sarcoidosis. Respir Investig 2012;50(3):104–9.

27. Drake WP, Dhason MS, Nadaf M, et al. Cellular recognition of Mycobacterium tuberculosis ESAT-6 and KatG peptides in systemic sarcoidosis. Infect Immun 2007;75(1):527–30.

28. Launois P, DeLeys R, Niang MN, et al. T-cell-epitope mapping of the major secreted mycobacterial antigen Ag85A in tuberculosis and leprosy. Infect Immun 1994;62(9):3679–87.

29. Hajizadeh R, Sato H, Carlisle J, et al. Mycobacterium tuberculosis antigen 85A induces Th-1 immune responses in systemic sarcoidosis. J Clin Immunol 2007;27(4):445–54.

30. Carlisle J, Evans W, Hajizadeh R, et al. Multiple Mycobacterium antigens induce interferon-gamma production from sarcoidosis peripheral blood mononuclear cells. Clin Exp Immunol 2007; 150(3):460–8.

31. Edwards KM, Cynamon MH, Voladri RK, et al. Iron-cofactored superoxide dismutase inhibits host responses to Mycobacterium tuberculosis. Am J Respir Crit Care Med 2001;164(12):2213–9.

32. Rigel NW, Gibbons HS, McCann JR, et al. The accessory SecA2 system of mycobacteria requires ATP binding and the canonical SecA1. J Biol Chem 2009;284(15):9927–36.

33. Braunstein M, Espinosa BJ, Chan J, et al. SecA2 functions in the secretion of superoxide dismutase A and in the virulence of Mycobacterium tuberculosis. Mol Microbiol 2003;48(2):453–64.

34. Chen ES, Wahlstrom J, Song Z, et al. T cell responses to mycobacterial catalase-peroxidase profile a pathogenic antigen in systemic sarcoidosis. J Immunol 2008;181(12):8784–96.

35. Pathan AA, Wilkinson KA, Klenerman P, et al. Direct ex vivo analysis of antigen-specific IFN-gamma-secreting CD4 T cells in Mycobacterium tuberculosis-infected individuals: associations with clinical disease state and effect of treatment. J Immunol 2001;167(9):5217–25.

36. Oswald-Richter KA, Culver DA, Hawkins C, et al. Cellular responses to mycobacterial antigens are present in bronchoalveolar lavage fluid used in the diagnosis of sarcoidosis. Infect Immun 2009;77(9): 3740–8.

37. Andersen P. The T cell response to secreted antigens of Mycobacterium tuberculosis. Immunobiology 1994;191(4–5):537–47.

38. Andersen P, Askgaard D, Ljungqvist L, et al. T-cell proliferative response to antigens secreted by Mycobacterium tuberculosis. Infect Immun 1991; 59(4):1558–63.

39. Essone PN, Chegou NN, Loxton AG, et al. Host cytokine responses induced after overnight stimulation with novel M. tuberculosis infection phase-dependent antigens show promise as diagnostic candidates for TB disease. PLoS One 2014;9(7):e102584.

40. de Beer FC, Nel AE, Gie RP, et al. Serum amyloid A protein and C-reactive protein levels in pulmonary tuberculosis: relationship to amyloidosis. Thorax 1984;39(3):196–200.

41. Shinozuka N, Kasamatsu N, Seto T, et al. A fatal case of pulmonary non-tuberculous mycobacteriosis with reactive AA amyloidosis. Nihon Kokyuki Gakkai Zasshi 2007;45(8):636–42 [in Japanese].

42. McAdam KP, Foss NT, Garcia C, et al. Amyloidosis and the serum amyloid A protein response to muramyl dipeptide analogs and different mycobacterial species. Infect Immun 1983;39(3):1147–54.

43. Chen ES, Moller DR. Etiologic role of infectious agents. Semin Respir Crit Care Med 2014;35(3): 285–95.

44. Chen ES, Moller DR. Etiologies of sarcoidosis. Clin Rev Allergy Immunol 2015;49(1):6–18.

45. Haggmark A, Hamsten C, Wiklundh E, et al. Proteomic profiling reveals autoimmune targets in sarcoidosis. Am J Respir Crit Care Med 2015;191(5):574–83.

46. Wahlstrom J, Dengjel J, Persson B, et al. Identification of HLA-DR-bound peptides presented by human bronchoalveolar lavage cells in sarcoidosis. J Clin Invest 2007;117(11):3576–82.

47. Wherry EJ. T cell exhaustion. Nat Immunol 2011; 12(6):492–9.

48. Singh A, Dey AB, Mohan A, et al. Programmed death-1 receptor suppresses gamma-IFN producing NKT cells in human tuberculosis. Tuberculosis (Edinb) 2014;94(3):197–206.

49. Singh A, Mohan A, Dey AB, et al. Inhibiting the programmed death 1 pathway rescues Mycobacterium tuberculosis-specific interferon gamma-producing T cells from apoptosis in patients with pulmonary tuberculosis. J Infect Dis 2013;208(4):603–15.

50. Henao-Tamayo M, Irwin SM, Shang S, et al. T lymphocyte surface expression of exhaustion markers as biomarkers of the efficacy of chemotherapy for tuberculosis. Tuberculosis (Edinb) 2011;91(4):308–13.

51. Colley DG, Sasser LE, Reed AM. PD-L2+ dendritic cells and PD-1+ CD4+ T cells in schistosomiasis correlate with morbidity. Parasite Immunol 2005; 27(1–2):45–53.

52. Braun NA, Celada LJ, Herazo-Maya JD, et al. Blockade of the programmed death-1 pathway restores sarcoidosis CD4(+) T-cell proliferative capacity. Am J Respir Crit Care Med 2014;190(5):560–71.

53. Patsoukis N, Sari D, Boussiotis VA. PD-1 inhibits T cell proliferation by upregulating p27 and p15 and suppressing Cdc25A. Cell Cycle 2012;11(23): 4305–9.

54. Patsoukis N, Brown J, Petkova V, et al. Selective effects of PD-1 on Akt and Ras pathways regulate molecular components of the cell cycle and inhibit T cell proliferation. Sci Signal 2012;5(230):ra46.

55. Sheppard KA, Fitz LJ, Lee JM, et al. PD-1 inhibits T-cell receptor induced phosphorylation of the ZAP70/CD3zeta signalosome and downstream signaling to PKCtheta. FEBS Lett 2004;574(1–3):37–41.

56. Kato T, Nishida T, Ito Y, et al. Correlations of programmed death 1 expression and serum IL-6 level with exhaustion of cytomegalovirus-specific T cells after allogeneic hematopoietic stem cell transplantation. Cell Immunol 2014;288(1–2):53–9.

57. Dirks J, Tas H, Schmidt T, et al. PD-1 analysis on CD28(-) CD27(-) CD4 T cells allows stimulation-independent assessment of CMV viremic episodes in transplant recipients. Am J Transplant 2013; 13(12):3132–41.

58. Sester U, Presser D, Dirks J, et al. PD-1 expression and IL-2 loss of cytomegalovirus- specific T cells correlates with viremia and reversible functional anergy. Am J Transplant 2008;8(7):1486–97.

59. Yonemaru M, Kasuga I, Kusumoto H, et al. Elevation of antibodies to cytomegalovirus and other herpes viruses in pulmonary fibrosis. Eur Respir J 1997; 10(9):2040–5.

60. Rottoli P, Bianchi Bandinelli ML, Rottoli L, et al. Sarcoidosis and infections by human lymphotropic viruses. Sarcoidosis 1990;7(1):31–3.

61. Sheu J, Saavedra AP, Mostaghimi A. Rapid response of tattoo-associated cutaneous sarcoidosis to minocycline: case report and review of the literature. Dermatol Online J 2014;20(8):1–5.

62. Steen T, English JC. Oral minocycline in treatment of cutaneous sarcoidosis. JAMA Dermatol 2013; 149(6):758–60.

63. Baba K, Yamaguchi E, Matsui S, et al. A case of sarcoidosis with multiple endobronchial mass lesions that disappeared with antibiotics. Sarcoidosis Vasc Diffuse Lung Dis 2006;23(1):78–9.

64. Miyazaki E, Ando M, Fukami T, et al. Minocycline for the treatment of sarcoidosis: is the mechanism of action immunomodulating or antimicrobial effect? Clin Rheumatol 2008;27(9):1195–7.

65. Takemori N, Nakamura M, Kojima M, et al. Successful treatment in a case of propionibacterium acnes-associated sarcoidosis with clarithromycin administration: a case report. J Med Case Rep 2014;8:15.

66. Tercelj M, Stopinsek S, Ihan A, et al. In vitro and in vivo reactivity to fungal cell wall agents in sarcoidosis. Clin Exp Immunol 2011;166(1):87–93.

67. Drake WP, Oswald-Richter K, Richmond BW, et al. Oral antimycobacterial therapy in chronic cutaneous sarcoidosis: a randomized, single-masked, placebo-controlled study. JAMA Dermatol 2013; 149(9):1040–9.

68. Drake W, Richmond BW, Oswald-Richter K, et al. Effects of broad-spectrum antimycobacterial therapy on chronic pulmonary sarcoidosis. Sarcoidosis Vasc Diffuse Lung Dis 2013;30(3):201–11.

69. Swigris JJ, Olson AL, Huie TJ, et al. Sarcoidosis-related mortality in the United States from 1988 to 2007. Am J Respir Crit Care Med 2011;183(11): 1524–30.

Genetics of Sarcoidosis

Tasha E. Fingerlin, PhD[a],*, Nabeel Hamzeh, MD[b,c],
Lisa A. Maier, MD, MSPH[b,c]

KEYWORDS

- Sarcoidosis • Genetic epidemiology • Immune-mediated disease • HLA region

KEY POINTS

- Sarcoidosis is a disease with highly variable presentation and progression; although it is hypothesized that disease phenotype is related to genetic variation, how much of this variability is driven by genetic factors is not known.
- The HLA region is the most strongly and consistently associated genetic risk factor for sarcoidosis, supporting the notion that sarcoidosis is an exposure-mediated immunologic disease.
- Genome-wide association studies have identified limited reproducibly-associated gene regions with sarcoidosis.
- Candidate gene studies have contributed important information on other genes likely associated with sarcoidosis or sarcoidosis phenotypes.
- Most of the genetic etiology of sarcoidosis remains unknown in terms of the specific variants that increase risk in various populations, their biologic functions, and how they interact with environmental exposures.

INTRODUCTION

Sarcoidosis is a multisystem, T-helper 1 (Th1) cell biased granulomatous disorder that develops in genetically predisposed individuals who are exposed to yet unknown environmental trigger(s) acting as antigens.[1] The lungs are involved in more than 90% of cases, although sarcoidosis can affect any organ in the body, demonstrating variable manifestations and disease course. The disparity in prevalence and variability of organ involvement between ethnic groups,[1] and the familial clustering of sarcoidosis cases strongly support a genetic basis for sarcoidosis and its phenotypes.[2] Current studies suggest that an antigen(s) is presented to naïve T cells by the major histocompatibility complex II (MHC-II), which subsequently leads to T-cell activation and production of a cascade of cytokines and chemokines leading to further immune cell recruitment and activation and the ultimate formation of granulomas.[3] It is plausible that genetic polymorphisms in the genes involved in the immune response impact the extent and type of immune response, which ultimately affects the disease phenotype. Others have posited that different antigens impact disease course and organ involvement, as different HLA genes are associated with different disease phenotypes and organ involvement, including those with systemic symptoms, acute arthritis, erythema nodosum, and bilateral hilar lymphadenopathy, more commonly known as Lofgren syndrome (LS).[1]

SUMMARY OF APPROACHES TAKEN IN GENETIC EPIDEMIOLOGY OF SARCOIDOSIS

A number of genetic epidemiologic research methods have been used in an attempt to define genetic susceptibility for sarcoidosis, including familial aggregation, familial linkage, candidate gene

[a] National Jewish Health, 1400 Jackson Street, Denver, CO 80206, USA; [b] Division of Environmental Occupational Health and Sciences, National Jewish Health, 1400 Jackson Street, Denver, CO 80206, USA; [c] Division of Pulmonary and Critical Care Sciences, Department of Medicine, School of Medicine, University of Colorado, Aurora, CO, USA
* Corresponding author.
E-mail address: FingerlinT@NJhealth.org

Clin Chest Med 36 (2015) 569–584
http://dx.doi.org/10.1016/j.ccm.2015.08.002
0272-5231/15/$ – see front matter © 2015 Elsevier Inc. All rights reserved.

and genome-wide association studies. A challenge for all of these studies is the heterogeneity in sarcoidosis presentation and course, both of which may reflect differences in underlying genetic susceptibility, environmental triggers, and the interaction between the two. To identify robust genetic associations in the presence of this disease, and presumably underlying genetic heterogeneity, requires collection and characterization of large numbers of patients with sarcoidosis and controls. We review the literature on genetic risk factors for sarcoidosis, focusing on studies in which reproducible associations have been obtained while recognizing that some studies lack replication because of an inability to replicate the subjects and/or conditions of the study. The ultimate goal is to understand both the predictive ability of genetic factors for disease risk and course and the mechanisms by which the genetic risk factors impact disease. Specifically, functional genetic polymorphisms may influence the immune system's response or function, leading to development of disease or disease phenotypes, such as active, progressive disease versus self-resolving, limited disease, or fibrotic disease.

Familial Heritability Studies

A common first approach to investigating the potential for genetic risk factors for disease is to examine the risk of disease among relatives of those with disease. Although each study needs to be interpreted carefully because familial aggregation of disease can occur for nongenetic reasons (eg, household proximity to industrial exposures or other shared exposures), a collection of studies showing evidence for higher risk among family members can provide compelling evidence for a genetic contribution to disease. Based on this type of study, there is strong evidence for the importance of genetic risk factors for sarcoidosis. Among Irish sarcoidosis cases, 9.6% had a first-degree relative with sarcoidosis[4]; familial sarcoidosis was present in 3.6% and 4.3% of Finnish and Japanese cases, respectively,[5] prevalences that are markedly higher than the prevalence estimates in the general population of each of these race groups. Among the cases in the *A Case Control Etiologic Study of Sarcoidosis* (ACCESS) sample, the familial relative risk (RR) of sarcoidosis was 2.8 among African Americans, and was markedly higher, 18, among Non-Hispanic Whites.[2] Although some of the differences noted across racial and ethnic groups may be attributed to underdiagnosis or overdiagnosis or differential exposure characteristics, to a greater degree these differences likely reflect differences in genetic

susceptibility related to varied genetic backgrounds. As such, investigations aimed at identifying specific genetic risk factors need to carefully consider race and ethnicity in the design and analysis phases of study.

Familial Linkage Studies

Three genome-wide linkage studies have been conducted in sarcoidosis, one in a sample of African American families[6] and 2 in a German sample of families.[7,8] These studies examined affected relatives to identify regions in which those relatives shared more alleles from a common ancestor than would be expected based on their relationships. Two loci were identified as at least suggestive of linkage in both African American and German families: the HLA region on Chromosome 6p21 and a region on Chromosome 9q33.1. Although the HLA region has been investigated in several other studies described later in this article, to our knowledge, there is no additional information about the specific genes or variants that might underlie the 9q33.1 locus. However, recent studies have noted associations with Toll-like receptor (TLR) genes that are found in this region (see later in this article).

Genome-wide Association Studies

Genome-wide association studies (GWAS) are currently considered the gold standard for identifying associations between disease and common (>1%) variants; as resequencing studies become less expensive, genome-wide resequencing studies will become the gold standard. Like the familial linkage studies, GWAS have been conducted among German[9–13] and African American[14,15] study populations. These studies are the largest genetic association studies to date but still lacked power to detect variants of very modest effect due to the need to correct for so many statistical tests across the genome.

Candidate Gene Studies

Despite the superiority of GWAS over candidate gene studies in terms of their ability to agnostically scan the entire genome rather than rely on a priori hypotheses about disease etiology, for a given sample size, GWAS do have less power than a candidate gene study given the large number of statistical tests undertaken genome-wide. Replication of results is still important for candidate gene studies, however, and later in this article we note where there is particularly strong evidence for the involvement of particular genes not yet implicated in a genome-wide study. There is likely also a publication bias, as nonreplicating or negative study results are often not published. We also discuss candidate gene association studies with sarcoidosis phenotypes, which are even more difficult to study via GWAS given the challenges in achieving large sample sizes with consistency in definition of disease phenotypes.

Admixture Mapping Studies

Admixture mapping studies take advantage of known differences in disease risk between ancestral populations that make up an admixed population.[16,17] This approach is particularly applicable to African American sarcoidosis study populations, in which individuals have a range of European and African ancestry; the risk of disease is approximately 2 to 3 times as high for African Americans compared with Europeans. Under the hypothesis that the differences in risk between the ancestral populations is due to genetic differences, the basis of the approach is to find regions of the genome that show a higher proportion of African ancestry among cases compared with controls to find risk alleles. This approach has been used to identify new variants in the HLA region relevant for African American risk and a gene that was not identified by any of the other methods on Chromosome 17p13.[16]

GENES AND REGIONS ASSOCIATED WITH SARCOIDOSIS

Using the study designs outlined previously, numerous genes and regions have been studied as risk factors for sarcoidosis, although the consistency of these results varies. The strongest and most consistent region associated with sarcoidosis risk and disease severity is the MHC region and the HLA-DRB1 variants. Other genes with functional implications, such as cytokines, cell surface markers, signaling molecules, and others, have been associated with sarcoidosis in candidate gene and GWAS. In the following sections, we present the studies investigating the association of genetic markers with the risk of developing sarcoidosis, some of which are distinguished as either Lofgren syndrome (LS) or non-LS sarcoidosis, and then review the findings with each of these genes/regions with sarcoidosis manifestations, such as disease course and/or organ involvement. The results of many of these studies are summarized in **Table 1** for classic HLA variants, **Table 2** for genes associated with sarcoidosis risk, and **Table 3** for associations noted with various disease phenotypes.

Cell Surface Immune Receptors

HLA region
The HLA system plays an important role in the ability to recognize antigen and initiate an immune response. The HLA genes are encoded on chromosome 6 and consist of more than 200 genes.[18] HLA class I molecules, HLA-A, B, and C, are expressed by most somatic cells and are important in the immune response to a number of pathogens.[18] They are composed of an α polypeptide chain, which is coded by the class I genes, and a β chain, which is coded by the β_2-microglobulin gene on chromosome 15.[18] The HLA class II genes code for the α and β polypeptides of the class II molecule.[19] The HLA class II molecules are designated by 3 letters, the first (D) represents the class, the second (M,O,P,Q, or R) represents the family, and the third (A or B) represents the α or β chains.[19] The numbers that precede the asterisk indicate the gene (eg, 1, 2, 3) and the numbers following the asterisk represent the allelic variant of that gene (such as *0101).[19] For example, HLA-DRB1*0301 refers to an HLA class II molecule, D class, R family, β chain, gene 1, with allelic variant 0301. This region of the genome demonstrates strong and long-range linkage disequilibrium or LD, indicating that alleles at 2 loci are not independent of each other. As such, when one genetic marker is identified as associated with a disease or trait, then any allele in strong LD with that marker could be the actual link to the disease. For example, some HLA-DRB1 variants are always inherited with specific HLA-DQB1 variants. This makes study of this region complex. However, as HLA class II molecules are primarily expressed on immune cells, and are known to play an important role in the immune response, presenting antigens to the effector cells and induce activation of the immune cells, they have been well-studied in sarcoidosis.[19]

Several HLA alleles have been associated with LS. HLA-DRB1 is the most common and has been reported in white Dutch and UK cohorts,[20] Spanish and Swedish cohorts,[21] a Scandinavian cohort,[22] and a Dutch cohort with associations noted in HLA-DRB1*03 or *0301.[23] In addition, HLA-DQB1*0201 has been reported in white UK and Dutch cohorts,[23] although HLA-DRB1*03 and HLA-DQB1*02 are in strong LD.[23] In addition, 2 single nucleotide polymorphisms (SNPs) (rs3087456 and rs11074932) in the MHC class II transactivator (MHC2TA) gene, which acts as a master regulator for the expression of MHC class II molecules, have been associated with LS independent of HLA-DRB1*03,[24] suggesting that (1) these findings are not due to LD with the DRB1*0301 allele and that there may be other genes in the HLA region associated with sarcoidosis in addition to the classic HLA genes.

Several HLA alleles also have been associated with increased risk of developing non-LS

Table 1
Association of HLA genetic markers with risk of developing sarcoidosis and sarcoidosis phenotypes

Disease Risk Phenotype	Allele	Population	OR	CI	P	Reference
Increased risk of Lofgren syndrome	DRB1*03	White UK/Dutch	7.97	4.16–15.26	<.0001	20
	DRB1*0301	White Spanish	3.52	1.83–6.79	.0004	21
	DRB1*0301	White Swedish	7.71	4.63–12.84	<.0001	21
	DRB1*03	White Swedish	6.71	NR	<.0001	22
	DRB1*03-DQB1*0201	White Dutch	12.5	5.69–27.52	<.0001	26
	DRB1*0301	Finnish	2.46	1.11–5.45	.044	27
	DRB1*0301	Portuguese	4.01	1.88–8.56	<.01	115
	DRB1*1501	Finnish	2.16	1.06–4.41	.037	27
Increased risk of non-Lofgren syndrome	DQB1*0602-DRB1*15	White Dutch	2.27	1.46–3.54†	.0032	116
	DRB1*12	White UK/Dutch	2.5	1.26–4.96	.003	20
	DRB1*12	UK	3.7	1.73–7.94	.001	26
	DRB1*12	Japanese	2.5	1.17–5.21	.03	26
	DRB1*1201	US white/AA	2.13	1.14–4.12	.015	28
	DRB1*10	White UK/Dutch	2.4	1.00–5.88	.01	20
	DRB1*14	White UK/Dutch	3.1	1.7–5.57	.0003	—
	DRB1*14	White Swedish	1.79	NR	.017	22
	DRB1*1401	US white/AA	2.29	1.21–4.34	.011	28
	DRB1*14	UK	2.54	1.47–4.41	.001	26
	DRB1*14	Portuguese	4.07	1.0–23.6	Sig	115
	DQB1*0503/4	Dutch	2.4	1.11–5.18	.04	26
	DRB1*15	Finnish	1.67	1.12–2.5	.011	27
	DRB1*1501	US white/AA	1.7	1.18–2.46	.003	28
	DRB1*1101	US white/AA	1.98	1.37–2.9	<.001	28
	DRB3*0101	US white/AA	1.6	1.16–2.2	.004	28
	DRB1*1201	US AA	2.67	1.2–6.52	.014	28
	DPB1*0101	US AA	1.72	1.14–2.62	.008	28
	DRB1*0402	US white	2.57	1.02–7.28	.043	28
	DRB1*1501	US white	2.08	1.39–3.15	<.001	28
	DRB1*13	Czech	2.4	1.43–4.03	<.02	70
	HLA-B (rs4143332/ HLA-B*0801)	European/AA	—	—	—	9
	HLA-DPB1 (rs9277542),	European/AA	—	—	—	9
Decreased disease risk	DRB1*01	White Swedish	0.61	NR	.003	22
	DRB1*01	White UK/Dutch	0.5	0.35–0.82	.001	20
	DRB1*01	UK	0.5	0.34–0.76	.001	26
	DRB1*01	Dutch	0.4	0.23–0.76	.006	26
	DRB1*01	Japanese	0.12	0.03–0.52	.001	26
	DRB1*01	Finnish	0.43	0.26–0.72	.001	27
	DRB1*04	White UK/Dutch	0.6	0.46–0.92	.02	20
	DRB1*0401	US white/AA	0.48	0.28–0.8	.003	28
	DRB1*04	UK	0.54	0.35–0.84	.008	26
	DQB1*0301	UK	0.69	0.51–0.94	.02	26
	DQB1*0603	US males	0.5	NR	NR	28
	DRB1*1503	US AA	0.56	0.3–0.99	.44	28
	DRB1*0401	Us white	0.44	0.25–0.77	.003	28
	DRB1*07	Czech	0.40†	0.21–0.76†	.0031	70
Progressive pulmonary disease	DQB1*0602	AA	NR	NR	.032	30
	DRB1*07	Scandinavian	0.44	NR	.009	22
	DRB1*14	Scandinavian	2.14	NR	.005	22
	DRB1*15	Scandinavian	1.55	NR	.011	22
	DRB1*01	Scandinavian	0.41	NR	<.001	22
	DRB1*03	Scandinavian	5.42	NR	<.001	22
	DRB1*03	Finnish	2.22	1.20–4.1	.011	27
	HLA-B*07	Scandinavian	2.7	1.1–6.2	—	33
	HLA-B*08	Scandinavian	2.2	0.8–6.1	—	33
	A*03,B*07, DRB1*15	Scandinavian	4.7	2.2–10.2	—	33

(continued on next page)

Table 1
(continued)

Disease Risk Phenotype	Allele	Population	OR	CI	P	Reference
Resolving disease	DRB1*03	Scandinavian	5.42	NR	<.001	22
	HLA-B*08	Scandinavian	2.4	0.7–8.0	?	33
	HLA-B*07	Scandinavian	1.9	1.0–3.7	—	33
Ophthalmic	DRB1*0401	AA/White	3.49	1.62–7.54	<.0008	28
	DRB1*0401-DQB10301	UK	3.4	1.64–7.08	.001	26
	DRB1*03-DQB1*0201	UK	0.21	0.08–0.54	<.0001	26
Hypercalcemia	HLA-DPB1-0101	US white	4.28	1.45–12.6	.005	28
Arthritis	HLA-B8	Icelandic	—	—	.003	117
	HLA-B14	Icelandic	—	—	.04	117
	HLA-DRB1*03	Icelandic	—	—	.0002	117

† Values calculated by authors from raw data provided in original manuscripts.

Abbreviations: AA, African American; CI, confidence interval; NR, not reported; OR, odds ratio; UK, United Kingdom; US, United States.

sarcoidosis.[25] HLA-DRB1*14, *12, and *10 have been associated with increased risk of sarcoidosis in a white Dutch and British cohort,[20] and HLA-DRB1*12 and DRB1*14 in cohorts from the UK, Netherlands, and Japan,[26] whereas HLA-DRB1*1501 was associated with risk of sarcoidosis in a Finnish cohort.[27] HLA-DRB1*1201, *1401, *1501, *1101, and HLA-DRB3*0101 were associated with sarcoidosis in the ACCESS cohort in the United States.[28]

In contrast, HLA alleles that have been associated with decreased risk (protective) for sarcoidosis included HLA-DRB1*01 and *04 in white Dutch and UK cohorts[20] and HLA-DRB1*01 in cohorts from the United Kingdom, Netherlands, and Japan[26] and HLA-DRB1*0101 was protective in a Finnish cohort.[27] In the ACCESS cohort, HLA-DRB1*0401 was protective for the overall cohort (African Americans and Non-Hispanic Whites).[28] It has been posited that these variants may be less likely to bind putative sarcoidosis antigens and thus reduce the risk of disease. Understanding this effect and the function of these variants may help us prevent disease development.

Some HLA markers are gender-specific or ethnic-specific in their association with sarcoidosis. In the ACCESS cohort, HLA-DRB1*1101 was associated with increased risk more in male than female individuals, whereas HLA-DRB1*0401 was associated with decreased risk more in male than female individuals,[28] HLA-DQB1*0603 was a risk factor for female individuals but a protective factor for male individuals.[28] For black participants in the ACCESS cohort, HLA-DRB1*1201 and HLA-DPB1*1503 were associated with increased risk of sarcoidosis and HLA-DRB1*1503 was associated with decreased risk

of sarcoidosis,[28] whereas in white participants, HLA-DRB1*0402 and DRB1*1501 were associated with increased risk and HLA-DRB1*0401 was protective against sarcoidosis.[28] The finding of the risk associated with the HLA-DRB1*12:01 and HLA-DRB1*11:01 alleles was confirmed in a larger study of African American individuals,[29] although this may be related to use of some of the same subjects. Finally, in a recent admixture mapping study, SNP rs74318745 in the HLA-DRA gene was identified as a risk factor among African American individuals[16]; how this relates to any specific alleles is as-yet unknown, although it may be that there are also variants in the alpha chain of HLA-DR that are related to sarcoidosis in African American individuals.

In addition to disease risk, HLA genetic markers have been associated with sarcoidosis disease course, severity, and/or organ involvement. HLA-DQB1*0602 was associated with radiographic progression in an African American cohort,[30] and advanced pulmonary disease and uveitis in Dutch cohorts.[23,31] In a Scandinavian cohort, HLA-DRB1*07,*14, and *15 were associated with progressive pulmonary disease, whereas *01 and *03 were associated with nonprogressive disease[24]; note that HLA-DRB1 is a protective variant for disease. In a Finnish cohort, HLA-DRB1*03 also was associated with resolving disease.[27] Similarly, among an African American cohort, the HLA-DRB1*0301 allele was associated with decreased risk of persistent disease[29] and this association appears to be conditional on local ancestry at the locus. These results are also in keeping with the associations noted previously between DRB1*0301 and LS, which is usually a self-limiting disease, unless associated with

Table 2
Association of non-HLA genetic markers with risk of developing sarcoidosis

Phenotype Gene	Polymorphism	Population	OR	CI	P	Reference
Lofgren syndrome						
MHC2TA	rs3087456G	White Swedish	1.31[e]	1.04–1.65[e]	.019	22
	rs11074932C	White Swedish	1.27[e]	1.02–1.58[e]	.026	22
BTNL2	rs3117099T	White UK/Dutch	3.05	2.01–4.62	<.0001	20
CCR2	Haplotype 2[c]	White Dutch	4.4	1.9–9.7	<.0001	50
	Haplotype 2[c]	Spanish	2.03	1.11–3.73	.041	21
	Haplotype 2[c]	Swedish	3.02	1.65–5.52	.0027	21
CCR5	rs2040388A	German/Female	1.93	1.35–2.77	.0003	62
	rs2856757C	German/Female	1.65	1.17–2.33	.004	62
TNF[d]	TNF-α 308AA rs1800629	US white	8.182	2.45–27.34	.027	69
	TNF-α 308A rs1800629	Polish	2.3	1.23–4.32	<.01	82
	TNF-α 308A	UK/Dutch	3.1[e]	1.33–7.20[e]	.006	76
	TNF-α 308A	German	NR	NR	.0078	77
	LTA-252G rs909253	Polish	2.98	1.67–5.29	<.001	82
	LTA-252GG rs909253	US white females	11.33	3.18–40.37	.027	69
ANXA11	rs1049550TT	Czech	0.31	0.11–0.84	.02	98
Osteosarcoma amplified 9 (OS9)	rs1050045	German/Czech/ Swedish	1.41	1.05–1.88	.044	11
Increased risk of non-Lofgren syndrome						
BTNL-2	rs2076530A	German	2.31	1.27–4.23	<.006	39
	rs2076530A	White UK/Dutch	1.49	1.20–1.86	.002	20
	rs2076530A	White Dutch	1.85	1.19–2.88	.007	40
	rs2076530A	White US	2.03	1.32–3.12	NR	41
	rs2294878C	White UK/Dutch	1.54	1.24–1.92	.001	20
	rs2076530A	Portuguese	1.49	1.06–2.10	.01	115
TNF	LTA-252G rs909253	Czech	2.63	1.63–4.25	<.00001	70
	TNF-α 308A rs1800629	Polish	2.167	1.17–4.01	<.05	82
	TNF-α -857T	UK/Dutch	NR	NR	.002	76
	TNF-α 308A	European (meta-analysis)	1.445	1.010–2.065	.044	—
	LTA-252G	European (meta-analysis)	1.307	1.045–1.635	.019	—
IL-23	rs12069782	German/European Caucasian GWAS	1.24	1.16–1.33	3.07×10^{-10}	9
TLR-10	rs1109695C	Dutch	NR	NR	.002	48
	rs7658893A	Dutch	NR	NR	.001	48
TLR-1	rs5743604G	Dutch	NR	NR	.003	48
	rs5743594G	Dutch	NR	NR	.049	48
SLC11A1	Allele 2[a]	US AA	0.48	0.28–0.81	.014	64
	Allele 3[b]	Polish	1.68	1.01–2.81	.04	67
	Allele 3[b]	Turkish	2.69	1.61–4.47	<.001	66
	Allele 3[b]	Greek	1.52	1.08–4.52	.015	68
	INT4	Turkish	2.75	1.68–4.52	<.001	66
ANXA11	rs1049550C	German	1.54	1.23–1.92	.00014	97
	rs1049550T	Czech	0.77	NR	.04	98
	rs2573346C	German	1.55	1.24–1.92	.00008	97

(continued on next page)

Table 2
(continued)

Phenotype Gene	Polymorphism	Population	OR	CI	P	Reference
NOTCH4	rs715299T/G	AA	1.3	—	—	14
Decreased risk						
CCR2	CCR2-64I	Japanese	0.37	0.21–0.67	.0007	52
GWAS	Rs479777	European	—	—	<.001	100
FCGR3A	158FF – stage I	European	1.94	1.01–3.85	.05	118
	158VV – stage II	European	1.96	0.89–4.3	.06	118
	158F stage I vs II	European	2.73	1.30–5.76	.007	118

Abbreviations: AA, African American; ANXA11, Annexin A11; CCR, chemokine receptor; CI, confidence interval; GWAS, genome-wide association studies; IL, interleukin; NR, not reported; OR, odds ratio; TLR, Toll-like receptor; TNF, tumor necrosis factor; UK, United Kingdom; US, United States.
  [a] Allele 2: T $(GT)_5AC$ $(GT)_5AC$ $(GT)_{10}$.
  [b] Allele 3: T $(GT)_5AC$ $(GT)_5AC$ $(GT)_9$.
  [c] Haplotype 2: (A at -6752, A at 3000, T at 3547, and T at 4385).
  [d] TNF association with erythema nodosum.
  [e] Values calculated by authors from raw data provided in original article.

HLA-DRB1*1501 or a non-0301 variant.[32,33] Thus, whereas there is significant variation in HLA disease associations, the consensus of the studies to date support that HLA-DRB1*0301 is associated with a more benign form of disease in European (LS and resolving disease) and African American individuals.

Specific HLA variants have been associated with organ involvement in sarcoidosis. In the ACCESS study, HLA-DRB3 was associated with bone marrow involvement in black individuals, HLA-DPB1*0101 with hypercalcemia in white individuals, and HLA-DRB1*0401 with parotid and salivary gland involvement in black individuals, and HLA-DRB1*0401 was found to have possible association with eye involvement.[28] In a cohort from the United Kingdom, HLA-DRB1*0401-DQB1*0301 was associated with increased risk of uveitis, whereas HLA-DRB1*03 and DQB1*0201 were protective for uveitis.[26] In a Japanese cohort,

Table 3
Association of genetic markers with sarcoidosis disease course, severity, and/or organ involvement

Phenotype Gene	Polymorphism	Population	OR	CI	P	Reference
Progressive pulmonary disease						
BTNL 2	rs2076530	Dutch	1.84	1.06–3.21	.03	71
CCR5	HHC haplotype	British	6.8[a]	2.5–18.0	.0045	63
	HHC haplotype	Dutch	9[a]	3.5–23.1	.0009	63
IL23	Rs11209026A	German	0.63	0.5–0.79	<.001	96
TNF	TNF-α 308A	Dutch	0.43	0.31–0.61	<.001	71
	TNF-α 308T	Italian	3.53	1.66–7.5	<.001	82
TGF-β						
TGF-β1	rs1800469	US white	2.5	1.3–4.5	.005	92
TGF-β3	rs3917165A	US white	7.9	2.1–30.9	.01	92
TGF-β3	rs3917200C	US white	5.1	1.6–17.7	.05	92
GREM1	rs1919364CC	Dutch	6.37	2.89–14.1	<.001	119
ANXA11	rs1049550T	Czech	0.61	0.41–0.89	.01	98
Ophthalmic						
Complement factor H	rs1061170C	US	1.72	1.09–2.78	.018	120

Abbreviations: ANXA11, Annexin A11; CCR5, chemokine receptor type 5; CI, confidence interval; IL, interleukin; OR, odds ratio; TGF, transforming growth factor; TNF, tumor necrosis factor; US, United States.
  [a] OR at 4 years.

HLA-DRB1*15 and DQB1*0602 were associated with skin disease and HLA-DRB1*0803 with neurosarcoidosis.[26]

In addition to HLA-DRB1, other classic HLA genes and variants have been associated with sarcoidosis disease risk. For example, HLA-B*07 and -*08 have been associated with disease risk in Scandinavian individuals, in those with persistent and resolving disease, independent of Class II genotypes. However, a haplotype of HLA-A*03, B*07, DRB1*15 was associated with persistent disease, whereas HLA-A*01, B*08, DRB1*03 was associated with resolving disease in Sweden. Interestingly, a very recent study using a panel of immune SNPs noted associations with HLA-B*0801, confirming the Swedish findings, as well as finding an association with HLA-DPB1, independent of other HLA associations.[9] Interestingly, other studies have not noted these associations with DPB1.[34]

Overall, HLA-DRB1 likely plays an important role in the pathogenesis of sarcoidosis by recognizing specific antigen(s), blocking recognition of antigen, or dictating different immune responses to different antigen(s). Thus it is likely that if there are multiple exposures or antigens that trigger sarcoidosis, there may be multiple and corresponding HLA variants associated with disease and disease phenotype, if the latter is determined by exposure. For example, an in silico assessment of antigen binding suggested that mycobacterial antigens would bind a subset of the disease-associated HLA variants in a study of African American individuals.[29] In other diseases, evaluating specific amino acids that bind peptide in the HLA pockets has defined specific potential antigens for a similar disease: chronic beryllium disease.[35] A better understanding of the role of HLA molecules in the pathogenesis of sarcoidosis will move us a step closer to potentially identifying the antigen(s) that trigger sarcoidosis.[36] However, studying this region is complicated from a genetic standpoint because of the number of important immune-related genes and the significant LD that likely complicates associations noted to date, especially in non-Hispanic white individuals.

Butyrophilinlike 2

The butyrophilinlike 2 gene (BTNL2) belongs to the immunoglobulin gene superfamily, is related to the CD80 and CD86 costimulatory receptors, and is found in the MHC region on chromosome 6.[37] BTNL-2 was first linked to sarcoidosis via the first genome-wide familial linkage study involving 63 German families with sarcoidosis identified linkage to chromosome 6p21.[8] Further investigation defined an association between SNP rs2076530A in the BTNL2 gene and sarcoidosis.[37] In a mouse model, BTNL2 was shown to bind activated T cells and inhibit their proliferation.[38] Thus, it is possible that variants that alter BTNL-2 function could result in an increased T-cell immune response, as seen in sarcoidosis. Indeed, the rs2076530A variant produces an alternative splice site that results in an early stop codon and a truncated, nonfunctional protein as a final product.[37] The association between BTNL2 and sarcoidosis has been replicated in another German sarcoidosis cohort,[39] as well as Caucasian British and Dutch cohorts, although in the latter study, haplotype 4 (which included rs2076530G and rs2294878A) had a protective association.[20] The SNP rs2076530A was associated with non-Lofgren sarcoidosis and a gene dose effect was detected (AG vs GG odds ratio [OR] 1.98, AA vs GG OR 2.63).[20] There is strong LD between BTNL2 haplotype 2 and HLA-DRB1*03 and between BTNL2 haplotype 4 and HLA-DRB1*01 and thus questions have been raised regarding the primary association.[20] When the association of rs2076530A with the risk of sarcoidosis was analyzed in the context of HLA-DRB1, the rs2076530A association no longer held, whereas the association of HLA-DRB1*12 and *14 with the risk of sarcoidosis persisted.[20] In the same cohort, BTNL2 rs3117099T was associated with LS, with a similar but stronger association detected for haplotype 2, which contains rs3117099T.[20] The association of both haplotype 2 and HLA-DRB1*03 with LS remained significant after adjusting for each other and was stronger when both were present and protective against sarcoidosis when both were absent.[20] In a Dutch cohort, BTNL2 was associated with sarcoidosis but was also in LD with HLA-DRB1*15.[40] Although the rs2076530A conferred increased risk of sarcoidosis in an American Non-Hispanic White cohort, in an African American cohort, the BTNL2 gene risk and the HLA-DRB1 gene risk negated each other.[20,41] Although independence of BTNL2 and HLA genes was noted in a recent large study of immune variants,[9] it is not clear how many of these patients overlapped with the studies noted previously. Thus, the association between sarcoidosis and BTNL2 and its independence of the HLA genes nearby remains controversial and difficult to sort out.

Toll-like receptors

TLRs are transmembrane proteins that are critical in the innate immune system[42] and are also known as pattern recognition receptors, as they recognize specific microbial structures.[42] So far, 11 TLRs have been recognized.[42] Several studies in German and Dutch cohorts have investigated the potential association of polymorphisms in the TLR4, TLR2, and TLR9 genes with sarcoidosis, but found no association with the risk of sarcoidosis.[43–47] In a Dutch cohort, SNPs rs1109695 and rs7658893 in the TLR-10 gene and rs57436004 and rs5743594 in the TLR-1 gene were associated with the risk of sarcoidosis.[48] Interestingly, the study of the German cohort suggested an association with a chronic sarcoidosis phenotype,[43] whereas in the Dutch cohort, the SNPs in the TLR-10 gene and the TLR-1 gene associated with the risk of sarcoidosis did not differ between remitting and chronic disease but they did differ significantly between healthy controls and patients with sarcoidosis with chronic/progressive disease.[48] It is possible that there was some misclassification in individuals that confounded the association, although further study is needed to clarify this relationship.

Chemokine receptor type 2

Chemokine receptor type 2 (CCR2) is a receptor for the chemokines CCL5, CCL2, and CCL3 that play an important role in recruiting monocytes, T cells, and other inflammatory cells.[49,50] A study of 8 SNPs in the CCR2 gene revealed that a haplotype consisting of 4 unique alleles (A at -6752, A at 3000, T at 3547, and T at 4385) was associated with LS; this association remained significant after adjustment for HLA-DRB1*0301-DQB1*0201 and female gender (both of which have been associated with LS).[50] No difference was seen between non-LS sarcoidosis cases and controls.[50] This association and independence from HLA-DRB1 was confirmed in Swedish and Spanish sarcoidosis cohorts,[21] with similar findings noted in a Czech cohort that did not reach statistical significance.[49] However, no association was detected between 3 SNPs in CCR2 and sarcoidosis in a German cohort.[51] In contrast to the previously mentioned studies, the CCR2-64I mutation (A substitution mutation where isoleucine replaces valine in the transmembrane region) was found it to be protective against sarcoidosis in a Japanese cohort.[52] These findings have not been replicated in another cohort, although it is worth noting that Japanese sarcoidosis cases demonstrate different disease manifestations than European and American cases.

Chemokine receptor type 5

The CCR5 gene is located on the short arm of chromosome 3,[53] codes for a receptor for several chemokines, including CCL3, CCL4, CCL5, and CCL8.[54] These chemokines play an important role in lymphocyte and monocyte recruitment and activation in sarcoidosis[55,56] and CCR5 expression is upregulated in bronchoalveolar

lavage (BAL) macrophages and lymphocytes.[57,58] Levels of the CCR5 ligands, CCL3 and CCL5, correlate with risk of disease progression.[59–61] The CCR5Δ32 null allele results a 32-bp deletion in the CCR5 gene and produces a nonfunctional receptor that is unable to bind to it ligands; this variant was first discovered as it was associated with resistance to HIV infection. Variants that are part of a haplotype (HHC), were associated with LS in a German cohort, particularly in female subjects.[62] No association between 8 SNPs in the CCR5 gene and risk of sarcoidosis was detected in white Dutch and UK cohorts, but an association was observed with severity of lung disease with the haplotype HHC (-5663A, -3900C, -3458T, -2459G, -2135T, -2086G, -1835C, Δ32 wt) and increased chest radiographic abnormalities and worse lung function in British and Dutch cohorts.[63] Also supporting a more severe phenotype association, the CCR5Δ32 null allele was associated with the need for immunosuppressive therapy in a Czech cohort.[49]

SLC11A1 (NRAMP1, NATURAL RESISTANCE-ASSOCIATED MACROPHAGE PROTEIN GENE)

The SLC11A1 gene encodes a macrophage-specific membrane protein involved in transport, which appears to be important in the early stages of macrophage activation.[64] This gene was associated with an infectious granulomatous disease, tuberculosis.[65] Because of this association, the gene was studied in US African American individuals, and allele 2 of the gene was found to be protective for sarcoidosis.[64] This finding was replicated in Polish, Turkish, and Greek cohorts, where the alternative polymorphism (allele 3) was associated with increased risk of sarcoidosis,[66–68] whereas in a polymorphism in intron 4 was associated with risk of sarcoidosis in a Turkish cohort, a finding not present in the other cohorts.[66]

Cytokines

As increased Th1 cytokine production is noted in sarcoidosis lung and bronchoalveolar lavage cells, and these factors are known to be important in disease pathogenesis, many genetic studies have focused on the association of variants in cytokines and sarcoidosis.

Tumor necrosis factor-α and lymphotoxin-A, tumor necrosis factor-β

Tumor necrosis factor (TNF)-α and lymphotoxin-A (LTA) genes are located within the MHC class III region on chromosome 6p21.3.[69–71] TNF-α plays a pivotal role in granulomatous inflammation, and high levels of TNF-α released from sarcoidosis lung cells correlates with disease severity.[72] Furthermore, treatment with blocking of this cytokine with biologics has been an effective treatment for some patients with sarcoidosis.[72] The relationship between serum TNF-α levels and genotypes is unclear, as one study found an increased serum TNF-α level with the TNF-α-307G and the TNF-α-238A alleles in a sarcoidosis population but not healthy controls,[73] whereas another study did not detect any association between lung or blood cell TNF and the TNF-α 308 genotype.[74] It has been postulated that the TNF-α-863 A allele variant inhibits the binding of NF-kB p50-p50, leading to a higher production of TNF-α.[75]

Several loci in the TNF-α gene have been studied in association with sarcoidosis and an association between TNF-α 308A (rs1800629) allele and LS and between TNF-α-857T allele and non-LS sarcoidosis was found in a British and Dutch cohort[76] and German cohorts,[77–79] with a marginal association with the TNF-1031A noted in an Indian cohort.[80] It is possible that the variability in the association between the TNF-α and sarcoidosis is due to LD with other genes in the HLA region, such as LTA. For example, the TNF-α-308 (rs1800629) and LTA252G (rs909253) SNPs were associated with erythema nodosum in US Non-Hispanic White women[69] with no association noted in African American individuals.[81] Furthermore, LTA-252G (rs909253) and TNF-α-308A were associated with sarcoidosis in Czech and Polish cohorts.[82] There is strong LD between the TNF-α 308A, LTA252G alleles and HLA-DRB1*03, which has been associated with LS.[70] In fact, a meta-analysis failed to find evidence for an association between any of the previously mentioned alleles with sarcoidosis while reporting an association with the LTA-252A allele.[83]

Transforming growth factor-β

Transforming growth factor-β (TGF-β) is a growth factor with 3 isoforms: TGF-β1, TGF-β2, and TGF-β3. They have nearly identical biological properties but the functional properties are usually attributed to TGF-β1.[84] TGF-β induces the synthesis of extracellular matrix and decreases matrix degradation, is thought to be important in pulmonary fibrosis, and has immunomodulatory properties acting as a mediator regulating chemotaxis and fibroblasts as well as Treg cells.[84,85] The variant allele C of -509T/C and C of codon 10 are associated with higher TGF-β1 protein levels in the serum and the codon 10 variant is associated with increased mRNA levels in PBMC.[86,87] TGF-β1 levels in the BAL and alveolar macrophage supernatant are higher in patients with active

sarcoidosis and especially in those with pulmonary function changes,[88] and there is also a positive correlation with BAL lymphocytosis.[88]

No clear associations have been found between sarcoidosis and the TGF-β1 gene in a Japanese,[89] or German cohort,[90] or with the TGF-β1, TGF-β2, and TGF-β3 genes in a white Dutch cohort.[91] However, in this white Dutch cohort, there was an increased frequency of the A allele in rs3917165 and C allele in rs3917200 in the TGF-β3 gene in a fibrotic group compared with acute/chronic groups.[91] In the Japanese group, no relationship was noted with Scadding chest x-ray stage and the TGF-β1 variants,[89] although white American patients with sarcoidosis who had CC homozygosity at position -509 (rs1800469) were more likely to have parenchymal disease,[92] suggesting that TGF-β may be a disease-modifiying gene.

Interleukin-23

Interleukin (IL)-23 is a proinflammatory cytokine that stimulates Th-17 cells to produce IL-17 and other cytokines, and has a role in a number of autoimmune diseases, including Crohn disease (CD).[93,94] Polymorphisms in rs11209026 in these genes appear to affect serum IL-17A levels in patients with rheumatoid arthritis (RA).[95] In a German cohort and family-based study, rs11209026A was protective against chronic sarcoidosis,[96] but not disease overall. Using this cohort, as well as other cases in a recent immune SNP study, an association was noted with IL-23R with genome-wide significance in the discovery group (rs12069782). This SNP was replicated in European populations ($P = 3.07 \times 10^{-10}$, OR = 1.24, confidence interval 1.16–1.33). Interestingly, no association was noted in the African American cohort or German family; there was a question whether there was sufficient power in this group.[9]

Signaling Molecules

Annexin A11

The Annexin A11 (ANXA11) gene plays a role in the apoptosis pathway and depletion or dysfunction of the Annexin A11 protein may impair cell apoptosis and the downregulation of the immune response.[13] It is thought to be important in other immune-mediated diseases, including RA, systemic lupus erythematosus (SLE), and Sjogren syndrome (SS), playing a role in autoantibody formation.[92] A GWAS analysis in a German sarcoidosis cohort found a strong association between several SNPs in the ANXA11 gene on chromosome 10 (10q22.3) and the risk of sarcoidosis.[13] This association was confirmed in a separate German cohort where the C alleles of both rs1049550 and rs2573346 were associated with the development of sarcoidosis.[97] The association of rs1049550 with risk of sarcoidosis was also confirmed in a Czech cohort.[98] In this Czech cohort, the rs1049550 T-allele was protective against parenchymal disease (Scadding stages II-IV).[98]

Others Genes Associated with Sarcoidosis in Recent Genome-wide Association Studies

Neurogenic locus notch homolog protein 4

The neurogenic locus notch homolog protein 4 (NOTCH 4) is involved in T-cell immune response and has been associated with other immune-mediated diseases, including SLE as well as systemic sclerosis. In a recent GWAS, a locus in the HLA region at the NOTCH4 gene was found to be associated with sarcoidosis in African American individuals ($P = 6.5 \times 10^{-10}$), although it was only marginally associated in the Non-Hispanic White American population.[14] This has not been confirmed in other studies to date.

Osteosarcoma amplified 9

In a German GWAS, an association was found at 12q13.3-q14.1,[11] which was validated in another German cohort. The most likely gene was the osteosarcoma amplified 9 (OS9) gene; this gene was associated with sarcoidosis in a replication study of subjects from Germany, Czech Republic, and Sweden (OR 1.14). Of note, there appeared to be a stronger association noted with acute sarcoidosis than sarcoidosis overall. From a functional standpoint, OS9 is a protein that responds to endoplasmic reticulum stress and exposure to noxious stimulants, although its roles in sarcoidosis pathogenesis are not clear.

X-linked inhibitor of apoptosis associated factor

Fine-mapping of an admixture signal identified an SNP in the intron of the X-linked inhibitor of apoptosis associated factor (XFA1) gene that accounted for most of the admixture association signal.[16] Follow-up immunohistochemistry of sarcoidosis granulomas indicated that a decrease in XFA1 protein was associated with an increase in a downstream target of XFA1, suggesting a potential functional role of the variant that will require further study.[16]

A number of other candidate genes have been studied (see **Tables 2** and **3**), with some showing association with disease and/or disease phenotype and others not in relatively small samples. Similarly, other GWAS studies have noted associations with regions (10p12.2),[10,99] and genes such as the coiled-coil domain containing 88B (CCDC88B)[100] and 4q24 (rs223498; MANBA/NFKB1)[9] that have and have not been verified in independent studies; these studies ultimately need follow-up studies to understand whether or not there is robust evidence for a role in sarcoidosis risk and to understand the potential functional role of genes that are robustly associated.

GENE ENVIRONMENT INTERACTIONS IN SARCOIDOSIS

Several environmental and infectious agents have been proposed to be associated with sarcoidosis but none are definitively proven yet. The ACCESS study group identified 5 occupations and 5 exposures that were more prevalent in subjects with sarcoidosis than in controls.[101] These exposures included agricultural employment, physicians, jobs raising birds, jobs in automotive manufacturing, and middle/secondary school teachers, employment in pesticide- or insecticide-using industries, occupational exposure to mold and mildew, occupational exposure to musty odors and use of home central air-conditioning.[101] In contrast, smoking was found to be protective against sarcoidosis in this study and others.[101,102] Infectious agents, particularly *Mycobateria*, are re-emerging as a potential etiologic antigen in sarcoidosis with studies detecting mycobacterial proteins in tissues from patients with sarcoidosis, antibodies to mycobacterial protein noted in serum, and T cells from patients with sarcoidosis responding to stimulation by mycobacterial antigens.[103–109] Recent studies have also demonstrated an interaction between HLA-DRB1*1101 and in vitro immune responses to specific mycobacterial antigens, further supporting the gene-environment interaction theory.[108] Similarly, an in silico evaluation of antigens binding to HLA variants associated with sarcoidosis also demonstrated that mycobacterial peptides were prime candidates.[29]

SARCOIDOSIS GENETICS: A FINGERPRINT OF IMMUNE-MEDIATED DISEASE

Although numerous sarcoidosis genetic associations have been reported so far, further research is still needed to clarify the associations of the various genetic markers with risk and prognosis of disease. In addition, the interaction between 2 or more distinct SNPs or haplotypes in sarcoidosis has yet to be studied.[110] In general, the studies mentioned previously confirm that sarcoidosis is an immune-mediated disease. Interestingly, a pattern is emerging from these studies and those of other immune-mediated diseases, suggesting that many of these diseases share immune-mediated loci. Specifically, BTNL2, IL-23R,

NOTCH4, and the locus at 11q13.1 containing CCDC88B have all been associated with other immune-mediated diseases, including RA, ulcerative cholitis (UC) for BTNL2, CD, UC, RA, and ankylosing spondylitis for IL-23, SLE, SS for NOTCH4 and psoriasis for the 11q13.1 region.[111]

Currently, genetic testing is being used in Sweden, where the risk of progression versus remission is well predicted by the HLA-DRB1*0301 allele.[112] Ideally, similar markers will be available in this or other countries in the future, although currently there are no recommendations to use these or other markers in clinical practice in the United States. Studies of genome-wide transcription are beginning to show promise in this regard.[113] Although the odds of a first-degree or second-degree relative of a patient with sarcoidosis also having sarcoidosis has been reported to be 4.6, with a larger familial relative risk noted in siblings than in parents and in White than African American individuals,[2] the absolute risk and attributable risk for a sibling or parent of a patient with sarcoidosis is approximately 1% and, as such, screening family members, clinically or genetically, is not currently recommended.[2] However, as genetic research progresses and expands to include epigenetics, our understanding of the interaction of various pathways and networks will further expand, leading to the discovery and development of genetic panels and biomarkers that will serve as prognostic indicators of the disease. This will aid physicians in determining the extent and intensity of their workup and follow-up of patients with sarcoidosis. In addition, the potential role for pharmacogenomics in guiding immunomodulatory therapy has begun to be explored and further work is still needed.[114] However, at this time, this will need to be left to the clinician's knowledge and expertise to determine the optimal approach in the management of patients with sarcoidosis.

REFERENCES

1. Statement on sarcoidosis. Joint Statement of the American Thoracic Society (ATS), the European Respiratory Society (ERS) and the World Association of Sarcoidosis and Other Granulomatous Disorders (WASOG) adopted by the ATS Board of Directors and by the ERS Executive Committee, February 1999. Am J Respir Crit Care Med 1999; 160:736–55.
2. Rybicki BA, Iannuzzi MC, Frederick MM, et al. Familial aggregation of sarcoidosis. A case-control etiologic study of sarcoidosis (ACCESS). Am J Respir Crit Care Med 2001;164:2085–91.
3. Gerke AK, Hunninghake G. The immunology of sarcoidosis. Clin Chest Med 2008;29:379–90, vii.
4. Brennan NJ, Crean P, Long JP, et al. High prevalence of familial sarcoidosis in an Irish population. Thorax 1984;39:14–8.
5. Pietinalho A, Ohmichi M, Hirasawa M, et al. Familial sarcoidosis in Finland and Hokkaido, Japan–a comparative study. Respir Med 1999;93:408–12.
6. Iannuzzi MC, Fontana JR. Sarcoidosis: clinical presentation, immunopathogenesis, and therapeutics. JAMA 2011;305:391–9.
7. Fischer A, Nothnagel M, Schurmann M, et al. A genome-wide linkage analysis in 181 German sarcoidosis families using clustered biallelic markers. Chest 2010;138:151–7.
8. Schurmann M, Reichel P, Muller-Myhsok B, et al. Results from a genome-wide search for predisposing genes in sarcoidosis. Am J Respir Crit Care Med 2001;164:840–6.
9. Fischer A, Ellinghaus D, Nutsua M, et al. Identification of immune-relevant factors conferring sarcoidosis genetic risk. Am J Respir Crit Care Med 2015. [Epub ahead of print].
10. Franke A, Fischer A, Nothnagel M, et al. Genome-wide association analysis in sarcoidosis and Crohn's disease unravels a common susceptibility locus on 10p12.2. Gastroenterology 2008;135: 1207–15.
11. Hofmann S, Fischer A, Nothnagel M, et al. Genome-wide association analysis reveals 12q13.3–q14.1 as new risk locus for sarcoidosis. Eur Respir J 2013;41:888–900.
12. Hofmann S, Fischer A, Till A, et al. A genome-wide association study reveals evidence of association with sarcoidosis at 6p12.1. Eur Respir J 2011;38: 1127–35.
13. Hofmann S, Franke A, Fischer A, et al. Genome-wide association study identifies ANXA11 as a new susceptibility locus for sarcoidosis. Nat Genet 2008;40:1103–6.
14. Adrianto I, Lin CP, Hale JJ, et al. Genome-wide association study of African and European Americans implicates multiple shared and ethnic specific loci in sarcoidosis susceptibility. PLoS One 2012;7: e43907.
15. Li J, Yang J, Levin AM, et al. Efficient generalized least squares method for mixed population and family-based samples in genome-wide association studies. Genet Epidemiol 2014;38:430–8.
16. Levin AM, Iannuzzi MC, Montgomery CG, et al. Admixture fine-mapping in African Americans implicates XAF1 as a possible sarcoidosis risk gene. PLoS One 2014;9:e92646.
17. Rybicki BA, Levin AM, McKeigue P, et al. A genome-wide admixture scan for ancestry-linked genes predisposing to sarcoidosis in African-Americans. Genes Immun 2011;12:67–77.

18. Klein J, Sato A. The HLA system. First of two parts. N Engl J Med 2000;343:702–9.
19. Klein J, Sato A. The HLA system. Second of two parts. N Engl J Med 2000;343:782–6.
20. Spagnolo P, Sato H, Grutters JC, et al. Analysis of BTNL2 genetic polymorphisms in British and Dutch patients with sarcoidosis. Tissue Antigens 2007;70: 219–27.
21. Spagnolo P, Sato H, Grunewald J, et al. A common haplotype of the C-C chemokine receptor 2 gene and HLA-DRB1*0301 are independent genetic risk factors for Lofgren's syndrome. J Intern Med 2008;264:433–41.
22. Grunewald J, Brynedal B, Darlington P, et al. Different HLA-DRB1 allele distributions in distinct clinical subgroups of sarcoidosis patients. Respir Res 2010;11:25.
23. Sato H, Grutters JC, Pantelidis P, et al. HLA-DQB1*0201: a marker for good prognosis in British and Dutch patients with sarcoidosis. Am J Respir Cell Mol Biol 2002;27:406–12.
24. Grunewald J, Idali F, Kockum I, et al. Major histocompatibility complex class II transactivator gene polymorphism: associations with Löfgren's syndrome. Tissue Antigens 2010;76:96–101.
25. Voorter CEM, Drent M, van den Berg-Loonen EM. Severe pulmonary sarcoidosis is strongly associated with the haplotype HLA-DQB1*0602-DRB1*150101. Hum Immunol 2005;66:826–35.
26. Sato H, Woodhead FA, Ahmad T, et al. Sarcoidosis HLA class II genotyping distinguishes differences of clinical phenotype across ethnic groups. Hum Mol Genet 2010;19:4100–11.
27. Wennerstrom A, Pietinalho A, Vauhkonen H, et al. HLA-DRB1 allele frequencies and C4 copy number variation in Finnish sarcoidosis patients and associations with disease prognosis. Hum Immunol 2012;73(1):93–100.
28. Rossman MD, Thompson B, Frederick M, et al. HLA-DRB1*1101: a significant risk factor for sarcoidosis in blacks and whites. Am J Hum Genet 2003;73(4):720–35.
29. Levin AM, Adrianto I, Datta I, et al. Association of HLA-DRB1 with sarcoidosis susceptibility and progression in African Americans. Am J Respir Cell Mol Biol 2014;53(2):206–16.
30. Iannuzzi MC, Maliarik MJ, Poisson LM, et al. Sarcoidosis susceptibility and resistance HLA-DQB1 alleles in African Americans. Am J Respir Crit Care Med 2003;167:1225–31.
31. van den Berg-Loonen EM, Voorter CEM, Drent M. Strong association of severe pulmonary sarcoidosis with HLA DQB1*0602. Hum Immunol 2004; 65:826–35.
32. Grunewald J, Eklund A. Lofgren's syndrome: human leukocyte antigen strongly influences the disease course. Am J Respir Crit Care Med 2009;179:307–12.
33. Grunewald J, Eklund A, Olerup O. Human leukocyte antigen class I alleles and the disease course in sarcoidosis patients. Am J Respir Crit Care Med 2004;169:696–702.
34. Maliarik MJ, Rybicki BA, Malvitz E, et al. Angiotensin-converting enzyme gene polymorphism and risk of sarcoidosis. Am J Respir Crit Care Med 1998;158:1566–70.
35. Clayton GM, Wang Y, Crawford F, et al. Structural basis of chronic beryllium disease: linking allergic hypersensitivity and autoimmunity. Cell 2014;158: 132–42.
36. Dai S, Murphy GA, Crawford F, et al. Crystal structure of HLA-DP2 and implications for chronic beryllium disease. Proc Natl Acad Sci U S A 2010;107:7425–30.
37. Valentonyte R, Hampe J, Huse K, et al. Sarcoidosis is associated with a truncating splice site mutation in BTNL2. Nat Genet 2005;37:357–64.
38. Nguyen T, Liu XK, Zhang Y, et al. BTNL2, a butyrophilin-like molecule that functions to inhibit T cell activation. J Immunol 2006;176:7354–60.
39. Li Y, Wollnik B, Pabst S, et al. BTNL2 gene variant and sarcoidosis. Thorax 2006;61:273–4.
40. Wijnen PA, Voorter CE, Nelemans PJ, et al. Butyrophilin-like 2 in pulmonary sarcoidosis: a factor for susceptibility and progression? Hum Immunol 2011;72(4):342–7.
41. Rybicki BA, Walewski JL, Maliarik MJ, et al. The BTNL2 gene and sarcoidosis susceptibility in African Americans and Whites. Am J Hum Genet 2005;77:491–9.
42. West AP, Koblansky AA, Ghosh S. Recognition and signaling by Toll-like receptors. Annu Rev Cell Dev Biol 2006;22:409–37.
43. Pabst S, Baumgarten G, Stremmel A, et al. Toll-like receptor (TLR) 4 polymorphisms are associated with a chronic course of sarcoidosis. Clin Exp Immunol 2006;143:420–6.
44. Schurmann M, Kwiatkowski R, Albrecht M, et al. Study of Toll-like receptor gene loci in sarcoidosis. Clin Exp Immunol 2008;152:423–31.
45. Veltkamp M, Grutters JC, van Moorsel CH, et al. Toll-like receptor (TLR) 4 polymorphism Asp299Gly is not associated with disease course in Dutch sarcoidosis patients. Clin Exp Immunol 2006;145:215–8.
46. Veltkamp M, Van Moorsel CH, Rijkers GT, et al. Toll-like receptor (TLR)-9 genetics and function in sarcoidosis. Clin Exp Immunol 2010;162:68–74.
47. Veltkamp M, Wijnen PA, van Moorsel CH, et al. Linkage between Toll-like receptor (TLR) 2 promotor and intron polymorphisms: functional effects and relevance to sarcoidosis. Clin Exp Immunol 2007;149:453–62.
48. Veltkamp M, van Moorsel CH, Rijkers GT, et al. Genetic variation in the Toll-like receptor gene cluster (TLR10-TLR1-TLR6) influences disease course in sarcoidosis. Tissue Antigens 2011;79:25–32.

49. Petrek M, Drabek J, Kolek V, et al. CC chemokine receptor gene polymorphisms in Czech patients with pulmonary sarcoidosis. Am J Respir Crit Care Med 2000;162:1000–3.

50. Spagnolo P, Renzoni EA, Wells AU, et al. C-C chemokine receptor 2 and sarcoidosis: association with Lofgren's syndrome. Am J Respir Crit Care Med 2003;168:1162–6.

51. Valentonyte R, Hampe J, Croucher PJP, et al. Study of C-C chemokine receptor 2 alleles in sarcoidosis, with emphasis on family-based analysis. Am J Respir Crit Care Med 2005;171:1136–41.

52. Hizawa N, Yamaguchi E, Furuya KEN, et al. The role of the C-C chemokine receptor 2 gene polymorphism V64I (CCR2-64I) in sarcoidosis in a Japanese population. Am J Respir Crit Care Med 1999;159:2021–3.

53. Samson M, Soularue P, Vassart G, et al. The genes encoding the human CC-chemokine receptors CC-CKR1 to CC-CKR5 (CMKBR1-CMKBR5) are clustered in the p21.3-p24 region of chromosome 3. Genomics 1996;36:522–6.

54. Blanpain C, Migeotte I, Lee B, et al. CCR5 binds multiple CC-chemokines: MCP-3 acts as a natural antagonist. Blood 1999;94:1899–905.

55. Baggiolini M, Loetscher P. Chemokines in inflammation and immunity. Immunol Today 2000;21: 418–20.

56. Ziegenhagen MW, Schrum S, Zissel G, et al. Increased expression of proinflammatory chemokines in bronchoalveolar lavage cells of patients with progressing idiopathic pulmonary fibrosis and sarcoidosis. J Investig Med 1998;46:223–31.

57. Capelli A, Di Stefano A, Lusuardi M, et al. Increased macrophage inflammatory protein-1alpha and macrophage inflammatory protein-1beta levels in bronchoalveolar lavage fluid of patients affected by different stages of pulmonary sarcoidosis. Am J Respir Crit Care Med 2002; 165:236–41.

58. Katchar K, Eklund A, Grunewald J. Expression of Th1 markers by lung accumulated T cells in pulmonary sarcoidosis. J Intern Med 2003;254:564–71.

59. Iida K, Kadota J, Kawakami K, et al. Analysis of T cell subsets and beta chemokines in patients with pulmonary sarcoidosis. Thorax 1997;52:431–7.

60. Keane MP, Standiford TJ, Strieter RM. Chemokines are important cytokines in the pathogenesis of interstitial lung disease. Eur Respir J 1997;10: 1199–202.

61. Petrek M, Pantelidis P, Southcott AM, et al. The source and role of RANTES in interstitial lung disease. Eur Respir J 1997;10:1207–16.

62. Fischer A, Valentonyte R, Nebel A, et al. Female-specific association of C-C chemokine receptor 5 gene polymorphisms with Lofgren's syndrome. J Mol Med (Berl) 2008;86:553–61.

63. Spagnolo P, Renzoni EA, Wells AU, et al. C-C chemokine receptor 5 gene variants in relation to lung disease in sarcoidosis. Am J Respir Crit Care Med 2005;172:721–8.

64. Maliarik MJ, Chen KM, Sheffer RG, et al. The natural resistance-associated macrophage protein gene in African Americans with sarcoidosis. Am J Respir Cell Mol Biol 2000;22:672–5.

65. Bellamy R, Ruwende C, Corrah T, et al. Variations in the NRAMP1 gene and susceptibility to tuberculosis in West Africans. N Engl J Med 1998;338: 640–4.

66. Akcakaya P, Azeroglu B, Even I, et al. The functional SLC11A1 gene polymorphisms are associated with sarcoidosis in Turkish population. Mol Biol Rep 2012;39:5009–16.

67. Dubaniewicz A, Jamieson SE, Dubaniewicz-Wybieralska M, et al. Association between SLC11A1 (formerly NRAMP1) and the risk of sarcoidosis in Poland. Eur J Hum Genet 2005;13: 829–34.

68. Gazouli M, Koundourakis A, Ikonomopoulos J, et al. The functional polymorphisms of NRAMP1 gene in Greeks with sarcoidosis. Sarcoidosis Vasc Diffuse Lung Dis 2007;24:153–4.

69. McDougal KE, Fallin MD, Moller DR, et al. Variation in the lymphotoxin-alpha/tumor necrosis factor locus modifies risk of erythema nodosum in sarcoidosis. J Invest Dermatol 2009;129:1921–6.

70. Mrazek F, Holla LI, Hutyrova B, et al. Association of tumour necrosis factor-alpha, lymphotoxin-alpha and HLA-DRB1 gene polymorphisms with Lofgren's syndrome in Czech patients with sarcoidosis. Tissue Antigens 2005;65:163–71.

71. Wijnen PA, Nelemans PJ, Verschakelen JA, et al. The role of tumor necrosis factor alpha G-308A polymorphisms in the course of pulmonary sarcoidosis. Tissue Antigens 2010;75(3):262–8.

72. Ziegenhagen MW, Benner UK, Zissel G, et al. Sarcoidosis: TNF-alpha release from alveolar macrophages and serum level of sIL-2R are prognostic markers. Am J Respir Crit Care Med 1997;156: 1586–92.

73. Sharma S, Ghosh B, Sharma SK. Association of TNF polymorphisms with sarcoidosis, its prognosis and tumour necrosis factor (TNF)-alpha levels in Asian Indians. Clin Exp Immunol 2008;151:251–9.

74. Somoskovi A, Zissel G, Seitzer U, et al. Polymorphisms at position -308 in the promoter region of the TNF-alpha and in the first intron of the TNF-beta genes and spontaneous and lipopolysaccharide-induced TNF-alpha release in sarcoidosis. Cytokine 1999;11:882–7.

75. Udalova IA, Richardson A, Denys A, et al. Functional consequences of a polymorphism affecting NF-kappaB p50-p50 binding to the TNF promoter region. Mol Cell Biol 2000;20:9113–9.

76. Grutters JC, Sato H, Pantelidis P, et al. Increased frequency of the uncommon tumor necrosis factor -857T allele in British and Dutch patients with sarcoidosis. Am J Respir Crit Care Med 2002; 165:1119–24.

77. Seitzer U, Swider C, Stuber F, et al. Tumour necrosis factor alpha promoter gene polymorphism in sarcoidosis. Cytokine 1997;9:787–90.

78. Swider C, Schnittger L, Bogunia-Kubik K, et al. TNF-alpha and HLA-DR genotyping as potential prognostic markers in pulmonary sarcoidosis. Eur Cytokine Netw 1999;10:143–6.

79. Labunski S, Posern G, Ludwig S, et al. Tumour necrosis factor—a promoter polymorphism in erythema nodosum. Acta Derm Venereol 2001;81:18–21.

80. Sharma OP. Sarcoidosis around the world. Clin Chest Med 2008;29:357–63.

81. Rybicki BA, Maliarik MJ, Poisson LM, et al. Sarcoidosis and granuloma genes: a family-based study in African-Americans. Eur Respir J 2004;24:251–7.

82. Kieszko R, Krawczyk P, Chocholska S, et al. TNF-alpha and TNF-beta gene polymorphisms in Polish patients with sarcoidosis. Connection with the susceptibility and prognosis. Sarcoidosis Vasc Diffuse Lung Dis 2010;27:131–7.

83. Feng Y, Wang L, Zeng J, et al. FoxM1 is overexpressed in *Helicobacter pylori*-induced gastric carcinogenesis and is negatively regulated by miR-370. Mol Cancer Res 2013;11:834–44.

84. Border WA, Noble NA. Transforming growth factor beta in tissue fibrosis. N Engl J Med 1994;331: 1286–92.

85. Moses HL, Yang EY, Pietenpol JA. TGF-beta stimulation and inhibition of cell proliferation: new mechanistic insights. Cell 1990;63:245–7.

86. Grainger DJ, Heathcote K, Chiano M, et al. Genetic control of the circulating concentration of transforming growth factor type beta1. Hum Mol Genet 1999;8:93–7.

87. Yamada Y, Miyauchi A, Goto J, et al. Association of a polymorphism of the transforming growth factor-beta1 gene with genetic susceptibility to osteoporosis in postmenopausal Japanese women. J Bone Miner Res 1998;13:1569–76.

88. Salez F, Gosset P, Copin MC, et al. Transforming growth factor-beta1 in sarcoidosis. Eur Respir J 1998;12:913–9.

89. Niimi T, Sato S, Sugiura Y, et al. Transforming growth factor-beta gene polymorphism in sarcoidosis and tuberculosis patients. Int J Tuberc Lung Dis 2002;6:510–5.

90. Murakozy G, Gaede KI, Zissel G, et al. Analysis of gene polymorphisms in interleukin-10 and transforming growth factor-beta 1 in sarcoidosis. Sarcoidosis Vasc Diffuse Lung Dis 2001;18:165–9.

91. Kruit A, Grutters JC, Ruven HJT, et al. Transforming growth factor-β2 gene polymorphisms in sarcoidosis patients with and without fibrosis. Chest 2006;129:1584–91.

92. Jonth AC, Silveira L, Fingerlin TE, et al. TGF-beta1 variants in chronic beryllium disease and sarcoidosis. J Immunol 2007;179:4255–62.

93. Weaver CT, Harrington LE, Mangan PR, et al. Th17: an effector CD4 T cell lineage with regulatory T cell ties. Immunity 2006;24:677–88.

94. Hoeve MA, Savage ND, de Boer T. Divergent effects of IL-12 and IL-23 on the production f IL-17 by human T cells. Eur J Immunol 2006;36:661–70.

95. Hazlett J, Stamp LK, Merriman T, et al. IL-23R rs11209026 polymorphism modulates IL-17A expression in patients with rheumatoid arthritis. Genes Immun 2012;13:282–7.

96. Fischer A, Nothnagel M, Franke A, et al. Association of inflammatory bowel disease risk loci with sarcoidosis, and its acute and chronic subphenotypes. Eur Respir J 2011;37:610–6.

97. Liu Y, Helms C, Liao W, et al. A genome-wide association study of psoriasis and psoriatic arthritis identifies new disease loci. PLoS Genet 2008;4: e1000041.

98. Mrazek F, Stahelova A, Kriegova E, et al. Functional variant ANXA11 R230C: true marker of protection and candidate disease modifier in sarcoidosis. Genes Immun 2011;12:490–4.

99. Cozier YC, Ruiz-Narvaez EA, McKinnon CJ, et al. Fine-mapping in African-American women confirms the importance of the 10p12 locus to sarcoidosis. Genes Immun 2012;13:573–8.

100. Fischer A, Schmid B, Ellinghaus D, et al. A novel sarcoidosis risk locus for Europeans on chromosome 11q13.1. Am J Respir Crit Care Med 2012; 186(9):877–85.

101. Newman LS, Rose CS, Bresnitz EA, et al. A case control etiologic study of sarcoidosis: environmental and occupational risk factors. 10.1164/rccm.200402-249OC. Am J Respir Crit Care Med 2004;170:1324–30.

102. Gerke AK, van Beek E, Hunninghake GW. Smoking inhibits the frequency of bronchovascular bundle thickening in sarcoidosis. Acad Radiol 2011;18: 885–91.

103. Song Z, Marzilli L, Greenlee BM, et al. Mycobacterial catalase-peroxidase is a tissue antigen and target of the adaptive immune response in systemic sarcoidosis. J Exp Med 2005;201:755–67.

104. Dubaniewicz A, Dubaniewicz-Wybieralska M, Sternau A, et al. Mycobacterium tuberculosis complex and mycobacterial heat shock proteins in lymph node tissue from patients with pulmonary sarcoidosis. J Clin Microbiol 2006;44:3448–51.

105. Carlisle J, Evans W, Hajizadeh R, et al. Multiple *Mycobacterium* antigens induce interferon-gamma production from sarcoidosis peripheral blood mononuclear cells. Clin Exp Immunol 2007;150:460–8.

106. Drake WP, Dhason MS, Nadaf M, et al. Cellular recognition of *Mycobacterium tuberculosis* ESAT-6 and KatG peptides in systemic sarcoidosis. Infect Immun 2007;75:527–30.

107. Allen S, Evans W, Carlisle J, et al. Superoxide dismutase a antigens derived from molecular analysis of sarcoidosis granulomas elicit systemic Th-1 immune responses. Respir Res 2008;9:36.

108. Chen ES, Wahlstrom J, Song Z, et al. T-cell responses to mycobacterial catalase-peroxidase profile a pathogenic antigen in systemic sarcoidosis. J Immunol 2008;181:8784–96.

109. Oswald-Richter KA, Culver DA, Hawkins C, et al. Cellular responses to mycobacterial antigens are present in bronchoalveolar lavage fluid used in the diagnosis of sarcoidosis. Infect Immun 2009; 77:3740–8.

110. Zhang L, Liu R, wang z, et al. Modeling haplotype-haplotype interactions in case-control genetic association studies. Front Genet 2012;3(2).

111. Fischer A, Grunewald J, Spagnolo P, et al. Genetics of sarcoidosis. Semin Respir Crit Care Med 2014;35:296–306.

112. Grunewald J. HLA associations and Lofgren's syndrome. Expert Rev Clin Immunol 2012;8:55–62.

113. Su R, Li MM, Bhakta NR, et al. Longitudinal analysis of sarcoidosis blood transcriptomic signatures and disease outcomes. Eur Respir J 2014;44(4): 985–93.

114. Wijnen PA, Cremers JP, Nelemans PJ, et al. Association of the TNF-alpha G-308A polymorphism with TNF-inhibitor response in sarcoidosis. Eur Respir J 2014;43(6):1730–9.

115. Morais A, Lima B, Peixoto MJ, et al. BTNL2 gene polymorphism associations with susceptibility and phenotype expression in sarcoidosis. Respir Med 2012;106:1771–7.

116. Voorter CE, Drent M, Hoitsma E, et al. Association of HLA DQB1 0602 in sarcoidosis patients with small fiber neuropathy. Sarcoidosis Vasc Diffuse Lung Dis 2005;22:129–32.

117. Petursdottir D, Haraldsdottir SO, Bjarnadottir K, et al. Sarcoid arthropathy and the association with the human leukocyte antigen. The Icelandic sarcoidosis study. Clin Exp Rheumatol 2013; 31(5):711–6.

118. Typiak MJ, Rębała K, Dudziak M, et al. Polymorphism of FCGR3A gene in sarcoidosis. Hum Immunol 2014;75(4):283–8.

119. Heron M, van Moorsel CHM, Grutters JC, et al. Genetic variation in GREM1 is a risk factor for fibrosis in pulmonary sarcoidosis. Tissue Antigens 2010;77:112–7.

120. Thompson IA, Liu B, Sen HN, et al. Association of complement factor h tyrosine 402 histidine genotype with posterior involvement in sarcoid-related uveitis. Am J Ophthalmol 2013;155: 1068–74.e1.

The Diagnosis of Sarcoidosis

Praveen Govender, MB BCh, Jeffrey S. Berman, MD*

KEYWORDS

- Sarcoidosis • Differential diagnosis • Organ involvement • Lofgren's syndrome • Hilar adenopathy
- Heerfordt syndrome • Biopsy

KEY POINTS

- Sarcoidosis is a diagnosis of exclusion; cornerstones of diagnosis are careful history and physical examination looking for "footprints" of sarcoidosis or features that suggest alternative diagnoses.
- Some presentations are classic (eg, asymptomatic bilateral hilar adenopathy, Heerfordt syndrome and Lofrgren syndrome) and do not require tissue confirmation.
- A tissue biopsy should be performed if doubt exists and at an easily accessible site associated with the least morbidity.
- Sampling intrathoracic disease by bronchoscopy with transbronchial biopsy, or ultrasound-guided biopsy of mediastinal lymph nodes provide high diagnostic yield with low complication rates.
- Even with tissue confirmation diagnosis is never secure and follow-up over a number of years is required to be fully confident of the diagnosis.

NATURE OF THE PROBLEM

The diagnosis of sarcoidosis is never secure, but is made arbitrarily when the statistical likelihood of alternative diagnoses becomes too small to warrant further investigation.[1] The diagnosis of sarcoidosis can be challenging because symptoms and signs are nonspecific, are shared with other illnesses, and the finding of granulomatous inflammation in a tissue is itself nonspecific. There exists neither a pathognomonic clinical feature nor a perfect diagnostic test to aid in the diagnosis. As a result, missed diagnosis and overdiagnosis are often seen. Diagnosis of sarcoidosis requires pathologic examination of tissue from affected organs. However, tissue granulomas alone are not sufficient to diagnose sarcoidosis, which requires the presence of a consistent clinical syndrome and characteristic evolution over time. Thus, "definitive" diagnosis of sarcoidosis is not possible in some cases, particularly those in which the clinical evidence of disease is confined to 1 organ, until several years of follow-up.

DEFINITION

Sarcoidosis is a systemic granulomatous disease of unknown cause with variable symptoms and presentations.[2] The primary objective of the diagnostic evaluation is to support a compatible clinicoradiographic presentation with pathologic evidence of non-necrotizing granulomas, ideally in 2 or more organs, and to exclude other disorders with similar presentations or histopathology. The confidence that you have achieved this objective varies and diagnostic certainty can be stratified into highly probable, probable, possible, or unlikely[3] (**Box 1**). The highest level of confidence in a diagnosis of sarcoidosis has been changed from a definite diagnosis of sarcoidosis to highly probable diagnosis of sarcoidosis, acknowledging that absolute certainty in diagnosis is not achievable.[4]

Disclosure Statement: The authors have nothing to disclose.
Sarcoidosis Center, Boston University Medical Center, Boston, MA, USA
* Corresponding author. The Pulmonary Center, 72 East Concord Street, R-304, Boston, MA 02118.
E-mail address: jsberman@bu.edu

Clin Chest Med 36 (2015) 585–602
http://dx.doi.org/10.1016/j.ccm.2015.08.003

Box 1
Levels of confidence in diagnosis of sarcoidosis

Level of Confidence	Explanation
Highly probable (previously definite)	This is the highest level of confidence and is defined by a consistent clinical presentation, typically multisystemic, and is supported with positive histology in presenting/symptomatic organ.
Probable	This intermediate level of confidence is defined by a consistent clinical presentation, but supportive histology is from asymptomatic often non-presenting organ.
Possible	This is the lowest level of confidence where the clinical presentation is suggestive of the diagnosis, but supportive positive histology is unobtainable/not obtained and alternative explanations are not identifiable/identified.
Unlikely	Clinical presentation is suggestive, but histology is incompatible or absent and/or alternative diagnosis is revealed.

Adapted from Judson MA, Baughman RP, Teirstein AS, et al. Defining organ involvement in sarcoidosis: the ACCESS proposed instrument. ACCESS Research Group. A Case Control Etiologic Study of Sarcoidosis. Sarcoidosis Vasc Diffuse Lung Dis 1999;16(1):75–86; with permission.

APPROACH TO DIAGNOSIS

Sarcoidosis is a diagnosis of exclusion. There is no single approach to the diagnosis of sarcoidosis. Because clinical manifestations are protean, a general strategy should be adopted, but adapted on a case-to-case basis. **Fig. 1** outlines a strategy to use in diagnosis of sarcoidosis.[5] Fifty percent of cases achieve a diagnosis within 3 months of onset of symptoms, but 10% of cases can experience a delay of up to 2 years until definitive diagnosis is established.[6]

To work through the algorithm in **Fig. 1**, a series of questions should be answered during the diagnostic evaluation.

1. Does the clinical presentation justify consideration of diagnosis of sarcoidosis? (see **Fig. 1**, Box 1)
2. When and where is a tissue biopsy considered to support the diagnosis? (see **Fig. 1**, Boxes 2 and 3)
3. Have alternative explanations for the clinical presentation been excluded? (see **Fig. 1**, Box 4)

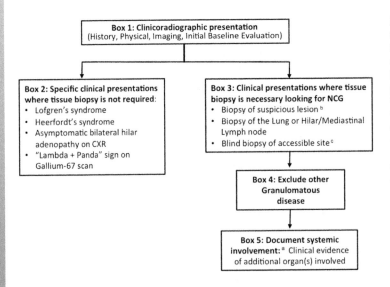

Fig. 1. Diagnostic algorithm for sarcoidosis. The diagnosis of sarcoidosis starts with a detailed clinical evaluation (Box 1). Diagnosis may be established without performing a tissue biopsy (Box 2). This requires the presence of specific clinical findings that are highly specific for the diagnosis. If none of these specific clinical presentations occurs, then the diagnosis requires tissue biopsy confirmation of granulomatous inflammation (Box 3), exclusion of alternative causes for the granulomatous inflammation (Box 4), and documentation that the disease is systemic and is, therefore, not confined to a single organ (Box 5). CXR, chest radiograph; NCG, noncaseating granulomas.

[a] Controversial criterion. [b] For example, abnormal skin, conjunctiva, lacrimal gland, or lymph node. [c] For example, conjunctiva, lacrimal gland, minor salivary gland, liver, lymph node. (*Adapted from* Judson MA. Advances in the diagnosis and treatment of sarcoidosis. F1000Prime Rep 2014;6:89. Available at: http://f1000.com/prime/reports/m/6/89.)

4. Is there any evidence of additional organ involvement? (see **Fig. 1**, Box 5)

Essentially, the diagnostic algorithm starts with a clinical presentation that is either highly specific for a diagnosis of sarcoidosis such that tissue biopsy is not required, or one that is consistent with a diagnosis of sarcoidosis, but needs tissue confirmation. Next efforts should focus on excluding alternative explanations for the clinical presentation and establishing further organ involvement. The subsequent sections of this article discuss aspects of this algorithm in more detail.

Does the Clinical Presentation Justify Consideration of Diagnosis of Sarcoidosis?

Sarcoidosis can affect any organ and present in virtually any manner (see **Fig. 1**, Box 1). However, up to 50% of patients are asymptomatic (eg, asymptomatic bilateral hilar adenopathy detected on chest radiograph [CXR] done for other purposes). Common symptoms at presentation are persistent cough, fever, arthralgias, visual changes, and skin lesions, and in up to 70% of cases fatigue.[7] Despite the seeming multitude of possible presentations of sarcoidosis, several are typical whereas others are less common to rare.[8] Knowledge a priori of the commonest organs involved in sarcoidosis and their associated symptoms is useful when considering a diagnosis of sarcoidosis. **Table 1** shows the observed frequency of organ involvement within 6 months of diagnosis in the 736 patients enrolled in the ACCESS study[9] and **Table 2** shows the commonest presenting symptoms of the various organ systems.

However, symptoms alone are not sufficient to justify the consideration of a diagnosis of sarcoidosis and other clinical variables should be incorporated to either strengthen or weaken the confidence in a diagnosis of sarcoidosis and justify the need to pursue further evaluation. **Table 3** reviews important clinical variables to consider: (1) at-risk populations based on age, ethnicity, occupational and nonoccupational exposures, and family history, (2) the physical examination, and (3) initial serologic and radiographic findings.

At-risk populations

Sarcoidosis affects people of all racial and ethnic groups and usually develops before the age of 50 years, with the incidence peaking at 20 to 39 years. In Scandinavia, the incidence in women seems to be bimodal, with 1 peak at 25 to 29 years of age and another at 65 to 69 years of age.[10] If

Table 1 Organ involvement within 6 months of presentation		
Organ	**n**	**%**
Lungs	699	95.0
Skin[a]	117	15.9
Lymph node	112	15.2
Eye	87	11.8
Liver	85	11.5
Erythema nodosum	61	8.3
Spleen	49	6.7
Neurologic	34	4.6
Parotid/salivary	29	3.9
Bone marrow	29	3.9
Calcium	27	3.7
ENT	22	3.0
Cardiac	17	2.3
Renal	5	0.7
Bone/joint	4	0.5
Muscle	3	0.4

Abbreviation: ENT, ear, nose, throat.
[a] Excluding erythema nodosum.
Adapted from Baughman RP, Teirstein AS, Judson MA, et al. Clinical characteristics of patients in a case control study of sarcoidosis. Am J Respir Crit Care Med 2001;164(10 Pt I):1886; with permission of the American Thoracic Society.

patients present at extremes of age, an alternative diagnosis should be considered.

The incidence of sarcoidosis is more common among persons of Scandinavian, Irish, German, and West Indian descent and is relatively rare in Japan, Spain, and Portugal.[11] In the United States, African-American patients have an estimated 2.4% lifetime risk for sarcoidosis compared with 0.85% of white Americans. Although the age-adjusted incidence of sarcoidosis in the United States is 10 to 35 per 100 000, a recent prospective cohort study found a yearly incidence of 71 per 100,000 in African-American women.[12]

Smoking status and whether family members have a diagnosis of sarcoidosis should be elicited. The relative risk of development of sarcoidosis is increased and in nonsmokers[13] and in first-degree and second-degree family members.[14]

A comprehensive environmental and occupational exposure history should be obtained, because it may lead to consideration of an alternative diagnosis. A history of exposure to inorganic particles that can cause granulomatous disease, such as silica, silicates, zirconium, and in

Table 2
Symptoms associated with specific organ involvement at presentation

Symptom	Grade
Lung	
No symptoms	+++
Cough	+++
Dyspnea	+++
Wheeze	+++
Pleuritic chest pain	++
Hemoptysis	+[a]
Eye	
No symptoms	+++
Red eye	+++
Painful eye	+++
Photophobia	+++
Dry eye	+++
Floaters	+++
Visual loss	++[b]
Loss of color vision	+[b]
Blindness	+[b]
Skin	
Painful lesion	+
Pruritic lesion	+
Cardiac	
No symptoms	+++
Palpitations	++
Heart failure symptoms	++
Syncope	+
Sudden death	+
Chest pain	VR
Neurosarcoidosis	
Facial nerve palsy	+++
Other cranial nerve deficits	+++
Headache	++
Meningismus	+
Peripheral neuropathy	+
Distal painful neuropathy	++[c]
Sweating, tachycardia	++[c]
Seizures	+
Mental status change	+
Psychosis	VR
Vitamin D dysregulation	
No symptoms	+++
Hematuria	++
Nephrolithiasis	++

(continued on next page)

Table 2
(continued)

Symptom	Grade
Liver	
No symptoms	+++
Nausea	++
Pruritus	++
Abdominal pain	++
Vomiting	+
Malaise	+
Fever	+
Sarcoidosis of upper respiratory tract	
Nasal congestion	+++
Nasal crusting	+++
Epistaxis	+++
Hoarseness	++
Tongue/pharyngeal lesion	VR
Peripheral lymph node	
Painful lymph node	VR
Bone	
No symptoms	+++
Painful lesion	VR[d]
Joints	
Arthralgias	+++[e]
Arthritis	VR
Muscle	
Pain	+++
Weakness	++
Mass lesion	VR
Gastrointestinal tract	
No symptoms	+++
Abdominal pain	VR
Hematemesis	VR
Blood per rectum	VR
Non–organ specific	
Fatigue	+++
Weight loss	++[f]
Night sweats	++
Other	
Tendonitis	+
Breast mass	+

Abbreviations: +++, common; ++, occasional; +, seldom; VR, very rare.
[a] Usually with stage 4 (fibrocystic disease) from bronchiectasis or mycetoma. Rarely caused by a granulomatous lesion.
[b] Usually related to optic neuritis.
[c] Related to small fiber neuropathy; distribution of pain may be patchy and in other locations.
[d] Usually related to vertebral or digit involvement.
[e] Including periarticular swelling with Lofrgren syndrome.
[f] Usually limited to 2–6 kg during the 10–12 wk before presentation.
Adapted from Judson MA. The clinical features of sarcoidosis: a comprehensive review. Clin Rev Allergy Immunol 2015;49(1):72; with permission.

Table 3
Findings on history, physical, and initial baseline evaluation that increases or decreases confidence in diagnosis of sarcoidosis

	Increases Confidence	Decreases Confidence
Demographics	United States African American Northern European	Age <18 y Age >50 y in males
Medical history	Non-smoking No symptoms (in patients with CXR findings) Positive family history of sarcoidosis Symptoms involving >2 organs commonly involved with sarcoidosis (eg, lung and eyes)	Exposure to tuberculosis (positive TST) Exposure to organic bioaerosol Exposure to beryllium Intravenous drug abuse
Physical examination	Lupus pernio Uveitis Facial nerve palsy (especially if bilateral)	Rales/crackles Clubbing Weight loss >10% Tender lymphadenopathy
Laboratory data	Elevated SACE, especially if >2× ULN	Low immunoglobulin levels
Radiographic findings	CXR: Bilateral hilar adenopathy (especially if without symptoms) HRCT: Disease along the bronchovascular bundle (perilymphatic distribution)	Asymmetrical bilateral hilar adenopathy

Abbreviations: CXR, chest radiograph; HRCT, high-resolution computed tomography; SACE, serum angiotensin converting enzyme; TST, tuberculin skin test; ULN, upper limit of normal.
Adapted from Judson MA. The diagnosis of sarcoidosis. Clin Chest Med 2008;29(3):417; with permission.

particular beryllium, should be sought. Chronic beryllium disease can be misdiagnosed as sarcoidosis in up to 40% of cases according to 1 series.[15] Exposure to beryllium can occur in diverse industries, for example, aerospace, automotive, biomedical (dental), x-ray tubes manufacturing, defense, and telecommunications (see ref[16] for comprehensive listing of beryllium exposures). Environmental exposures to organic bioaerosols should not be overlooked, because hypersensitivity pneumonitis is an important differential to exclude. Important clinical clues are bird (including feathered pillow), hot tub, and mold exposure. Finally, an exposure history to infectious agents particularly tuberculosis and travel to fungal endemic regions should be elicited.

The physical examination: "Footprints of sarcoidosis"

A complete physical examination should be performed looking for "footprints" of multisystemic involvement, which would strengthen the diagnosis of sarcoidosis. A close working relationship between pulmonary, cardiology, dermatology, ophthalmology, and neurology subspecialty clinics is helpful in these evaluations.

There are no pathognomonic clinical findings to diagnosis sarcoidosis. However, lupus pernio, uveitis, and bilateral facial nerve palsy are among the most useful clinical findings on physical

examination to support a diagnosis of sarcoidosis. Conversely, digital clubbing and crackles on pulmonary auscultation are uncommon clinical findings. In cases of sarcoidosis, crackles are heard in less than 2% of patients without pulmonary fibrosis[17] and in 28% with pulmonary fibrosis.[18] Digital clubbing is present during the course of disease in 3% to 6% of patients with sarcoidosis,[18,19] but is a rarer finding at diagnosis. Thus, if found on examination alternative causes should be excluded before assigning a diagnosis of sarcoidosis. Similarly, weight loss of greater than 10% of body weight[2] and tender lymphadenopathy should prompt consideration of an alternative diagnosis first.

Serologic and radiographic findings

Beyond the clinical evaluation, a series of investigations should be done at initial evaluation (**Box 2**). As mentioned, there is no absolutely reliable diagnostic test for sarcoidosis, but over time a number of tests have evolved a role in the diagnosis of the disease: serum angiotensin-converting enzyme (SACE) levels, tuberculin skin test anergy, asymptomatic bilateral hilar adenopathy, and disease detected along the bronchovascular bundle of computed tomography (CT).

Serum angiotensin-converting enzyme SACE levels are increased in 60% of patients with acute sarcoidosis and in 10% of patients with chronic

---

Box 2
Recommended initial evaluation of patients with sarcoidosis

History and Physical Examination (attention to environmental and occupational exposure and family history)

Posteroanterior chest radiography

Pulmonary functions tests: spirometry with bronchodilator, lung volumes, and diffusion capacity

Electrocardiogram

Complete blood count with differential cell count, serum calcium, creatinine, alkaline phosphatase, alanine aminotransferase, and aspartate aminotransferase levels

Tuberculin skin test

Complete ophthalmologic evaluation (slit lamp, tonometric, and fundoscopic examinations)

Adapted from Statement on sarcoidosis. Am J Respir Crit Care Med 1999;160(2):744; with permission of the American Thoracic Society.

---

disease.[20] Although levels greater than 2 times the upper limit of normal are rarely seen in other diseases[21] (**Table 4**) and are not often seen in cancer or lymphoma, serum levels of these enzymes in isolation are neither specific nor sensitive for a diagnosis of sarcoidosis.[22] This lack of sensitivity and specificity, taken together with genetic polymorphisms in angiotensin-converting enzyme gene and the low prevalence of sarcoidosis in both the general population and in patients with nonspecific symptoms, makes SACE activity poorly suited as a screening test for sarcoidosis.[23]

Tuberculin skin test and interferon-gamma release assay A tuberculin skin test should be considered as part of the workup for newly diagnosed sarcoidosis. Because almost all patients with active sarcoidosis are anergic to purified protein derivative, a positive test suggests a diagnosis other than sarcoidosis.[24] Despite the increasing use of interferon-gamma release assays (IGRAs) for diagnosis of latent tuberculosis infection, little is known of their use in the diagnostic evaluation of patients with sarcoidosis. Experience with IGRA use is limited to 3 case series: 3.3% of patients with a diagnosis of sarcoidosis in a Japanese series[25] and 25% to 29% of patients with a diagnosis of sarcoidosis in 2 series from India were tuberculin skin test negative, but IGRA positive.[26,27] These small series suggest that IGRAs are potentially

more sensitive than skin testing in identifying patients with sarcoidosis who have been infected previously with *Mycobacterium tuberculosis*, although the additive information, both in pathogenesis of disease and importance in diagnosis, provided by this new assay is not clear.

Asymptomatic bilateral hilar adenopathy on chest radiography During the course of the disease, more than 90% of patients with sarcoidosis manifest abnormalities on CXR. In 1961, Scadding[28] classified these changes on CXR at diagnosis: stage 0, normal appearances; stage I, bilateral hilar lymphadenopathy; stage II, bilateral hilar lymphadenopathy with pulmonary infiltrates; stage III, parenchymal infiltrates alone; and stage IV, pulmonary fibrosis with parenchymal distortion or bullae. This classification has stood the test of time and continues to provide useful clinical information. In 1973, Winterbauer and colleagues[29] further reported in a seminal study that CXR stage I (the presence of bilateral hilar with right paratracheal lymphadenopathy) in an asymptomatic individual was sufficiently specific for a diagnosis of sarcoidosis that histologic confirmation was not required. A clinical diagnosis based on this presentation is a cost-effective strategy to diagnose sarcoidosis because the pretest probability approaches 99.95%.[30,31]

Abnormalities in perilymphatic distribution on computed tomography Although thoracic CT is ordered frequently and is a superior imaging modality to detect intrathoracic lymphadenopathy and lung parenchymal changes, overall CT adds little clinically useful information to the standard CXR at initial assessment.[32] Current consensus statements[2] do not recommend routine use of CT. However, if CT is performed, a pattern of nodularity along the bronchovascular bundle (perilymphatic distribution) does increase the confidence of a diagnosis of sarcoidosis, especially if seen in conjunction with bilateral hilar and mediastinal lymphadenopathy. A more detailed discussion of imaging in pulmonary disease is presented by Grutters[33] and Valeyre.[34] Indications for performing a high-resolution CT include (1) atypical clinical presentations, (2) differentiation of sarcoidosis from other pulmonary conditions (eg, idiopathic pulmonary fibrosis), (3) guiding choices for tissue sampling, and (4) helping to increase confidence in the diagnosis in situations of high clinical suspicion, but a normal initial CXR.

Other tests Although it is recommended at initial evaluation to perform a complete blood count with differential white cell count analysis and serum chemistries for calcium and liver

Table 4
SACE in diseases other than sarcoidosis

Disease	N	No. (%) of Measurements >2 SD of Controls, n (%)
SACE in diseases that may confused with sarcoidosis		
Miliary tuberculosis	9	8 (89)
Silicosis	65	30 (45)
Primary biliary cirrhosis	55	11 (20)
Asbestosis	32	6 (19)
Leprosy	111	21 (18)
Histoplasmosis	50	7 (14)
Atypical mycobacteria	39	5 (13)
Berylliosis	25	3 (12)
Treated tuberculosis	132	13 (10)
Coccidioidomycosis	18	1 (6)
Hodgkin's disease	108	7 (6)
Lung fibrosis	161	9 (5)
Active tuberculosis	388	15 (4)
Extrinsic allergic alveolitis	67	3 (4)
Lung cancer	374	2 (<1)
SACE in other conditions		
Gaucher's disease	22	19 (80)
Hyperthyroidism	87	51 (61)
Alcoholic liver disease	151	43 (28)
Diabetes mellitus	265	48 (18)
Bronchial asthma	288	4 (1)
Bronchitis and emphysema	374	2 (<1)

Abbreviation: SACE, serum angiotensin converting enzyme.
Adapted from Studdy PR, Bird R. Serum angiotensin converting enzyme in sarcoidosis–its value in present clinical practice. Ann Clin Biochem 1989;26 (Pt I):17; with permission.

transaminases (see **Box 2**), findings of peripheral blood lymphopenia, hypercalcemia, and abnormal liver function testing (elevated alkaline phosphatase most common) are nonspecific.

Additional testing should be guided by the clinical presentation that is, echocardiography and advanced cardiac imaging (MRI or fasting PET) for cardiac sarcoidosis, right heart catheterization for pulmonary hypertension, and 25-OH and 1,25-diOH vitamin D levels, serum parathyroid hormone, and urine collection for hypercalcuria to characterize serum hypercalcemia. Up to 10% of patients with common variable immunodeficiency develop a sarcoidlike illness. In atypical presentations, common variable immunodeficiency can be screened with measurement of serum immunoglobulin levels or inferred from a low serum total protein to albumin ratio.[35]

When and Where to Consider a Tissue Biopsy to Support a Diagnosis of Sarcoidosis

Classic presentations where biopsy is not required

In patients with classical Lofgren's syndrome, Heerfordt syndrome, or asymptomatic bilateral hilar lymphadenopathy, a clinical diagnosis without tissue confirmation may be reasonable given the high likelihood of self-limited disease and lack of benefit of biopsy to justify the risk (see **Fig. 1**, **Box 2**). The presence of all features of Lofgren's syndrome (fever, bilateral hilar lymphadenopathy, ankle arthralgia (swelling), and erythema nodosum) has a 95% diagnostic specificity for sarcoidosis, allowing a clinical diagnosis to be made without biopsy. Heerfordt syndrome (uveoparotid fever—fever, uveitis, and parotitis with or without VII nerve palsy), is a classic but relatively rare presentation of sarcoidosis. As mentioned, if bilateral hilar lymphadenopathy is present on CXR and the patient is asymptomatic, the diagnosis is sarcoidosis in approximately 95% of cases.[29,36] Lacrimal and parotid uptake ("panda sign") combined with right paratracheal and hilar uptake ("lambda sign") on gallium scanning is a specific but insensitive pattern for diagnosis of sarcoidosis.[37] Although this distinct pattern has diagnostic potential, gallium scans are not recommended for routine use.[11]

Selecting a Site for Biopsy

In the absence of the classic presentations described, a diagnosis should not be made on clinical grounds alone, especially if the presentation is not typical of sarcoidosis, treatment with systemic corticosteroids is required, or the clinical course does not stabilize or improve over 3 to 6 months.[11] In these situations, a tissue biopsy should be performed at an easily accessible site associated with the least morbidity (see **Fig. 1**, Box 3).[38]

After the initial evaluation, typically 3 diagnostic options become apparent for tissue biopsy.

Option 1: Sample easily accessible sites first
Often, biopsy of a suspicious lesion based on clinical examination such as skin lesions (including subcutaneous or tattoo), nasal or conjunctiva nodules, an enlarged peripheral lymph node or an enlarged lacrimal gland can safely establish diagnosis. If these clinical findings are not present, the second option usually considered is biopsy of intrathoracic lymph nodes or the lung owing to the high prevalence of lung involvement.

Option 2: Sample intrathoracic disease
The gold standard approach to sampling the lung and mediastinal or hilar lymph nodes is surgical lung biopsy and cervical mediastinoscopy, respectively. However, the diagnostic yield from endoscopic procedures transbronchial lung biopsy (TBLB), endobronchial biopsy (EBB), blind (conventional) transbronchial needle aspiration (TBNA or cTBNA) and ultrasound-guided TBNA via bronchoscopy (EBUS-TBNA) or esophagoscopy (EUS-NA) have decreased the need for invasive surgical procedures in the majority of cases.[39,40]

Reported diagnostic yields of these procedures in sarcoidosis are variable: TBLB yield range is 40% to 90%[41]; EBB yield range is 40% to 60%[42]; cTBNA yield as reported by meta-analysis ranged 6% to 90%, with pooled diagnostic efficacy of 62% (95% CI, 52%–71%)[43] and EBUS-TBNA yield as reported by meta-analysis ranged

54% to 93% with pooled diagnostic efficacy of 79% (95% CI, 71%–86%).[44] The variability of diagnostic yields can be explained by a number of factors ranging from different Scadding CXR stages biopsied, to endoscopic technique (eg, needle size, number of biopsies or aspirates, number of nodes sampled, abnormal vs normal tissue sampled, operator experience) and to pathology issues (rapid on site "pathologic" evaluation [ROSE]) versus non-ROSE, processing samples, experience in detecting and differentiating tissue granulomas. There is currently no consensus on which is the "recommended" endoscopic sampling method for optimal diagnostic yield.

The recent GRANULOMA trial[45] tried to answer the practical question: Which is the better place to sample, the lung or lymph nodes, in stage I and II disease? In this prospective study, 304 patients were randomized to ultrasound-guided needle aspiration (via bronchoscopy or esophagoscopy) of mediastinal or hilar lymph nodes versus TBLB/EBB (conventional bronchoscopy) of the lung with suspected stage I and II sarcoidosis. Two hundred seventy-eight patients were diagnosed with sarcoidosis. The diagnostic yield of ultrasound guided needle aspiration was 74% (stage I, 84%; stage II, 77%) and for conventional bronchoscopy was 48% (stage I, 38%; stage II, 66%). The difference was statistically significant in overall comparison and stage I disease, but not in stage II disease. Ultrasound guided need aspiration via esophagoscopy performed better than EBUS-TBNA with a diagnostic yield of 88% versus 66% (P<.01). There were more adverse events with TBLB and EBB compared with US-guided node biopsy. This rate is consistent with other recent studies that support an approach to mediastinal and hilar lymph node biopsy using TBNA with endoscopic ultrasonography versus TBLB and EBB in stage I and II sarcoidosis.[46,47]

Another recent study randomized 130 patients with stage I and II disease to either EBUS-TBNA or cTBNA sampling of mediastinal lymph nodes. All patients had TBLB and EBB performed. Eighty percent of cases were stage I disease. The diagnostic yield of EBUS-TBNA (74.5%) was superior to cTBNA (48.4%) and EBB (36.3%), but TBLB did have a similar yield (69.6%). Thus, the evidence in aggregate suggests the modality with the greatest diagnostic yield in stage I and II sarcoidosis is EBUS-TBNA, but for optimal yield it should be combined with TBLB.[48]

Bronchoalveolar lavage fluid cellular analysis has been used as an adjunct to diagnosis with or without TBLB or lymph node TBNA. The finding of greater than 15% lymphocytes in bronchoalveolar lavage fluid has a sensitivity of 90% for the diagnosis of sarcoidosis. However, fewer than one-half of patients with sarcoidosis have this degree of CD4 lymphocytosis in lavage samples.[49] A lymphocyte CD4/CD8 ratio of greater than 3.5 has a sensitivity of 53%, specificity of 94%, a positive predictive value of 76%, and a negative predictive value of 85% for the diagnosis of sarcoidosis.[50] Ultimately, the choice of procedure depends on the individual facility, and the knowledge and skill of the clinician involved in the various diagnostic techniques.

Option 3: Diagnostic dilemma—When a biopsy site is not easily accessible

Often patients present with isolated ocular, cardiac, or neurologic symptoms with no suspicious clinical findings or pulmonary manifestation to sample after initial evaluation. In this scenario, the third diagnostic option is blind biopsies of an accessible site, which could be done based on clinical necessity to establish tissue confirmation of the diagnosis.

One study of 60 patients with ocular findings suspicious for sarcoidosis, but without apparent extraocular manifestations such as bilateral hilar adenopathy on CXR, showed granulomas on TBLB in 37 patients (62%). It is not clear why these patients did not undergo blind conjunctival biopsy because the diagnostic yield of conjunctival biopsy without defined lesion is upward of 55%.[51] Other accessible locations for blind biopsies have shown similar yields: minor salivary glands, 20% to 58% yield[52,53]; scalene lymph nodes, 74% to 80%[38,54,55]; liver, 50% to 60%[56]; and gastrocnemius in setting of erythema nodosum, 90%.[38,57] These sites are rarely biopsied, but knowledge of their potential yield could help in particularly difficult or confusing cases. PET/CT is emerging as a tool in locating occult sites of active disease in which to potentially biopsy; however, routine use is not recommended currently.[58]

The Kveim test, a skin biopsy of a nodule that develops 4 to 6 weeks after intradermal inoculation of a suspension from a human spleen involved with sarcoidosis, is reportedly specific for a diagnosis of sarcoidosis. It is, however, little used as a diagnostic test for sarcoidosis primarily owing to reagent availability and it is not approved by the US Food and Drug Administration.[59]

Have Alternative Explanations for the Clinical Presentation Been Excluded?

Although the demonstration of tissue granulomas is necessary for a diagnosis of sarcoidosis, histology by itself is not enough to secure a diagnosis of sarcoidosis. **Table 5** shows the broad differential diagnosis of granulomatous inflammation for the common tissues biopsied after clinical evaluation, that is, skin, lymph node, and the lung (see **Fig. 1**, Box 4). Thus, the exclusion of these alternative causes of granulomatous inflammation requires careful examination of the histologic tissue by an experienced pathologist for infectious organisms and foreign particles that can induce granulomatous inflammation.

Pathology of sarcoidal granulomas

There are no specific diagnostic features of a sarcoidal granuloma. The classic histologic lesion described in sarcoidosis is multiple, discrete, well-formed, non-necrotizing granulomas with a compact cluster of epithelioid and multinucleated histiocytes with minimal or no central necrosis. There is often a peripheral rim of lymphocytes and, as the lesion ages, concentric hyalinization is seen.[60] In reality, there is a range of histopathologic findings in sarcoidosis.[61,62]

Inclusion bodies are often seen in sarcoidal granulomas: asteroid bodies are seen in 2% to 9% of granulomas. Schaumann's (conchoidal) bodies are seen 41% to 88% of granulomas, birefringent calcium oxalate crystals are seen up to two-thirds of open lung biopsies, and finally acid-fast staining, and periodic acid-Schiff–positive Hamazaki–Wesenberg bodies can be seen in 16% lung biopsies and 11% to 68% of lymph node biopsies.[63] It is important to recognize that these inclusions are not foreign bodies and, in the case of Hamazaki–Wesenberg bodies, are not viable infectious particles that could lead to a false or delayed diagnosis.

Both necrosis and vascular (both arterial and venous) involvement may be seen. Necrosis is seen up to 35% of cases[64] and vascular involvement (arterial and venous) can be seen on 53% of TBLB, 69% of open lung biopsies, and in 100% of autopsy samples.[63]

The anatomic location of the granuloma in the tissue is important in diagnosis. For example, bronchovascular distribution of granulomas[65] is an important histologic clue and correlates with the "perilymphatic distribution" seen on CT thorax (see **Table 3**).

Atypical pathologic presentations

Atypical or non-classic histologic features should not discourage a diagnosis of sarcoidosis; again, final diagnosis requires correlation with the clinical presentation and monitoring evolution over time. However, even with clinical correlation, there exist in the literature alternative, idiopathic, multiorgan granulomatous syndromes that can make confident diagnosis of sarcoidosis challenging. It is debated if necrotizing sarcoid granulomatosis

Table 5
Major pathologic differential diagnosis of sarcoidosis at biopsy

Lung	Lymph Node	Skin	Liver	Bone Marrow	Other Biopsy Sites
Tuberculosis	Tuberculosis	Tuberculosis	Tuberculosis	Tuberculosis	Tuberculosis
Atypical mycobacteriosis	Atypical mycobacteriosis	Atypical mycobacteriosis	Brucellosis	Histoplasmosis	Brucellosis
Fungi	Brucellosis	Fungi	Schistosomiasis	Infectious mononucleosis	Other infections
Pneumocystis carinii	Toxoplasmosis	Reaction to foreign bodies: beryllium, zirconium, tattooing, paraffin, etc	Primary biliary cirrhosis	Cytomegalovirus	Crohn's disease
Mycoplasma	Granulomatous histiocytic necrotizing Lymphadenitis (Kikuchi's disease)	Rheumatoid nodules	Crohn's disease	Hodgkin's disease	Giant cell myocarditis
Hypersensitivity pneumonitis	Cat-scratch disease		Hodgkin's disease	Non-Hodgkin's lymphoma	GLUS syndrome
Pneumoconiosis	Sarcoid reaction in regional lymph nodes to carcinoma		Non-Hodgkin's lymphoma	Drugs	
Beryllium (chronic beryllium disease)	Hodgkin's disease		GLUS syndrome	GLUS syndrome	
Titanium, aluminum	Non-Hodgkin's lymphoma		Drug reactions		
Drug reactions	GLUS syndrome				
Aspiration of foreign materials					
Granulomatous polyangiitis (GPA; sarcoid-type granulomas are rare)					
Necrotizing sarcoid granulomatosis (NSG); see text					

Abbreviation: GLUS, granulomatous lesions of unknown significance.
Adapted from Statement on sarcoidosis. Am J Respir Crit Care Med 1999;160(2):742; with permission of the American Thoracic Society.

Table 6
The WASOG sarcoidosis organ assessment instrument

	Highly Probable[a,b]	At Least Probable	Possible	No Consensus
Lung	CXR: Bilateral hilar adenopathy Chest CT: perilymphatic nodules Chest CT: symmetric hilar/mediastinal adenopathy PET/gallium-67: Mediastinal/hilar adenopathy enhancement	CXR: Diffuse infiltrates CXR: Upper lobe fibrosis Chest CT: peribronchial thickening BAL: Lymphocytic alveolitis BAL: Elevated CD4/CD8 ratio PET/gallium-67: Diffuse parenchymal lung enhancement TBNA: Lymphoid aggregates/giant cells	CXR: Localized infiltrate PFT: Obstruction	PFT: Restriction PFT: Isolated reduction in diffusing capacity
Skin	Lupus pernio	Subcutaneous nodules or plaques Inflammatory papules within a scar or tattoo Violaceous or erythematous annular lesions Violaceous or erythematous macular, papular lesions around the eyes, nose, or mouth	Atypical lesions: Ulcerative, erythrodermic, alopecic, ichthyosiform	Verrucous/scaly papules or plaques hypopigmented or hyperpigmented macules or patches
Eye	Uveitis Optic neuritis Mutton fat keratic precipitates Iris nodules Snowball/string of pearls (pars planitis)	Lacrimal gland swelling Trabecular meshwork nodules red/eye Retinitis Scleritis Multiple chorioretinal peripheral lesions Adnexal nodularity Candle wax drippings	Cataract Glaucoma Red eye	Blindness Painful eye Cystoid macular edema
Liver	—	Abdominal imaging demonstrating hepatomegaly Abdominal imaging demonstrating hepatic nodules	—	Hepatomegaly on physical examination Serum alkaline phosphate >3× the upper limit of normal
Spleen	—	Low attenuation nodules on CT PET/gallium-67 uptake in splenic nodules Splenomegaly on imaging or physical examination	—	—

Extrathoracic lymph node	—	Multiple enlarged palpable cervical or epitrochlear lymph nodes without B symptoms Enlarged lymph nodes identified by imaging in at least 2 peripheral or visceral lymph node stations without B symptoms	—	Multiple enlarged palpable peripheral or visceral lymph nodes with B symptoms Multiple palpable enlarged peripheral or visceral lymph nodes at sites other than cervical and epitrochlear
Nervous system	Clinical syndrome consistent with granulomatous inflammation of the meninges, brain, ventricular (CSF) system, cranial nerves, pituitary gland, spinal cord, cerebral vasculature or nerve roots Plus An abnormal MRI characteristic of neurosarcoidosis, defined as exhibiting abnormal enhancement after the administration of gadolinium or a CSF examination demonstrating inflammation	Isolated facial palsy, negative MRI Clinical syndrome consistent with granulomatous inflammation of the meninges, brain, ventricular (CSF) system, cranial nerves, pituitary gland, spinal cord, cerebral vasculature, nerve roots but without characteristic MRI or CSF findings	Seizures, negative MRI Cognitive decline, negative MRI	Peripheral neuropathy involving large fibers (including axonal and demyelinating polyneuropathies and multiple mononeuropathies) Cranial nerve palsies other than VII, negative MRI Pleocytosis in the CSF low CSF glucose
Cardiac	—	Treatment responsive CM or AVNB Decreased LVEF in the absence of other clinical risk factors Spontaneous or inducible sustained VT with no other risk factor Mobitz type II or third-degree heart block Patchy uptake on dedicated cardiac PET Delayed enhancement on CMRI Positive gallium uptake Defect on perfusion scintigraphy or SPECT scan T2 prolongation on CMRI	Decreased LVEF in the presence of other risk factors (eg, HTN, DM) Atrial dysrhythmias	Frequent ectopy (>5% QRS) Bundle branch block Impaired RV function with a normal PVR Fragmented QRS or pathologic Q waves in ≥2 anatomically contiguous leads At least 1 abnormal SAECG domain Interstitial fibrosis or monocyte infiltration

(continued on next page)

Table 6
(continued)

	Highly Probable[a,b]	At Least Probable	Possible	No Consensus
Salivary gland	Positive gallium-67 scan ("panda sign") Positive PET scan of the parotid glands	Symmetric parotitis with syndrome of mumps Enlarged salivary glands	Dry mouth	—
ENT	—	Granulomatous changes on direct laryngoscopy Consistent imaging studies (eg, sinonasal erosion, mucoperiosteal thickening, positive PET scan)	Chronic sinusitis	Nasal crusting, epistaxis, or anosmia associated with chronic sinus congestion
Calcium–vitamin D	Hypercalcemia plus all of the following: (a) a normal serum PTH level, (b) a Normal or increased 1,25-diOH vitamin D level, (c) a low 25-OH vitamin D level Hypercalciuria plus all of the following: (a) a Normal serum PTH level, (b) a normal or increased 1,25-diOH vitamin D level, c) a low 25-OH vitamin D level	Nephrolithiasis plus all of the following: (a) a normal serum PTH level, (b) a normal or increased 1,25-diOH vitamin D level, (c) a low 25-OH vitamin D level Hypercalciuria without serum PTH and 25-OH and 1,25-diOH vitamin D levels Nephrolithiasis with calcium stones, without serum PTH and 25-OH and 1,25-diOH vitamin D levels	Nephrolithiasis, no stone analysis	—

Bone–joint	Typical radiographic features (trabecular pattern, osteolysis, cysts/punched out lesions)	Dactylitis Nodular tenosynovitis Positive PET, MRI, or gallium-67	Arthralgias	Nonspecific arthritis
Bone marrow	PET displaying diffuse uptake	—		Leukopenia Anemia Thrombocytopenia
Muscle	—	Positive imaging (MRI, galium-67) Palpable muscle masses	Myalgias	Increased serum muscle enzymes
Kidney	—	Treatment-responsive renal failure with no other risk factors Treatment-responsive renal failure in patient with diabetes and/or hypertension	Renal failure with other potential risk factors	CT evidence of abnormal renal enhancement.
Other organs	—	Positive imaging	—	—

Abbreviations: AVNB, atrioventricular nodal block; B symptoms, fever, weight loss, or night sweats; BAL, bronchoalveolar lavage; CM, cardiomyopathy; CMRI, cardiovascular MRI; CSF, cerebrospinal fluid; CT, computed tomography; CXR, chest radiograph; diOH, dihydroxy; DM, diabetes mellitus; ENT, ear, nose, throat; gallium-67, gallium-67 nuclear scan; HTN, systemic hypertension; LVEF, left ventricular ejection fraction; OH, hydroxy; PFT, pulmonary function tests; PTH, serum parathyroid hormone; PVR, pulmonary vascular resistance; RV, right ventricular; SAECG, signal-averaged electrocardiogram; SPECT, single photon emission commuted tomography; TBNA, transbronchial needle aspiration (of a mediastinal lymph node); VT, ventricular tachycardia; WASOG, World Association for Sarcoidosis and Other Granulomatous Disorders.

[a] At least 70% agreement by the experts.

[b] For all clinical conditions: (a) biopsy of that organ demonstrating granulomatous inflammation of no alternate cause implies highly probable involvement, (b) another organ has demonstrated granulomatous inflammation of no alternate cause, (c) alternative causes for the clinical manifestation have been reasonable excluded.

Adapted from Judson MA, Costabel U, Drent M, et al. The WASOG sarcoidosis organ assessment instrument: an update of a previous clinical tool. Sarcoidosis Vase Diffuse Lung Dis 2014;31:22–4; with permission.

and nodular sarcoidosis should be considered distinct clinical syndromes or variants of sarcoidosis. The conclusion from an extensive review of the literature suggests that nodular sarcoidosis and necrotizing sarcoid granulomatosis are merely variant manifestations of sarcoidosis.[62] Granulomatous lesions of unknown significance (GLUS) syndrome is considered a distinct clinic entity, but its multisystemic clinic features of prolonged fever and involvement of the liver, spleen, lymph nodes, and bone marrow is difficult to separate clinically from sarcoidosis, except that SACE and calcium are never elevated and the Kveim is always negative.[66] Finally, common variable immunodeficiency can manifest with granulomatous lesions in multiple organs that can be misdiagnosed as sarcoidosis.[35] However, the history of recurrent infections, physical finding of crackles and hepatosplenomegaly, atypical CT findings and low bronchoalveolar lavage CD4:CD8 ratio suggests that this is an alternative diagnosis.[17]

Is There Any Evidence of Additional Organ Involvement?

Sarcoidosis, by definition,[2] is a systemic disease (see **Fig. 1**, Box 5). Whether demonstration of this criterion is required for diagnosis is controversial.[67] It is not uncommon for sarcoidosis to present with manifestations in only one organ, especially the brain, spinal cord or heart. Although the manifestation of sarcoidosis in a single organ does not exclude a diagnosis of sarcoidosis, the presence of multi-organ involvement does increase the confidence in a diagnosis of sarcoidosis (see **Table 3**).

However, what constitutes organ involvement in the absence of a tissue biopsy is still being clarified. **Table 6** is the updated organ assessment tool for sarcoidosis, which seeks to establish consensus for what defines organ involvement without biopsy.[4] The tool was created based on updated literature from the prior iteration from the ACCESS study and expert opinion. Similar to the confidence levels in diagnosis of the overall disease, the level of confidence that one has a second organ involved can be classified into highly probable, at least probable, possible, and undecided (no consensus).

SUMMARY

"Absolute certainty in diagnosis is unattainable, no matter how much information we gather, how many observations we make, or how many tests we perform. Our task is not to attain certainty, but rather to reduce the level of diagnostic uncertainty enough to make optimal therapeutic decisions."
— *JP Kassirer.[68]*

At times, confident diagnosis of sarcoidosis is elusive and seemingly unattainable. Although the defining feature of the disease is histopathologic, diagnosis during life depends largely on clinical and radiologic findings. Thus, diagnosis begins with a detailed review of the clinical presentation looking for "footprints" of sarcoidosis that will justify further evaluation. The amount of support required from histology varies from case to case. Although histology from 1 site cannot, in itself, establish the diagnosis of sarcoidosis, by definition a systemic disease, detailed histologic study of biopsy tissue makes an important and often essential contribution to diagnosis.[69] In atypical cases, subsequent surveillance, including possible response to treatment, may show a clinical course justifying a diagnosis of sarcoidosis. Patience is required in some cases, particularly those in which the clinical evidence of disease is confined to 1 organ, because diagnosis is likely to remain in doubt for long periods.

REFERENCES

1. Baughman RP, Culver DA, Judson MA. A concise review of pulmonary sarcoidosis. Am J Respir Crit Care Med 2011;183:573–81.
2. Statement on sarcoidosis. Joint Statement of the American Thoracic Society (ATS), the European Respiratory Society (ERS) and the World Association of Sarcoidosis and Other Granulomatous Disorders (WASOG) adopted by the ATS Board of Directors and by the ERS Executive Committee, February 1999. Am J Respir Crit Care Med 1999;160:736–55.
3. Judson MA, Baughman RP, Teirstein AS, et al. Defining organ involvement in sarcoidosis: the ACCESS proposed instrument. ACCESS Research Group. A case control etiologic study of sarcoidosis. Sarcoidosis Vasc Diffuse Lung Dis 1999;16:75–86.
4. Judson MA, Costabel U, Drent M, et al. The WASOG sarcoidosis organ assessment instrument: an update of a previous clinical tool. Sarcoidosis Vasc Diffuse Lung Dis 2014;31:19–27.
5. Judson MA. Advances in the diagnosis and treatment of sarcoidosis. F1000Prime Rep 2014;6:89.
6. Judson MA, Thompson BW, Rabin DL, et al. The diagnostic pathway to sarcoidosis. Chest 2003;123:406–12.
7. Valeyre D, Prasse A, Nunes H, et al. Sarcoidosis. Lancet 2014;383:1155–67.
8. Judson MA. The clinical features of sarcoidosis: a comprehensive review. Clin Rev Allergy Immunol 2014;49(1):63–78.

9. Baughman RP, Teirstein AS, Judson MA, et al. Clinical characteristics of patients in a case control study of sarcoidosis. Am J Respir Crit Care Med 2001;164:1885–9.

10. Iannuzzi MC, Rybicki BA, Teirstein AS. Sarcoidosis. N Engl J Med 2007;357:2153–65.

11. O'Regan A, Berman JS. Sarcoidosis. Ann Intern Med 2012;156:ITC5–1-15.

12. Cozier YC, Berman JS, Palmer JR, et al. Sarcoidosis in black women in the United States: data from the Black Women's Health Study. Chest 2011;139:144–50.

13. Valeyre D, Soler P, Clerici C, et al. Smoking and pulmonary sarcoidosis: effect of cigarette smoking on prevalence, clinical manifestations, alveolitis, and evolution of the disease. Thorax 1988;43:516–24.

14. Rybicki BA, Iannuzzi MC, Frederick MM, et al. Familial aggregation of sarcoidosis. A case-control etiologic study of sarcoidosis (ACCESS). Am J Respir Crit Care Med 2001;164:2085–91.

15. Muller-Quernheim J, Gaede KI, Fireman E, et al. Diagnoses of chronic beryllium disease within cohorts of sarcoidosis patients. Eur Respir J 2006;27:1190–5.

16. Kreiss K, Day GA, Schuler CR. Beryllium: a modern industrial hazard. Annu Rev Public Health 2007;28:259–77.

17. Bouvry D, Mouthon L, Brillet PY, et al. Granulomatosis-associated common variable immunodeficiency disorder: a case-control study versus sarcoidosis. Eur Respir J 2013;41:115–22.

18. Nardi A, Brillet PY, Letoumelin P, et al. Stage IV sarcoidosis: comparison of survival with the general population and causes of death. Eur Respir J 2011;38:1368–73.

19. Yancey J, Luxford W, Sharma OP. Clubbing of the fingers in sarcoidosis. JAMA 1972;222:582.

20. Lieberman J. Elevation of serum angiotensin-converting-enzyme (ACE) level in sarcoidosis. Am J Med 1975;59:365–72.

21. Studdy PR, Bird R. Serum angiotensin converting enzyme in sarcoidosis–its value in present clinical practice. Ann Clin Biochem 1989;26(Pt 1):13–8.

22. Baughman RP, Ploysongsang Y, Roberts RD, et al. Effects of sarcoid and steroids on angiotensin-converting enzyme. Am Rev Respir Dis 1983;128:631–3.

23. Stouten K, van de Werken M, Tchetverikov I, et al. Extreme elevation of serum angiotensin-converting enzyme (ACE) activity: always consider familial ACE hyperactivity. Ann Clin Biochem 2014;51:289–93.

24. Gupta D, Chetty M, Kumar N, et al. Anergy to tuberculin in sarcoidosis is not influenced by high prevalence of tuberculin sensitivity in the population. Sarcoidosis Vasc Diffuse Lung Dis 2003;20:40–5.

25. Inui N, Suda T, Chida K. Use of the QuantiFERON-TB Gold test in Japanese patients with sarcoidosis. Respir Med 2008;102:313–5.

26. Gupta D, Kumar S, Aggarwal AN, et al. Interferon gamma release assay (QuantiFERON-TB Gold in Tube) in patients of sarcoidosis from a population with high prevalence of tuberculosis infection. Sarcoidosis Vasc Diffuse Lung Dis 2011;28:95–101.

27. Vyas S, Thangakunam B, Gupta R, et al. Interferon gamma release assay and tuberculin skin test positivity in sarcoidosis. Lung India 2015;32:91–2.

28. Scadding JG. Prognosis of intrathoracic sarcoidosis in England. A review of 136 cases after five years' observation. Br Med J 1961;2:1165–72.

29. Winterbauer RH, Belic N, Moores KD. Clinical interpretation of bilateral hilar adenopathy. Ann Intern Med 1973;78:65–71.

30. Reich JM. Tissue confirmation of presumptive stage I sarcoidosis. J Bronchology Interv Pulmonol 2013;20:103–5.

31. Reich JM, Brouns MC, O'Connor EA, et al. Mediastinoscopy in patients with presumptive stage I sarcoidosis: a risk/benefit, cost/benefit analysis. Chest 1998;113:147–53.

32. Mana J, Teirstein AS, Mendelson DS, et al. Excessive thoracic computed tomographic scanning in sarcoidosis. Thorax 1995;50:1264–6.

33. Keijsers RG, Veltkamp M, Grutters JC. Chest imaging. Clin Chest Med 2015, in press.

34. Valeyre D, Bernaudin JF, Jeny F, et al. Pulmonary sarcoidosis. Clin Chest Med 2015, in press.

35. Fasano MB, Sullivan KE, Sarpong SB, et al. Sarcoidosis and common variable immunodeficiency. Report of 8 cases and review of the literature. Medicine 1996;75:251–61.

36. Pakhale SS, Unruh H, Tan L, et al. Has mediastinoscopy still a role in suspected stage I sarcoidosis? Sarcoidosis Vasc Diffuse Lung Dis 2006;23:66–9.

37. Sulavik SB, Spencer RP, Palestro CJ, et al. Specificity and sensitivity of distinctive chest radiographic and/or 67Ga images in the noninvasive diagnosis of sarcoidosis. Chest 1993;103:403–9.

38. Israel HL, Sones M. Selection of biopsy procedures for sarcoidosis diagnosis. Arch Intern Med 1964;113:255–60.

39. Navani N, Lawrence DR, Kolvekar S, et al. Endobronchial ultrasound-guided transbronchial needle aspiration prevents mediastinoscopies in the diagnosis of isolated mediastinal lymphadenopathy: a prospective trial. Am J Respir Crit Care Med 2012;186:255–60.

40. Ravini M, Ferraro G, Barbieri B, et al. Changing strategies of lung biopsies in diffuse lung diseases: the impact of video-assisted thoracoscopy. Eur Respir J 1998;11:99–103.

41. Gilman MJ. Transbronchial biopsy in sarcoidosis. Chest 1983;83:159.

42. Shorr AF, Torrington KG, Hnatiuk OW. Endobronchial biopsy for sarcoidosis: a prospective study. Chest 2001;120:109–14.

43. Agarwal R, Aggarwal AN, Gupta D. Efficacy and safety of conventional transbronchial needle aspiration in sarcoidosis: a systematic review and meta-analysis. Respir Care 2013;58:683–93.

44. Agarwal R, Srinivasan A, Aggarwal AN, et al. Efficacy and safety of convex probe EBUS-TBNA in sarcoidosis: a systematic review and meta-analysis. Respir Med 2012;106:883–92.

45. von Bartheld MB, Dekkers OM, Szlubowski A, et al. Endosonography vs conventional bronchoscopy for the diagnosis of sarcoidosis: the GRANULOMA randomized clinical trial. JAMA 2013;309:2457–64.

46. Plit M, Pearson R, Havryk A, et al. Diagnostic utility of endobronchial ultrasound-guided transbronchial needle aspiration compared with transbronchial and endobronchial biopsy for suspected sarcoidosis. Intern Med J 2012;42:434–8.

47. Oki M, Saka H, Kitagawa C, et al. Prospective study of endobronchial ultrasound-guided transbronchial needle aspiration of lymph nodes versus transbronchial lung biopsy of lung tissue for diagnosis of sarcoidosis. J Thorac Cardiovasc Surg 2012;143:1324–9.

48. Gupta D, Dadhwal DS, Agarwal R, et al. Endobronchial ultrasound-guided transbronchial needle aspiration vs conventional transbronchial needle aspiration in the diagnosis of sarcoidosis. Chest 2014;146:547–56.

49. Kantrow SP, Meyer KC, Kidd P, et al. The CD4/CD8 ratio in BAL fluid is highly variable in sarcoidosis. Eur Respir J 1997;10:2716–21.

50. Drent M, Mansour K, Linssen C. Bronchoalveolar lavage in sarcoidosis. Semin Respir Crit Care Med 2007;28:486–95.

51. Bonfioli AA, Orefice F. Sarcoidosis. Semin Ophthalmol 2005;20:177–82.

52. Nessan VJ, Jacoway JR. Biopsy of minor salivary glands in the diagnosis of sarcoidosis. N Engl J Med 1979;301:922–4.

53. Harvey J, Catoggio L, Gallagher PJ, et al. Salivary gland biopsy in sarcoidosis. Sarcoidosis 1989;6:47–50.

54. Stjernberg N, Truedson H, Bjornstad-Petersen H. Scalene node biopsy in sarcoidosis. Acta Med Scand 1980;207:111–3.

55. Truedson H, Stjernberg N, Thunell M. Scalene lymph node biopsy. A diagnostic method in sarcoidosis. Acta Chir Scand 1985;151:121–3.

56. Karagiannidis A, Karavalaki M, Koulaouzidis A. Hepatic sarcoidosis. Ann Hepatol 2006;5:251–6.

57. Andonopoulos AP, Papadimitriou C, Melachrinou M, et al. Asymptomatic gastrocnemius muscle biopsy: an extremely sensitive and specific test in the pathologic confirmation of sarcoidosis presenting with hilar adenopathy. Clin Exp Rheumatol 2001;19:569–72.

58. Teirstein AS, Machac J, Almeida O, et al. Results of 188 whole-body fluorodeoxyglucose positron emission tomography scans in 137 patients with sarcoidosis. Chest 2007;132:1949–53.

59. Siltzbach LE. The Kveim test in sarcoidosis. A study of 750 patients. JAMA 1961;178:476–82.

60. Ma Y, Gal A, Koss MN. The pathology of pulmonary sarcoidosis: update. Semin Diagn Pathol 2007;24:150–61.

61. Rosen Y. Pathology of sarcoidosis. Semin Respir Crit Care Med 2007;28:36–52.

62. Rosen Y. Four decades of necrotizing sarcoid granulomatosis: what do we know now? Arch Pathol Lab Med 2015;139:252–62.

63. Rossi G, Cavazza A, Colby TV. Pathology of sarcoidosis. Clin Rev Allergy Immunol 2015;49(1):36–44.

64. Ricker W, Clark M. Sarcoidosis; a clinicopathologic review of 300 cases, including 22 autopsies. Am J Clin Pathol 1949;19:725–49.

65. Myers JL, Tazelaar HD. Challenges in pulmonary fibrosis: 6–problematic granulomatous lung disease. Thorax 2008;63:78–84.

66. Judson MA. The diagnosis of sarcoidosis. Clin Chest Med 2008;29:415–27, viii.

67. Judson MA, Baughman RP. How many organs need to be involved to diagnose sarcoidosis?: an unanswered question that, hopefully, will become irrelevant. Sarcoidosis Vasc Diffuse Lung Dis 2014;31:6–7.

68. Kassirer JP. Our stubborn quest for diagnostic certainty. A cause of excessive testing. N Engl J Med 1989;320:1489–91.

69. Mitchell DN, Scadding JG, Heard BE, et al. Sarcoidosis: histopathological definition and clinical diagnosis. J Clin Pathol 1977;30:395–408.

Chest Imaging

Ruth G. Keijsers, MD, PhD[a], Marcel Veltkamp, MD, PhD[b],
Jan C. Grutters, MD, PhD[b,c],*

KEYWORDS

- Sarcoidosis • Chest radiography • HRCT • FDG PET/CT • Disease activity

KEY POINTS

- Staging pulmonary sarcoidosis has been performed using the chest radiograph Scadding criteria for more than 50 years.
- High-resolution computed tomography (HRCT) is an essential diagnostic modality in diagnosing sarcoidosis.
- Pulmonary sarcoidosis is notorious for mimicking many other interstitial lung diseases.
- Fluorodeoxyglucose F 18 (FDG) PET/computed tomography (CT) is able to image active sarcoidosis in mediastinal and hilar lymph nodes, lung parenchyma, and myocardium.
- FDG PET/CT can be used to evaluate sarcoidosis activity in patients with persistent symptoms, stage IV disease, and cardiac sarcoidosis and for treatment monitoring.
- Diffuse lung parenchymal activity in FDG PET/CT is associated with loss of pulmonary function after 1 year when untreated. In addition, a decrease in lung parenchymal FDG uptake correlates with lung functional improvement on immunosuppressive treatment.

INTRODUCTION

The clinical manifestations of sarcoidosis are highly variable and often nonspecific. Every organ can be affected, but thoracic involvement occurs in more than 90% of patients.[1] For pulmonary sarcoidosis, therefore, chest imaging by chest radiograph or HRCT, is important for diagnosing and management of this disease. In sarcoidosis patients with extrapulmonary manifestations, such as cardiac sarcoidosis or neurosarcoidosis, other imaging modalities are warranted. In these patients MRI and FDG-PET scanning are increasingly recognized as essential imaging techniques required for adequate diagnosing sarcoidosis localization and disease management.[2] The first publications on radiological findings on sarcoidosis date from the early twentieth century.[3] More than 50 years ago, Professor John Guyett Scadding proposed 5 stages of disease based on chest radiographs.[4] In the past decades, multiple scoring systems for sarcoidosis have been developed, but the Scadding stages still are the most used in clinical practice.[5,6]

RADIOGRAPHIC SCORING SYSTEMS: SCADDING STAGING

Sarcoidosis is commonly staged according to its appearance on the chest radiograph following the Scadding criteria (**Table 1**).[4] Stage 0 indicates no visible intrathoracic findings. Stage I represents bilateral hilar lymphadenopathy, which may be accompanied by paratracheal lymphadenopathy.

Disclosures: None.
[a] Department of Nuclear Medicine, St. Antonius Hospital, Koekoekslaan 1, Utrecht, Nieuwegein 3435 CM, The Netherlands; [b] ILD Center of Excellence, St. Antonius Hospital, Koekoekslaan 1, Utrecht, Nieuwegein 3435 CM, The Netherlands; [c] Division of Heart and Lungs, University Medical Center, Utrecht, The Netherlands
* Corresponding author. ILD Center of Excellence, St. Antonius Hospital, Koekoekslaan 1, Utrecht, Nieuwegein 3435 CM, The Netherlands.
E-mail address: j.grutters@antoniusziekenhuis.nl

Clin Chest Med 36 (2015) 603–619
http://dx.doi.org/10.1016/j.ccm.2015.08.004
0272-5231/15/$ – see front matter © 2015 Elsevier Inc. All rights reserved.

Table 1
Radiographic staging of sarcoidosis patients at presentation according to the Scadding criteria

Radiographic Stage	Chest Radiograph	Frequency (%)	Resolution (%)
0	Normal	5–15	
I	BHL	25–65	60–90
II	BHL and pulmonary infiltrates	20–40	40–70
III	Pulmonary infiltrates without BHL	10–15	10–20
IV	Advanced pulmonary fibrosis	5	0

The estimated frequency at presentation is given as well as the probability of spontaneous resolution during disease course.
Abbreviation: BHL, bilateral hilar lymphadenopathy.

Stage II represents bilateral hilar lymphadenopathy accompanied by parenchymal infiltration. Stage III represents parenchymal infiltration without hilar lymphadenopathy. Stage IV consists of advanced fibrosis with evidence of honeycombing, hilar retraction, bullae, cysts, and emphysema. Despite the nomenclature, patients do not all progress through stages I to IV and these stages have no sequential order. For example, a patient may present with stage III that normalizes during follow-up. Also, it can be seen that a patient who initially presents with stage I disease that normalizes can present later with parenchymal disease only (stage III).[7] Hillerdal and colleagues[8] found that in a cohort of patients presenting with stage I disease, 9% progressed to stage II compared with 1.6% who progressed to stage III or IV. Of patients presenting with stage II disease, only 5.5% progressed to stage III or IV disease.

An interesting feature of the Scadding criteria is that they give prognostic information.[9–11] In stage I disease, spontaneous resolution occurs in 60% to 90% of patients. Spontaneous resolution occurs in 40% to 70% of patients with stage II disease and in 10% to 20% of patients with stage III disease. A majority of spontaneous remissions occur within the first 2 years of disease presentation. There is no spontaneous resolution in patients with stage IV pulmonary sarcoidosis. An important limitation of the Scadding criteria is the great interobserver variability, especially between stages II and III and between stages III and IV.[7] Furthermore, stage IV fibrotic sarcoidosis does not always indicate end-stage disease. It has been demonstrated that in 50% of patients with stage IV pulmonary sarcoidosis, metabolic activity is present on FDG PET/CT.

LARGE AIRWAY INVOLVEMENT

Sarcoidosis of the upper respiratory tract may involve the nose, sinuses, larynx, oral cavity, ear, trachea, and bronchi.[12,13] The incidence of sarcoidosis of the upper respiratory tract is approximately 5%.[14] During bronchoscopy, common lesions in the trachea as well as in the bronchi are erythema, thickening of the mucosa, and a cobblestone appearance (**Fig. 1**), which yields a high number of granulomas on biopsy. A small study by Shorr and colleagues[15] showed that 71% of sarcoidosis patients undergoing bronchoscopy had bronchial abnormalities. Severe endoluminal stenosis of the trachea or main bronchi is rare in sarcoidosis, estimated as less than 1%.[16] When diagnosing sarcoidosis, even in patients with a normal-appearing airway, granulomas can be identified in approximately 30% of patients.[15]

MEDIASTINAL AND HILAR LYMPHADENOPATHY

Lymphadenopathy is the most common intrathoracic manifestation of sarcoidosis, occurring in approximately 80% of patients during their illness,

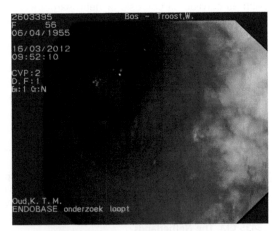

Fig. 1. Endobronchial cobblestone appearance in a 57-year-old sarcoidosis patient. Biopsy-proved multiple non-necrotizing granulomas.

irrespective of radiographic staging.[17–23] An overview of common and uncommon sites of thoracic lymphadenopathy in sarcoidosis is given in **Box 1**. In most cases, bilateral hilar lymphadenopathy is present (**Fig. 2**), with unilateral hilar adenopathy occurring in only 3% to 5% of patients.[17,24,25] When present, unilateral hilar lymphadenopathy is more common on the right side than on the left

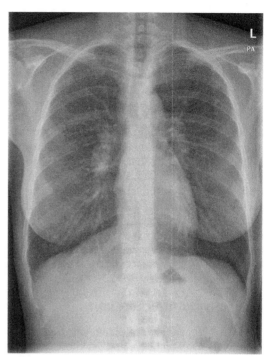

Fig. 2. Characteristic distribution of bilateral hilar lymphadenopathy in stage I sarcoidosis on a chest radiograph.

Box 1
Classical versus more uncommon features of pulmonary sarcoidosis seen on HRCT

Classic findings, potentially reversible

Lymphadenopathy: bilateral hilar, mediastinal, right paratracheal, subcarinal, aortopulmonary

Reticulonodular pattern: micronodules (2–4 mm, well defined, bilateral distribution)

Perilymphatic distribution of nodules (peribronchovascular, subpleural, interlobular septal)

Predominant upper and middle zones parenchymal abnormalities

Uncommon findings, potentially reversible

Lymphadenopathy: unilateral, isolated, anterior and posterior mediastinal, paracardiac

Reticular pattern

Isolated cavitations

Isolated ground glass opacities without micronodules

Mosaic attenuation pattern

Pleural disease (effusion, pleural thickening, chylothorax, pneumothorax)

Mycetoma

Macronodules (>5 mm, coalescing); galaxy sign and cluster sign

Classic findings reflecting irreversible fibrosis or chronic disease

Reticular opacities, predominantly middle and upper zones

Architectural distortion

Traction bronchiectasis

Volume loss, predominantly upper lobes

Calcified lymphnodes

Fibrocystic changes

Uncommon findings reflecting irreversible fibrosis or chronic disease

Honeycomb-like changes

Reticular opacities in predominantly lower lobes

---

side. Furthermore, besides the hilar region, lymphadenopathy in sarcoidosis is also seen in the right paratracheal, aortopulmonary window, and tracheobronchial regions.[20–23,26] A typical example of bilateral lymphadenopathy and right paratracheal lymphnode enlargement in sarcoidosis is known as Garland triad or 1-2-3 sign.

The groups of Niimi and colleagues[22] and Patil and colleagues[21] demonstrated that the most commonly involved nodal stations are Naruke 4R (right lower paratracheal), Naruke 10R (right hilar), Naruke 7 (subcarinal), Naruke 5 (aortopulmonary window), Naruke 11R (right interlobular), and Naruke 11L (left interlobular), as shown in **Box 1**.[21,22]

Massive hilar and/or mediastinal lymphadenopathy is often asymptomatic but can cause fatigue, retrosternal pain, dysphagia, and even pulmonary hypertension in some patients.

The differential diagnosis of hilar and mediastinal lymphadenopathy is broad, with the major diagnostic alternatives lymphoma, metastatic disease, and infections, especially tuberculosis. An important feature of lymphadenopathy in sarcoidosis is the symmetric distribution, which is unusual in these diagnostic alternatives. Lymphadenopathy can also be seen in other interstitial lung diseases, such as (idiopathic) interstitial pneumonitis and hypersensitivity pneumonitis. In diseases other than sarcoidosis, however, usually only 1 or 2 nodes are enlarged and their maximal short axis diameter is mostly less than 15 mm.[22] Mediastinal lymphadenopathy without hilar involvement is uncommon in sarcoidosis and a biopsy-proved diagnosis is warranted.

Lymph node calcification is visible at presentation in approximately 20% of patients, increasing to 44% during disease course.[27] The morphology of calcified lymph nodes is variable and nonspecific. Sometimes, the calcification can have an eggshell appearance.[28] Calcification of lymph nodes is linked to the duration of disease and can be seen in other granulomatous disorders, like tuberculosis or histoplasmosis, as well. When comparing calcified lymph nodes in sarcoidosis and tuberculosis, in sarcoidosis their diameter was significantly larger, calcium deposition more focal, and hilar distribution more bilaterally (65% vs 8%).[23]

PARENCHYMAL INVOLVEMENT

The HRCT appearance of pulmonary sarcoidosis has a great variability and is notorious for mimicking many other interstitial lung diseases. The most important 2 radiological patterns in sarcoidosis with involvement of the lung parenchyma are the nodular pattern and the reticulonodular pattern. The distribution of nodules on HRCT can follow 3 different patterns: random distribution, centrilobular distribution, and perilymphatic distribution.

Nodular and Reticulonodular Pattern

The nodular pattern is seen in approximately 90% of sarcoidosis patients with parenchymal involvement.[29,30] Sarcoid granulomas are microscopic in size but can aggregate to form small nodules that can be seen on HRCT. These small nodules are 1 to 10 mm in diameter, usually have irregular margins, and are predominantly present in the mid and upper zones of the lungs. The nodules are frequently found along the bronchovascular bundles and in the subpleural region after a perilymphatic distribution. Aggregated subpleural nodules account for the fissural thickening that can be seen on HRCT. The nodules adjacent to interfaces of vessels, airways, and septa give these structures an irregular or beaded appearance, implicating them as pathognomic for sarcoidosis (**Fig. 3**). This pattern is also seen in histologic specimens, where granulomas are found in association with lymphatics along vessels and airways and in the subpleural area.[31] This distribution of granulomas can also explain the high rate of success in diagnosing sarcoidosis by bronchial and transbronchial biopsy. Frequently, sarcoidosis

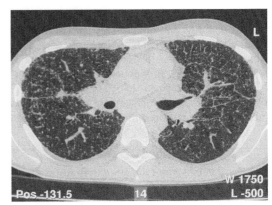

Fig. 3. HRCT with the classic perilymphatic distribution of nodules in a patient with sarcoidosis. Note the occurrence of small nodules along subpleural surface and fissures, along interlobular septa and the peribronchovascular bundles, giving these structures a beaded appearance. This is thought pathognomic for sarcoidosis.

causes nodular septal thickening defining the reticulonodular pattern. A reticular pattern is a descriptive term (*reticulum* means network) with several morphologic variations ranging from generalized thickening of interlobular septa to honeycomb lung destruction. A pure reticular pattern is rarely seen in sarcoidosis.[32]

Large Nodules and Alveolar Sarcoidosis

Sarcoid nodules can aggregate into pulmonary nodules (not >3 cm in diameter) or large masses. Such a presentation is uncommon in sarcoidosis and estimated as 2.4% to 4%.[17,25,33–35] In a retrospective analysis of African American patients, 82% had multiple masses/nodules and only 18% had a solitary lesion.[36] An air bronchogram was seen in 58% of the cases and the nodules tended to be more peripheral. The margins of the nodules are often irregular and hazy.[34] The nodules can remain stable for years; however, partial or complete regression has been described.[33] Cavitation is rarely seen in large pulmonary masses and is usually benign; however, hemoptysis can occur.[37,38] In approximately 10% to 20% of patients, massive consolidation with air bronchograms develops (**Fig. 4**).[39–42] The pathologic mechanism is loss of alveolar air due to compression of the alveoli by coalescent granulomas in the interstitium.[24] The alveolar opacities are usually present in the peripheral middle zones of the lung.[24,34]

Galaxy Sign, Cluster Sign, and (Reversed) Halo Sign

Recently, 3 CT signs have been reviewed in sarcoidosis involving a more atypical distribution

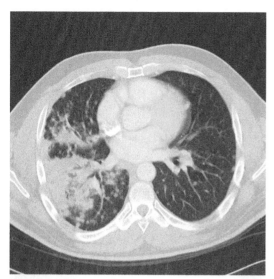

Fig. 4. Alveolar consolidation in the middle and right lower lobe of a sarcoidosis patient. Note the presence of air bronchograms in the major consolidation in the right lower lobe. Furthermore, multiple nodules with a mildly irregular outline are seen bilaterally.

of large and small nodules.[43] The sarcoid galaxy sign represents a large pulmonary nodule or mass surrounded by many small satellite nodules (**Fig. 5**). It is named after a galaxy where the stars are more concentrated to the galactic center than in the periphery. The sarcoid cluster sign is also characterized by clusters of multiple small nodules forming a pulmonary mass but, in contrast to the galaxy sign, the nodules do not tend to coalesce in the center (**Fig. 6**). The most important differential diagnosis for sarcoid galaxy sign or sarcoid cluster sign is tuberculosis. Clusters of small nodules can also be seen, however, in cryptococcus infection and silicosis.[43] The reversed halo sign is a far more nonspecific sign and describes a focal area of ground glass opacity surrounded by an almost complete ring of consolidation (**Fig. 7**). It was first described as a specific finding in patients with cryptogenic organizing pneumonia.[44] Later, several investigators described the reversed halo sign in various diseases, such as tuberculosis, aspergillosis, Wegener granulomatosis, and adenocarcinoma in situ (formerly known as bronchoalveolar carcinoma).[45] The reversed halo sign is also known as the atoll sign due to its resemblance of a ring-shaped coral reef that encloses a lagoon with shallow water.[46] A true halo sign, describing a pulmonary mass with a surrounding area of ground glass, has been rarely described in sarcoidosis.[47]

Ground Glass Opacities

Ground glass attenuation in HRCT is defined as areas of hazy increased attenuation with preservation of bronchial and vascular margins. In sarcoidosis patients, the prevalence of ground glass opacities is estimated at 40%, ranging from 16% to 83%.[27,39,42,48,49] Historically, it was believed to represent active alveolitis but now it is thought caused by small interstitial granulomas or fibrotic

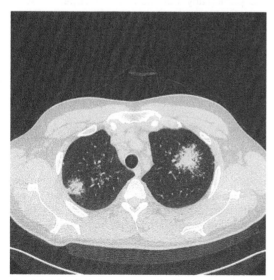

Fig. 5. Pulmonary mass with sarcoid galaxy sign in both left and right upper lobes in a 28-year-old sarcoidosis patient. In both upper lobes the mass is surrounded by multiple small satellite nodules.

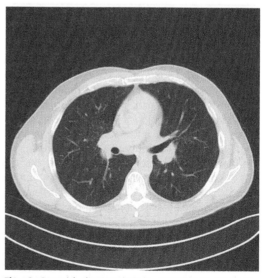

Fig. 6. Sarcoid cluster sign in sarcoidosis. Note the subtle clustering of micronodules without confluence in the right parahilar region.

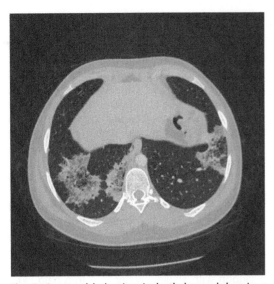

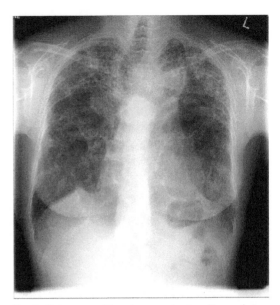

Fig. 7. Reversed halo sign in both lower lobes in a 32-year-old patient clinically and radiologically suspected of sarcoidosis. There is a focal area of ground glass opacity surrounded by an almost complete ring of consolidation. Lung biopsy of the mass in the right lower lobe revealed a histopathologic diagnosis of lymphocytic interstitial pneumonia.

Fig. 8. Pulmonary fibrosis on a chest radiograph in a 46-year-old sarcoidosis patient. Note that the hila are shifted upward.

lesions beyond the resolution of CT.[31] Ground glass is multifocal and often accompanied by subtle micronodularity.[50] Furthermore, it is most frequently seen at disease presentation.[40] The response to steroids depends on the presence of underlying fibrosis, with clearance more likely if it is of short duration.[42]

Fibrotic Sarcoidosis

At presentation, approximately 5% of sarcoidosis patients have fibrotic changes on their chest radiograph.[10,11] In an estimated 10% to 20% of patients, however, fibrosis develops or becomes more prominent during disease course.[51] On the chest radiograph, linear opacities radiating laterally from the hilum into the middle and upper zones is a characteristic finding.[24] The hila are shifted upward, and vessels and fissures are distorted (Fig. 8).[17] Due to compensatory hyperinflation, the lower lobes are sometimes transradiant. On HRCT, fibrotic changes are represented by fibrous bands, hilar retraction, displacement of fissures, traction bronchiectasis, honeycomb cysts, bullae, and irregular reticular opacities, including intralobular lines and irregular septal thickening. Fibrosis is seen predominantly in the upper and middle lobes, in a patchy distribution. A common feature of fibrotic sarcoidosis is the presence of conglomerated masses surrounding and encompassing vessels and bronchi. It occurs in 60% of fibrotic

sarcoidosis and is associated with bronchial distortion.[41]

Fibrotic cysts, bullae, traction bronchiectasis, and paracicatricial emphysema (air space enlargement and lung destruction developing adjacent to areas of pulmonary scarring) represent advanced fibrotic sarcoidosis (Fig. 9). Cystic abnormalities are particularly common in the upper lobes in advanced fibrotic sarcoidosis.[52] Honeycombing (subpleural clustering of cystic airspaces) is thought less common in sarcoidosis compared with other end-stage lung diseases.[53] If present, honeycomb-like cysts are most commonly found in the upper lobes but can also be seen in the lower lobes mimicking idiopathic pulmonary fibrosis.[32]

Mosaic Attenuation Pattern and Air Trapping

Mosaic attenuation is defined as a patchwork of regions with varied attenuation on HRCT. This pattern can represent patchy interstitial disease, vascular disease, or small airway disease. In patients with sarcoidosis, the presence of mosaic attenuation frequently results from small airway involvement by granulomas or fibrosis.[54,55] To verify that mosaic attenuation is caused by small airway disease, inspiratory images on CT must be compared with the parenchymal appearance on expiratory images to identify air trapping. Air trapping is a common but nonspecific feature of pulmonary sarcoidosis.[54,56]

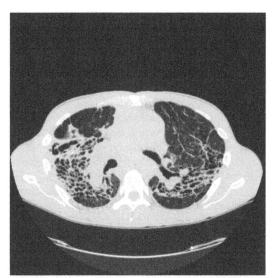

Fig. 9. Fibrotic pulmonary sarcoidosis on HRCT. The CT demonstrates parenchymal distortion and destruction. Multiple honeycomb cysts are noted throughout the upper lobes bilaterally.

MYCETOMAS

The formation of mycetomas occurs in approximately 2% of sarcoidosis patients, especially in stage IV cystic disease.[57] Fungal balls can develop in preexisting bullae or cysts that are colonized by fungi, usually *Aspergillus* species. The characteristic appearance of a pulmonary aspergilloma consists of a mobile opacity occupying part or most of the cavity. It is surrounded by a peripheral rim of air known as the air crescent sign or Monod sign **(Fig. 10)**.[58] A common symptom in patients with

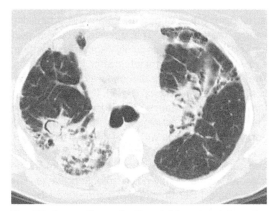

Fig. 10. Aspergilloma in the right upper lobe of a 57-year-old patient with advanced pulmonary sarcoidosis. The aspergilloma is surrounded by a peripheral rim of air known as the air crescent sign or Monod sign.

aspergillomas is hemoptysis and, when massive, can be life threatening.

PLEURAL INVOLVEMENT
Pleural Effusion

In sarcoidosis, granulomas can be found on both visceral and parietal pleura. This pleural localization as well as blockage of lymphatic channels by granulomas can result in pleural effusion. Pleural effusion, however, is an uncommon manifestation of sarcoidosis with an estimated incidence of 0.7% to 10% on chest radiograph.[59–64] In a more recent study, the occurrence of pleural effusion was studied with ultrasonography in 181 patients with sarcoidosis presenting at the outpatient clinic of a university hospital.[65] In 2.8% of patients, pleural fluid was detected, with some patients having a parapneumonic effusion and congestive heart failure. Therefore, in this study only 1.1% of patients had sarcoidosis-related pleural effusion demonstrated by biopsy-proved sarcoid pleural involvement. Sarcoidosis-related pleural effusion occurs more often in the right side of the lung compared with the left (45% vs 33%, respectively).[64] It mostly resolves spontaneously within 6 months, sometimes leaving residual pleural thickening.[24,62,66]

Chylothorax

The development of chylothorax is an exceptionally rare complication of sarcoidosis, with only a few case reports in the literature.[67–70] In 1 case report, chylothorax was the presenting feature of sarcoidosis.[68]

Pneumothorax

It has been estimated that pneumothorax has 2% to 3% prevalence in sarcoidosis patients.[71,72] Cases of spontaneous pneumothorax may develop due to rupture of a subpleural bleb, particularly in patients with advanced fibrocystic disease.[64] Bilateral pneumothorax in sarcoidosis has also been reported.[73]

NECROTIZING SARCOID GRANULOMATOSIS

Necrotizing Sarcoid Granulomatosis (NSG) is a rare entity and seen as a variant of sarcoidosis with, however, some uncertainty.[74] It is debated whether NSG is a manifestation of systemic sarcoidosis with necrotizing granulomata or a form of necrotizing angiitis with a sarcoid-like reaction.[75] NSG is defined by a granulomatous vasculitis, confluent non-necrotizing granulomas, and foci of infarct-like necrosis with variable degrees of fibrosis.[74,76] Since the first article describing NSG in 1973, approximately 135 cases have been described.[77,78] Recently, however, an excellent review was published providing reasonable evidence that NSG is a manifestation of sarcoidosis and essentially the same as nodular sarcoidosis.[79]

PULMONARY HYPERTENSION

It is estimated that 1% to 6% of patients with sarcoidosis have pulmonary hypertension, most patients having advanced stages on chest radiography (Scadding stages III and IV).[80,81] Fibrosis or extensive parenchymal abnormalities are not always present, however, and the absence should not exclude further evaluation for pulmonary hypertension.[82] Clinical characteristics are often atypical but some symptoms can suggest underlying pulmonary hypertension: dyspnea more severe compared with functional impairment, chest pain, and near-syncope on exertion. Also, approximately 25% of sarcoidosis patients with pulmonary hypertension present with signs of right-sided heart failure.[81,82] Diagnosing pulmonary hypertension in sarcoidosis solely with the use of CT is difficult and merely impossible. Severe pulmonary hypertension, however, is likely to be present when the diameter of the main pulmonary artery at the level of its bifurcation is greater than that of the adjacent ascending aorta or more than 29 mm.[83] In a study by Nunes and colleagues,[82] a higher frequency of ground glass attenuation and septal lines was found in sarcoidosis patients with pulmonary hypertension compared with sarcoidosis patients without pulmonary hypertension.

FLUORODEOXYGLUCOSE F 18 PET/ COMPUTED TOMOGRAPHY
Fluorodeoxyglucose F 18 Uptake in Sarcoidosis

FDG PET/CT is widely used in oncology. FDG is a glucose analogue that is transported through the cell membrane. Once in the cytosol, FDG is phosphorylated by hexokinase and metabolically trapped as FDG-6-phosphate. After annihilation, 2 gamma photons of 511 keV each are detected by the PET camera. The current resolution of PET cameras is up to 5 mm. FDG is a well-studied and practical tracer with various applications in medicine, without the need for an onsite cyclotron.

In sarcoidosis, the granuloma contains activated macrophages and CD4[+] T lymphocytes. Like malignant cells, macrophages and lymphocytes express glucose transporters (GLUTs),

specifically GLUT-1 and GLUT-3.[84] Analogous to glucose, FDG is transported into macrophages and activated leucocytes through GLUT-1 and GLUT-3. Therefore, FDG PET can be used in leukocyte-mediated processes, like sarcoidosis and other granulomatous diseases.[85] Lewis and Salama[86] were the first to report the use of FDG PET in sarcoidosis, and since then several important clinical studies have been performed.

The maximum standardized uptake value (SUV_{max}) represents the maximum amount of glucose, that is, activity, in 1 pixel. SUV_{max} has proved a powerful tool in oncology because it correlates with survival and can be used for treatment monitoring. In sarcoidosis, the SUV_{max} could be helpful for response assessment and correlates with recurrence. In contrast with tumors, however, sarcoidosis cannot be well demarcated and might diffusely affect organs. Therefore, the maximum activity in 1 pixel might be less appropriate.

Patient Preparation and Fluorodeoxyglucose F 18 PET/Computed Tomography Acquisition in Sarcoidosis

Prior to FDG injection, patients need to fast for 6 hours. In sarcoidosis, this fasting period is preceded by a carbohydrate-restricted diet for at least 24 hours. To reduce the radiation dose and accelerate FDG excretion by the kidneys, 20 mg of furosemide is injected intravenously. Subsequently, FDG is administered when the blood glucose level is less than 7 mmol/L. The dosage of FDG is based on a patient's body weight with a minimum of 37 MBq (Mega Becquerel) and a maximum of 400 MBq; 60 minutes after FDG administration, low-dose CT is performed from the subinguinal region to the head. Low-dose CT is used for attenuation correction and optimizing image interpretation. The emission scan is performed from the subinguinal region to the head and starts 55 to 65 minutes after FDG injection. The acquisition time is 2.5 minutes per bed position. Reconstruction of the PET images is performed in accordance with the 3D–row action maximum likelihood algorithm protocol (RAMLA), applying 4 iterations with a 144 × 144 matrix.

Mammalian metabolism depends on glucose and fatty acids.[87] Therefore, FDG uptake in the myocardium is simply a physiologic process. The physiologic FDG uptake can be reduced by the use of unfractioned heparin, prolonged fasting period, or a carbohydrate-restricted diet for at least 24 hours prior to acquisition.[88–93] The latter has proved the most effective method. Fat and proteins are allowed, whereas all carbohydrates, including fruit and vegetables, should be avoided. When carbohydrates are restricted, fatty acids are used and physiologic FDG uptake is absent. If so, only metabolic active processes, like granulomas, become evident. This is the basis of imaging active cardiac sarcoidosis with FDG PET/CT.

Radiation Dose of Fluorodeoxyglucose F 18 PET/Computed Tomography

The radiation dose of FDG is approximately 5.8 mSv for the first-generation PET cameras, without CT scan. Over time, the cameras have become more sensitive and, in the current PET/CT systems, the FDG dosage can be reduced. The dosage is based on a patient's body weight, in accordance with European guidelines.[94] A patient with a bodyweight of 80 kg receives a radiation dose of 3.8 mSv. Disease location is more accurate because of the concurrently obtained CT, also performed for attenuation correction. The low-dose CT adds approximately 2.9 mSv to the radiation dose. Therefore, the radiation dose of FDG PET/CT from the head to the subinguinal regions is approximately 6.7 mSv.

Although FDG PET/CT is a noninvasive technique, it should be performed with care. FDG PET/CT is more expensive than other tests or techniques and radiation exposure should be taken into account. Frequent, repetitive FDG PET/CT is, therefore, not recommended.

CHEST RADIOGRAPH AND FLUORODEOXYGLUCOSE F 18 PET/COMPUTED TOMOGRAPHY

Chest radiography is commonly performed at the initial presentation of sarcoidosis. It is cheap and widely available and in 85% to 95% of patients abnormal findings are present.[95]

Staging of pulmonary disease is based on the Scadding criteria for chest radiography. It describes the presence of bilateral hilar adenopathy, parenchymal involvement, and signs of fibrosis.[4,96,97] Although the staging system provides prognostic information, differentiating between active inflammation, fibrosis, and inactive disease is difficult. The Scadding stages do not correlate with disease activity imaged by FDG PET/CT.[98,99] Patients with stage 0 and stage IV disease frequently demonstrate disease activity in hila and/or lung parenchyma. Additionally, a majority of patients with stage I show active parenchymal disease. These data suggest that FDG PET/CT is more accurate than chest radiography in the evaluation of active parenchymal and/or lymph node involvement of sarcoidosis.

HIGH-RESOLUTION COMPUTED TOMOGRAPHY AND FLUORODEOXYGLUCOSE F 18 PET/COMPUTED TOMOGRAPHY

HRCT is able to assess the lung parenchyma meticulously due to its high spatial resolution. It is, therefore, superior to conventional radiography in detecting parenchymal distortion, nodules, and early fibrosis. Volumetric scanning with multidetector CT scans has become routine in most institutions and enables imaging of the whole lung in 1 single breath-hold.[98] It has become a powerful technique in the diagnosis of diffuse parenchymal lung disease. Compared with conventional chest radiography, HRCT is more accurate in diagnosing sarcoidosis and has a better interobserver agreement.[48]

The prognostic value of HRCT has been studied by evaluating serial HRCT scans. Architectural distortion, traction bronchiectasis, cysts, and honeycombing are irreversible but nodular disease is reversible in most patients. Ground glass, interlobular septal thickening, and irregular linear opacities, however, may or may not be reversible and can progress to fibrosis.[11,42,100–104]

In stage I sarcoidosis, no predictive value of parenchymal opacities in HRCT could be found during 2-year follow-up.[105]

Only a few studies have compared FDG PET/CT and HRCT. Ambrosini and colleagues[106] evaluated 35 scans in a heterogeneous group of 28 patients. FDG PET/CT was indicated for staging, assessment of disease activity, evaluation of disease activity during or after therapy, suspicion of cardiac sarcoidosis, or follow-up. Active disease at FDG PET/CT was defined by any pathologic FDG uptake. Their HRCT criteria for active disease were enlarged lymph nodes with or without calcifications, large or small nodules with perilymphatic distribution, diffuse or random distribution of nodules, consolidation or ground glass density, cluster sign, galaxy sign, halo sign, atoll sign, or airways abnormalities with or without air trapping on expiration. Active disease was present in 24 FDG PET/CT scans (69%) and 25 HRCT scans (71%). Only 10 scans, however, demonstrated corresponding active disease in the overall concordant group of 16.

Using a semiquantitative HRCT scoring system, Mostard and colleagues[107] compared HRCT and FDG PET in 95 sarcoidosis patients. HRCT features associated with increased FDG uptake are parenchymal consolidations in 48%, lymph nodes in 25%, intraparenchymal nodules in 21%, septal and nonseptal lines in 4%, and pleural thickening in 2%.

Signs of fibrosis on HRCT regularly show metabolic active lung parenchyma on FDG PET/CT. Although the amount of uptake is variable in fibrotic sarcoidosis, it is much higher than in idiopathic pulmonary fibrosis.[108] The significantly higher metabolism in sarcoidosis is suggested to reflect granulomatous inflammation, whereas the slightly increased FDG activity in idiopathic pulmonary fibrosis might be the result of increased glucose metabolism in fibroblasts. Because fibrotic changes on HRCT may vary in FDG activity, it seems that HRCT is not able to distinguish active, ongoing fibrogenesis and inactive, end-stage fibrosis.[2,83]

Pulmonary Function and Fluorodeoxyglucose F 18 PET/Computed Tomography

FDG PET/CT is able to demonstrate ongoing granulomatous inflammation in the lungs of patients with pulmonary sarcoidosis, representing active disease. Keijsers and colleagues[109] correlated baseline FDG PET with changes in vital capacity (VC), forced expiratory volume in the first second of expiration (FEV_1), and diffusion capacity of lung for carbon monoxide (DLCO) after 1 year in 43 newly diagnosed sarcoidosis patient. There was significant improvement of VC, FEV_1, and DLCO in patients with diffuse lung parenchymal activity receiving immunosuppressive therapy (n = 16). Patients with diffuse lung parenchymal activity without therapy (n = 11) showed a significant decrease in DLCO. On the other hand, there was no change in VC, FEV_1, and DLCO in patients without lung parenchymal activity and without treatment. In addition, the change in metabolic activity imaged by FDG PET was evaluated in 11 patients treated with infliximab and compared with pulmonary function tests.[110] Clinical improvement was associated with an overall reduced metabolic activity. In particular, the decrease in metabolic activity of the lung parenchyma, expressed as SUV_{max}, showed a significant correlation with the increase in VC (**Fig. 11**). These results suggest that the extent of active disease reflects the potential functional improvement that can be achieved and that lung parenchymal metabolic activity may have prognostic value.

From the authors' experience, the absence of FDG uptake in the lungs of patients with prolonged parenchymal sarcoidosis does indicate little or no lung functional improvement after initiation or intensification of immunosuppressive treatment (**Fig. 12**).

Fluorodeoxyglucose F 18 PET/Computed Tomography in Cardiac Sarcoidosis

Cardiac involvement in sarcoidosis may occur at any time and even without pulmonary or other systemic disease. Cardiac sarcoidosis may have major clinical consequences given the potential conduction defects and lethal arrhythmias. Accurate diagnosis of cardiac sarcoidosis is, therefore, of great importance.

Sarcoidosis can affect the pericardium, myocardium, and endocardium. Myocardial involvement is predominantly in the left ventricular wall followed by the papillary muscles, the interventricular septum, the right ventricular wall, and the atria.[111,112] The guidelines of the Japanese Ministry of Health and Welfare for the diagnosis of cardiac sarcoidosis are updated but FDG PET/CT is not included in the work-up.[113] FDG PET/CT has, however, been shown a promising tool to evaluate cardiac involvement[114] (**Fig. 13**).

Focal FDG uptake strongly suggests cardiac involvement, although a diffuse pattern may be seen as well.[89,90] Sensitivity of FDG PET in the diagnosis of cardiac sarcoidosis has been reported as high. A meta-analysis showed a pooled sensitivity of 89% and specificity of 78%.[115] A study comparing cardiac magnetic resonance (CMR) and FDG PET demonstrated a favorable sensitivity over MRI of 87.5% versus 75%, respectively.[114] On the other hand, Mehta and colleagues[116] found a higher sensitivity for FDG PET compared with MRI (86% vs 36%, respectively). Both MRI and PET scanning may be indicated in patients in whom the diagnosis of cardiac sarcoidosis is uncertain.[117]

Blankstein and colleagues[118] performed cardiac PET/CT in 118 patients with cardiac sarcoidosis. FDG PET/CT was performed to evaluate the presence of active inflammation. Rubidium Rb 82 PET/CT was carried out to assess perfusion defects and caused scarring. Patients were categorized by perfusion and/or metabolism abnormalities and outcome was measured; 47 patients had a normal and 71 had an abnormal cardiac PET. The presence of perfusion defects combined with increased metabolism was predictive of death or sustained ventricular tachycardia with a hazard ratio of 3.9.

In addition, an abnormal FDG PET scan is associated with an increased risk of major cardiac events.[118] Japanese criteria demonstrated poor sensitivity and had no significant association with adverse events, suggesting an important added value of FDG PET beyond the Japanese guidelines. In cardiac sarcoidosis patients with implantable cardioverter-defibrillators (ICDs), positive FDG PET scans for cardiac sarcoidosis in combination with positive MRI predicted a higher ventricular tachycardia and ventricular fibrillation risk than positive MRI alone.[119] Remarkably, 90% of FDG PET scans were positive versus 67% positive

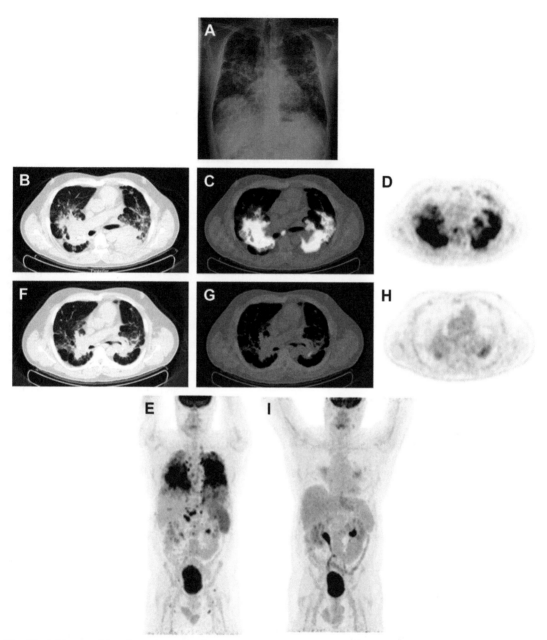

Fig. 11. A 51-year-old male patient was diagnosed with sarcoidosis 6 years prior to presentation at St. Antonius Hospital (The Netherlands). Initially, he was treated with prednisone, followed by methotrexate because of progressive dyspnea with pulmonary deterioration. With methotrexate, PFT remained decreased, but stable (VC 62% predicted, FEV_1 30% predicted, and DLCO 40% predicted). Chest radiography after 6 months demonstrated unchanged pulmonary infiltrates with signs of fibrosis (A). ACE was 85 U/L (normal 14–62 U/L) and sIL-2R was 10.500 pg/mL (normal <3000 pg/mL). FDG PET/CT was performed to evaluate the inflammation in the lung parenchyma. Widespread active disease was demonstrated in the lung parenchyma with active lymph nodes in the hila, mediastinum, abdomen, and inguinal regions (B–E). In addition, an active spleen was present. Infliximab was started and after 6 months, the fatigue and dyspnea were decreased. PFT was improved (VC 76% predicted, FEV_1 38% predicted, and DLCO 50% predicted), ACE remained unchanged, but sIL-2R dropped to 3814 pg/mL. FDG PET/CT showed a slight remaining metabolic activity in the perihilar regions (F–I). ACE, angiotensin converting enzyme; PFT, pulmonary function test; sIL-2R, soluble Interleukin-2 Receptor.

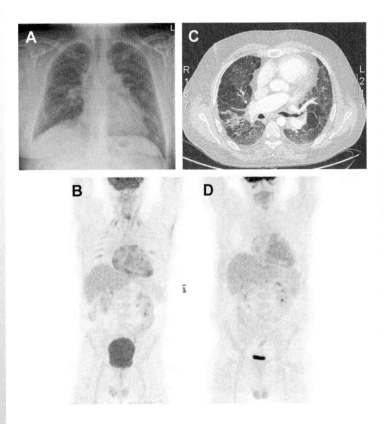

Fig. 12. A 39-year-old male patient was referred to St. Antonius Hospital (The Netherlands) because of pulmonary hypertension. He was diagnosed with sarcoidosis 2 years earlier and initially he was treated with prednisone followed by methotrexate. (*A*) Chest radiography showed mediastinal and hilar adenopathy with interstitial involvement. CMR showed a large right ventricle with signs of pulmonary hypertension but no cardiac sarcoidosis. Silfadenil was started but without improvement. PFT was invariably decreased (VC 61% predicted, FEV₁ 50% predicted, and DLCO 29% predicted). ACE was 50 U/L (24–82 U/L) and sIL-2R was 3538 pg/mL (normal <3000 pg/mL). (*B*) FDG PET/CT was performed to evaluate the inflammation in the lung parenchyma, but no active disease was present. The metabolic active right atrial and ventricle wall are due to the increased right ventricular pressure overload. (*C*) HRCT demonstrated mediastinal and hilar lymphnodes, traction bronchiectasis, and expanding areas of ground glass. Infliximab was started and after 6 cycles; ACE was 61 U/L and sIL-2R 4328 pg/mL. HRCT was unchanged and PFT was not improved (VC 60% predicted, FEV₁ 44% predicted, and DLCO 24% predicted). (*D*) FDG PET/CT was again normal. The results in this patient might indicate that the effect of immunosuppressive drugs is limited when active disease imaged by FDG PET/CT is absent. ACE, angiotensin converting enzyme; PFT, pulmonary function test; sIL-2R, soluble Interleukin-2 Receptor.

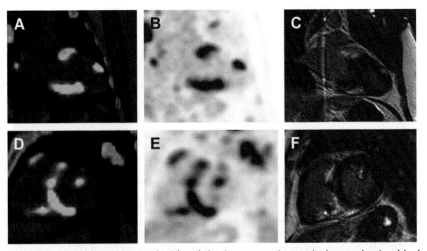

Fig. 13. A 47-year-old male patient presented with palpitations, an atrioventricular conduction block, and a right bundle branch block. He received a DDD pacemaker, compatible for MRI. Chest radiography after implantation showed hilar adenopathy and patchy consolidations, suspicious for sarcoidosis. During cardiac analysis at St. Antonius Hospital (The Netherlands), ventricular tachycardia occurred. FDG PET/CT ([*A* and *B*] long axis, [*D* and *E*] short axis) and CMR ([*C*] long axis, [*F*] short axis) demonstrates metabolic activity and corresponding enhancement in the right ventricle and right side of the interventricular septum and spread through the left ventricle. The left ventricular ejection fraction was 53%. The pacemaker was replaced by an ICD and prednisone was started.

MRI scans in the ICD treated group. Therefore, FDG PET seems particularly useful in patients with pacemakers or ICD or patients who cannot be evaluated with an MRI.[120]

Finally, follow-up studies demonstrated that FDG PET can detect changes in cardiac activity on treatment with corticosteroids 70.[121] This makes FDG PET useful for monitoring the effects of treatment in cardiac sarcoidosis patients.[119,122–124]

A recent consensus statement by the Heart Rhythm Society was published on the work-up in cardiac sarcoidosis.[125] In patients without symptoms and normal electrocardiogram and echocardiogram, the likelihood of cardiac involvement is low and additional testing is not recommended. In patients with 1 or more abnormalities, advanced cardiac imaging (ie, CMR and/or FDG PET/CT) can be useful.

When Should Fluorodeoxyglucose F 18 PET/Computed Tomography Be Used in Thoracic Sarcoidosis?

Besides conventional markers and imaging modalities used in the treatment of thoracic sarcoidosis, there is an emerging role of FDG PET/CT. From the current literature and the authors' experience, it can be suggested to use FDG PET/CT in the following situations:

- FDG PET/CT can guide in finding occult organ localizations when histologic proof is needed. Biopsy from metabolic active lesions is more likely to yield the diagnosis than biopsy from inactive lesions.
- In patients with persistent symptoms but without signs of disease activity based on conventional markers, FDG PET/CT is able to demonstrate ongoing disease activity. Mostard and colleagues[98] evaluated FDG PET/CT in 89 patients with unexplained persistent and disabling symptoms. They found metabolic active disease in 73% with normal serum markers in 20% of these patients.
- In patients suspected of having cardiac sarcoidosis, CMR is able to detect cardiac involvement and might give rise to the implantation of a cardiac defibrillator. FDG PET/CT, on the other hand, reveals the presence of active lesions in the myocardium, which helps indicating whether immunosuppressive treatment should be started or adjusted.
- In patients with prolonged and symptomatic pulmonary sarcoidosis with fibrosis, it can be difficult to determine the presence of ongoing parenchymal disease activity. When active pulmonary sarcoidosis is still present, immunosuppressive treatment might be started or adjusted. In 14 of 15 patients with stage IV disease, FDG PET/CT revealed persistent parenchymal disease activity.[98] In addition, patients with active metabolic parenchymal disease show a significant increase of their pulmonary function after treatment. Therefore, FDG PET/CT can be used to predict the potential functional improvement that can be achieved, even in patients with stage IV disease.

SUMMARY

Pulmonary sarcoidosis has a great variability and is notorious for mimicking many other interstitial lung diseases. Knowledge of pulmonary manifestations is important in diagnosing sarcoidosis because more than 90% of patients present with thoracic involvement. Both HRCT and FDG PET/CT are essential modalities in diagnosing and evaluation of pulmonary sarcoidosis. In addition, FDG PET/CT demonstrates extra pulmonary disease most accurate and has an important role in cardiac sarcoidosis.

REFERENCES

1. Lynch JP 3rd, Kazerooni EA, Gay SE. Pulmonary sarcoidosis. Clin Chest Med 1997;18(4):755–85.
2. Keijsers RG, van den Heuvel DA, Grutters JC. Imaging the inflammatory activity of sarcoidosis. Eur Respir J 2013;41(3):743–51.
3. DeRemee RA. The roentgenographic staging of sarcoidosis. Historic and contemporary perspectives. Chest 1983;83(1):128–33.
4. SCADDING JG. Prognosis of intrathoracic sarcoidosis in England. A review of 136 cases after five years' observation. Br Med J 1961; 2(5261):1165–72.
5. Van den Heuvel DA, de Jong PA, Zanen P, et al. Chest computed tomography-based scoring of thoracic sarcoidosis: inter-rater reliability of CT abnormalities. Eur Radiol 2015;25(9):2558–66.
6. Drent M, de Vries J, Lenters M, et al. Sarcoidosis: assessment of disease severity using HRCT. Eur Radiol 2003;13(11):2462–71.
7. Veltkamp M, van Moorsel CH, Rijkers GT, et al. Genetic variation in the Toll-like receptor gene cluster (TLR10-TLR1-TLR6) influences disease course in sarcoidosis. Tissue Antigens 2012;79(1):25–32.
8. Hillerdal G, Nou E, Osterman K, et al. Sarcoidosis: epidemiology and prognosis. A 15-year European study. Am Rev Respir Dis 1984;130(1):29–32.
9. Statement on sarcoidosis. Joint statement of the American thoracic society (ATS), the European Respiratory Society (ERS) and the World

Association of Sarcoidosis and Other Granuloma-tous Disorders (WASOG) adopted by the ATS Board of Directors and by the ERS Executive Committee, February 1999. Am J Respir Crit Care Med 1999;160(2):736–55.

10. Baughman RP, Teirstein AS, Judson MA, et al. Clinical characteristics of patients in a case control study of sarcoidosis. Am J Respir Crit Care Med 2001;164(10 Pt 1):1885–9.

11. Nunes H, Brillet PY, Valeyre D, et al. Imaging in sarcoidosis. Semin Respir Crit Care Med 2007; 28(1):102–20.

12. Baughman RP, Lower EE, Tami T. Upper airway. 4: sarcoidosis of the upper respiratory tract (SURT). Thorax 2010;65(2):181–6.

13. James DG, Barter S, Jash D, et al. Sarcoidosis of the upper respiratory tract (SURT). J Laryngol Otol 1982;96(8):711–8.

14. Panselinas E, Halstead L, Schlosser RJ, et al. Clinical manifestations, radiographic findings, treatment options, and outcome in sarcoidosis patients with upper respiratory tract involvement. South Med J 2010;103(9):870–5.

15. Shorr AF, Torrington KG, Hnatiuk OW. Endobronchial biopsy for sarcoidosis: a prospective study. Chest 2001;120(1):109–14.

16. Chambellan A, Turbie P, Nunes H, et al. Endoluminal stenosis of proximal bronchi in sarcoidosis: bronchoscopy, function, and evolution. Chest 2005;127(2):472–81.

17. Kirks DR, McCormick VD, Greenspan RH. Pulmonary sarcoidosis. Roentgenologic analysis of 150 patients. Am J Roentgenol Radium Ther Nucl Med 1973;117(4):777–86.

18. James DG, Neville E, Siltzbach LE. A worldwide review of sarcoidosis. Ann N Y Acad Sci 1976;278: 321–34.

19. Siltzbach LE, James DG, Neville E, et al. Course and prognosis of sarcoidosis around the world. Am J Med 1974;57(6):847–52.

20. Sider L, Horton ES Jr. Hilar and mediastinal adenopathy in sarcoidosis as detected by computed tomography. J Thorac Imaging 1990; 5(2):77–80.

21. Patil SN, Levin DL. Distribution of thoracic lymphadenopathy in sarcoidosis using computed tomography. J Thorac Imaging 1999;14(2):114–7.

22. Niimi H, Kang EY, Kwong JS, et al. CT of chronic infiltrative lung disease: prevalence of mediastinal lymphadenopathy. J Comput Assist Tomogr 1996; 20(2):305–8.

23. Gawne-Cain ML, Hansell DM. The pattern and distribution of calcified mediastinal lymph nodes in sarcoidosis and tuberculosis: a CT study. Clin Radiol 1996;51(4):263–7.

24. Rabinowitz JG, Ulreich S, Soriano C. The usual unusual manifestations of sarcoidosis and the "hilar haze"–a new diagnostic aid. Am J Roentgenol Radium Ther Nucl Med 1974;120(4):821–31.

25. Romer FK. Presentation of sarcoidosis and outcome of pulmonary changes. Dan Med Bull 1982;29(1):27–32.

26. Spann RW, Rosenow EC 3rd, DeRemee RA, et al. Unilateral hilar or paratracheal adenopathy in sarcoidosis: a study of 38 cases. Thorax 1971; 26(3):296–9.

27. Murdoch J, Muller NL. Pulmonary sarcoidosis: changes on follow-up CT examination. AJR Am J Roentgenol 1992;159(3):473–7.

28. McLoud TC, Putman CE, Pascual R. Eggshell calcification with systemic sarcoidosis. Chest 1974;66(5):515–7.

29. McLoud TC, Epler GR, Gaensler EA, et al. A radiographic classification for sarcoidosis: physiologic correlation. Invest Radiol 1982;17(2): 129–38.

30. Israel HL, Karlin P, Menduke H, et al. Factors affecting outcome of sarcoidosis. Influence of race, extrathoracic involvement, and initial radiologic lung lesions. Ann N Y Acad Sci 1986;465: 609–18.

31. Nishimura K, Itoh H, Kitaichi M, et al. Pulmonary sarcoidosis: correlation of CT and histopathologic findings. Radiology 1993;189(1):105–9.

32. Padley SP, Padhani AR, Nicholson A, et al. Pulmonary sarcoidosis mimicking cryptogenic fibrosing alveolitis on CT. Clin Radiol 1996;51(11):807–10.

33. Sharma OP, Hewlett R, Gordonson J. Nodular sarcoidosis: an unusual radiographic appearance. Chest 1973;64(2):189–92.

34. Battesti JP, Saumon G, Valeyre D, et al. Pulmonary sarcoidosis with an alveolar radiographic pattern. Thorax 1982;37(6):448–52.

35. McNicol MW, Luce PJ. Sarcoidosis in a racially mixed community. J R Coll Physicians Lond 1985; 19(3):179–83.

36. Malaisamy S, Dalal B, Bimenyuy C, et al. The clinical and radiologic features of nodular pulmonary sarcoidosis. Lung 2009;187(1):9–15.

37. Edelman RR, Johnson TS, Jhaveri HS, et al. Fatal hemoptysis resulting from erosion of a pulmonary artery in cavitary sarcoidosis. AJR Am J Roentgenol 1985;145(1):37–8.

38. Loh GA, Lettieri CJ, Shah AA. Bronchial arterial embolisation for massive haemoptysis in cavitary sarcoidosis. BMJ Case Rep 2013;2013:1–3.

39. Leung AN, Brauner MW, Caillat-Vigneron N, et al. Sarcoidosis activity: correlation of HRCT findings with those of 67Ga scanning, bronchoalveolar lavage, and serum angiotensin-converting enzyme assay. J Comput Assist Tomogr 1998;22(2):229–34.

40. Brauner MW, Grenier P, Mompoint D, et al. Pulmonary sarcoidosis: evaluation with high-resolution CT. Radiology 1989;172(2):467–71.

41. Abehsera M, Valeyre D, Grenier P, et al. Sarcoidosis with pulmonary fibrosis: CT patterns and correlation with pulmonary function. AJR Am J Roentgenol 2000;174(6):1751–7.

42. Remy-Jardin M, Giraud F, Remy J, et al. Pulmonary sarcoidosis: role of CT in the evaluation of disease activity and functional impairment and in prognosis assessment. Radiology 1994;191(3):675–80.

43. Marchiori E, Zanetti G, Barreto MM, et al. Atypical distribution of small nodules on high resolution CT studies: patterns and differentials. Respir Med 2011;105(9):1263–7.

44. Voloudaki AE, Bouros DE, Froudarakis ME, et al. Crescentic and ring-shaped opacities. CT features in two cases of bronchiolitis obliterans organizing pneumonia (BOOP). Acta Radiol 1996; 37(6):889–92.

45. Marchiori E, Zanetti G, Mano CM, et al. The reversed halo sign: another atypical manifestation of sarcoidosis. Korean J Radiol 2010;11(2): 251–2.

46. Zompatori M, Poletti V, Battista G, et al. Bronchiolitis obliterans with organizing pneumonia (BOOP), presenting as a ring-shaped opacity at HRCT (the atoll sign). A case report. Radiol Med 1999;97(4): 308–10.

47. Marten K, Rummeny EJ, Engelke C. The CT halo: a new sign in active pulmonary sarcoidosis. Br J Radiol 2004;77(924):1042–5.

48. Grenier P, Chevret S, Beigelman C, et al. Chronic diffuse infiltrative lung disease: determination of the diagnostic value of clinical data, chest radiography, and CT and Bayesian analysis. Radiology 1994;191(2):383–90.

49. Grenier P, Valeyre D, Cluzel P, et al. Chronic diffuse interstitial lung disease: diagnostic value of chest radiography and high-resolution CT. Radiology 1991;179(1):123–32.

50. Martin SG, Kronek LP, Valeyre D, et al. High-resolution computed tomography to differentiate chronic diffuse interstitial lung diseases with predominant ground-glass pattern using logical analysis of data. Eur Radiol 2010;20(6):1297–310.

51. Moller DR. Pulmonary fibrosis of sarcoidosis. New approaches, old ideas. Am J Respir Cell Mol Biol 2003;29(Suppl 3):S37–41.

52. Freundlich IM, Libshitz HI, Glassman LM, et al. Sarcoidosis. Typical and atypical thoracic manifestations and complications. Clin Radiol 1970;21(4): 376–83.

53. Primack SL, Hartman TE, Hansell DM, et al. End-stage lung disease: CT findings in 61 patients. Radiology 1993;189(3):681–6.

54. Davies CW, Tasker AD, Padley SP, et al. Air trapping in sarcoidosis on computed tomography: correlation with lung function. Clin Radiol 2000;55(3): 217–21.

55. Hansell DM, Milne DG, Wilsher ML, et al. Pulmonary sarcoidosis: morphologic associations of airflow obstruction at thin-section CT. Radiology 1998;209(3):697–704.

56. Bartz RR, Stern EJ. Airways obstruction in patients with sarcoidosis: expiratory CT scan findings. J Thorac Imaging 2000;15(4):285–9.

57. Pena TA, Soubani AO, Samavati L. Aspergillus lung disease in patients with sarcoidosis: a case series and review of the literature. Lung 2011;189(2):167–72.

58. Pesle GD, Monod O. Bronchiectasis due to aspergilloma. Dis Chest 1954;25(2):172–83.

59. Chusid EL, Siltzbach LE. Sarcoidosis of the pleura. Ann Intern Med 1974;81(2):190–4.

60. Sharma OP, Gordonson J. Pleural effusion in sarcoidosis: a report of six cases. Thorax 1975; 30(1):95–101.

61. Beekman JF, Zimmet SM, Chun BK, et al. Spectrum of pleural involvement in sarcoidosis. Arch Intern Med 1976;136(3):323–30.

62. Wilen SB, Rabinowitz JG, Ulreich S, et al. Pleural involvement in sarcoidosis. Am J Med 1974;57(2): 200–9.

63. Tommasini A, Di Vittorio G, Facchinetti F, et al. Pleural effusion in sarcoidosis: a case report. Sarcoidosis 1994;11(2):138–40.

64. Soskel NT, Sharma OP. Pleural involvement in sarcoidosis. Curr Opin Pulm Med 2000;6(5): 455–68.

65. Huggins JT, Doelken P, Sahn SA, et al. Pleural effusions in a series of 181 outpatients with sarcoidosis. Chest 2006;129(6):1599–604.

66. Littner MR, Schachter EN, Putman CE, et al. The clinical assessment of roentgenographically atypical pulmonary sarcoidosis. Am J Med 1977; 62(3):361–8.

67. Aberg H, Bah M, Waters AW. Sarcoidosis: complicated by chylothorax. Minn Med 1966;49(7): 1065–70.

68. Jarman PR, Whyte MK, Sabroe I, et al. Sarcoidosis presenting with chylothorax. Thorax 1995;50(12): 1324–5.

69. Lengyel RJ, Shanley DJ. Recurrent chylothorax associated with sarcoidosis. Hawaii Med J 1995; 54(12):817–8.

70. Parker JM, Torrington KG, Phillips YY. Sarcoidosis complicated by chylothorax. South Med J 1994; 87(8):860–2.

71. Hours S, Nunes H, Kambouchner M, et al. Pulmonary cavitary sarcoidosis: clinico-radiologic characteristics and natural history of a rare form of sarcoidosis. Medicine (Baltimore) 2008;87(3): 142–51.

72. Froudarakis ME, Bouros D, Voloudaki A, et al. Pneumothorax as a first manifestation of sarcoidosis. Chest 1997;112(1):278–80.

73. Akelsson IG, Eklund A, Skold CM, et al. Bilateral spontaneous pneumothorax and sarcoidosis. Sarcoidosis 1990;7(2):136–8.

74. Popper HH, Klemen H, Colby TV, et al. Necrotizing sarcoid granulomatosis–is it different from nodular sarcoidosis? Pneumologie 2003;57(5):268–71.

75. Koss MN, Hochholzer L, Feigin DS, et al. Necrotizing sarcoid-like granulomatosis: clinical, pathologic, and immunopathologic findings. Hum Pathol 1980;11(Suppl 5):510–9.

76. Rosen Y. Pathology of sarcoidosis. Semin Respir Crit Care Med 2007;28(1):36–52.

77. Liebow AA. The J. Burns Amberson lecture–pulmonary angiitis and granulomatosis. Am Rev Respir Dis 1973;108(1):1–18.

78. Yeboah J, Afkhami M, Lee C, et al. Necrotizing sarcoid granulomatosis. Curr Opin Pulm Med 2012;18(5):493–8.

79. Rosen Y. Four decades of necrotizing sarcoid granulomatosis: what do we know now? Arch Pathol Lab Med 2015;139(2):252–62.

80. Handa T, Nagai S, Miki S, et al. Incidence of pulmonary hypertension and its clinical relevance in patients with sarcoidosis. Chest 2006;129(5):1246–52.

81. Sulica R, Teirstein AS, Kakarla S, et al. Distinctive clinical, radiographic, and functional characteristics of patients with sarcoidosis-related pulmonary hypertension. Chest 2005;128(3):1483–9.

82. Nunes H, Humbert M, Capron F, et al. Pulmonary hypertension associated with sarcoidosis: mechanisms, haemodynamics and prognosis. Thorax 2006;61(1):68–74.

83. Nunes H, Uzunhan Y, Freynet O, et al. Pulmonary hypertension complicating sarcoidosis. Presse Med 2012;41(6 Pt 2):e303–16.

84. Fu Y, Maianu L, Melbert BR, et al. Facilitative glucose transporter gene expression in human lymphocytes, monocytes, and macrophages: a role for GLUT isoforms 1, 3, and 5 in the immune response and foam cell formation. Blood Cells Mol Dis 2004;32(1):182–90.

85. Satomi T, Ogawa M, Mori I, et al. Comparison of contrast agents for atherosclerosis imaging using cultured macrophages: FDG versus ultrasmall superparamagnetic iron oxide. J Nucl Med 2013;54(6):999–1004.

86. Lewis PJ, Salama A. Uptake of fluorine-18-fluorodeoxyglucose in sarcoidosis. J Nucl Med 1994;35(10):1647–9.

87. Frayn KN. The glucose-fatty acid cycle: a physiological perspective. Biochem Soc Trans 2003;31(Pt 6):1115–9.

88. Cheng VY, Slomka PJ, Ahlen M, et al. Impact of carbohydrate restriction with and without fatty acid loading on myocardial 18F-FDG uptake during PET: a randomized controlled trial. J Nucl Cardiol 2010;17(2):286–91.

89. Ishimaru S, Tsujino I, Takei T, et al. Focal uptake on 18F-fluoro-2-deoxyglucose positron emission tomography images indicates cardiac involvement of sarcoidosis. Eur Heart J 2005;26(15):1538–43.

90. Langah R, Spicer K, Gebregziabher M, et al. Effectiveness of prolonged fasting 18f-FDG PET-CT in the detection of cardiac sarcoidosis. J Nucl Cardiol 2009;16(5):801–10.

91. Ohira H, Tsujino I, Yoshinaga K. (1)(8)F-Fluoro-2-deoxyglucose positron emission tomography in cardiac sarcoidosis. Eur J Nucl Med Mol Imaging 2011;38(9):1773–83.

92. Okumura W, Iwasaki T, Toyama T, et al. Usefulness of fasting 18F-FDG PET in identification of cardiac sarcoidosis. J Nucl Med 2004;45(12):1989–98.

93. Williams G, Kolodny GM. Suppression of myocardial 18F-FDG uptake by preparing patients with a high-fat, low-carbohydrate diet. AJR Am J Roentgenol 2008;190(2):W151–6.

94. Boellaard R, Delgado-Bolton R, Oyen WJ, et al. FDG PET/CT: EANM procedure guidelines for tumour imaging: version 2.0. Eur J Nucl Med Mol Imaging 2015;42(2):328–54.

95. Keir G, Wells AU. Assessing pulmonary disease and response to therapy: which test? Semin Respir Crit Care Med 2010;31(4):409–18.

96. Miller BH, Putman CE. The chest radiograph and sarcoidosis. Reevaluation of the chest radiograph in assessing activity of sarcoidosis: a preliminary communication. Sarcoidosis 1985;2(2):85–90.

97. Prasse A, Katic C, Germann M, et al. Phenotyping sarcoidosis from a pulmonary perspective. Am J Respir Crit Care Med 2008;177(3):330–6.

98. Mostard RL, Voo S, van Kroonenburgh MJ, et al. Inflammatory activity assessment by F18 FDG-PET/CT in persistent symptomatic sarcoidosis. Respir Med 2011;105(12):1917–24.

99. Keijsers RG, Grutters JC, van Velzen-Blad H, et al. (18)F-FDG PET patterns and BAL cell profiles in pulmonary sarcoidosis. Eur J Nucl Med Mol Imaging 2010;37(6):1181–8.

100. Akira M, Kozuka T, Inoue Y, et al. Long-term follow-up CT scan evaluation in patients with pulmonary sarcoidosis. Chest 2005;127(1):185–91.

101. Brauner MW, Lenoir S, Grenier P, et al. Pulmonary sarcoidosis: CT assessment of lesion reversibility. Radiology 1992;182(2):349–54.

102. Lynch DA, Webb WR, Gamsu G, et al. Computed tomography in pulmonary sarcoidosis. J Comput Assist Tomogr 1989;13(3):405–10.

103. Wells AU, Rubens MB, du Bois RM, et al. Functional impairment in fibrosing alveolitis: relationship to reversible disease on thin section computed tomography. Eur Respir J 1997;10(2):280–5.

104. Wells AU, Rubens MB, du Bois RM, et al. Serial CT in fibrosing alveolitis: prognostic significance of the initial pattern. AJR Am J Roentgenol 1993;161(6): 1159–65.

105. Ziora D, Kornelia K, Jastrzebski D, et al. High resolution computed tomography in 2-year follow-up of stage I sarcoidosis. Adv Exp Med Biol 2013; 788:369–74.

106. Ambrosini V, Zompatori M, Fasano L, et al. (18)F-FDG PET/CT for the assessment of disease extension and activity in patients with sarcoidosis: results of a preliminary prospective study. Clin Nucl Med 2013;38(4):e171–7.

107. Mostard RL, van Kroonenburgh MJ, Drent M. The role of the PET scan in the management of sarcoidosis. Curr Opin Pulm Med 2013;19(5):538–44.

108. Groves AM, Win T, Screaton NJ, et al. Idiopathic pulmonary fibrosis and diffuse parenchymal lung disease: implications from initial experience with 18F-FDG PET/CT. J Nucl Med 2009;50(4):538–45.

109. Keijsers RG, Verzijlbergen EJ, van den Bosch JM, et al. 18F-FDG PET as a predictor of pulmonary function in sarcoidosis. Sarcoidosis Vasc Diffuse Lung Dis 2011;28(2):123–9.

110. Keijsers RG, Verzijlbergen JF, van Diepen DM, et al. 18F-FDG PET in sarcoidosis: an observational study in 12 patients treated with infliximab. Sarcoidosis Vasc Diffuse Lung Dis 2008;25(2): 143–9.

111. Roberts WC, McAllister HA Jr, Ferrans VJ. Sarcoidosis of the heart. A clinicopathologic study of 35 necropsy patients (group 1) and review of 78 previously described necropsy patients (group 11). Am J Med 1977;63(1):86–108.

112. Tavora F, Cresswell N, Li L, et al. Comparison of necropsy findings in patients with sarcoidosis dying suddenly from cardiac sarcoidosis versus dying suddenly from other causes. Am J Cardiol 2009;104(4):571–7.

113. Watanabe E, Kimura F, Nakajima T, et al. Late gadolinium enhancement in cardiac sarcoidosis: characteristic magnetic resonance findings and relationship with left ventricular function. J Thorac Imaging 2013;28(1):60–6.

114. Ohira H, Tsujino I, Ishimaru S, et al. Myocardial imaging with 18F-fluoro-2-deoxyglucose positron emission tomography and magnetic resonance imaging in sarcoidosis. Eur J Nucl Med Mol Imaging 2008;35(5):933–41.

115. Youssef G, Leung E, Mylonas I, et al. The use of 18F-FDG PET in the diagnosis of cardiac sarcoidosis: a systematic review and metaanalysis including the Ontario experience. J Nucl Med 2012;53(2):241–8.

116. Mehta D, Lubitz SA, Frankel Z, et al. Cardiac involvement in patients with sarcoidosis: diagnostic and prognostic value of outpatient testing. Chest 2008;133(6):1426–35.

117. Skali H, Schulman AR, Dorbala S. 18F-FDG PET/CT for the assessment of myocardial sarcoidosis. Curr Cardiol Rep 2013;15(4):352.

118. Blankstein R, Osborne M, Naya M, et al. Cardiac positron emission tomography enhances prognostic assessments of patients with suspected cardiac sarcoidosis. J Am Coll Cardiol 2014;63(4): 329–36.

119. Betensky BP, Tschabrunn CM, Zado ES, et al. Long-term follow-up of patients with cardiac sarcoidosis and implantable cardioverter-defibrillators. Heart Rhythm 2012;9(6):884–91.

120. Sekhri V, Sanal S, Delorenzo LJ, et al. Cardiac sarcoidosis: a comprehensive review. Arch Med Sci 2011;7(4):546–54.

121. Soussan M, Brillet PY, Nunes H, et al. Clinical value of a high-fat and low-carbohydrate diet before FDG-PET/CT for evaluation of patients with suspected cardiac sarcoidosis. J Nucl Cardiol 2013; 20(1):120–7.

122. Gyorik S, Ceriani L, Menafoglio A, et al. 18F-FDG PET scan as follow-up tool for sarcoidosis with symptomatic cardiac conduction disturbances requiring a pacemaker. Thorax 2007;62(6):560.

123. Smedema JP, White L, Klopper AJ. FDG-PET and MIBI-Tc SPECT as follow-up tools in a patient with cardiac sarcoidosis requiring a pacemaker. Cardiovasc J Afr 2008;19(6):309–10.

124. Mc Ardle BA, Leung E, Ohira H, et al. The role of F(18)-fluorodeoxyglucose positron emission tomography in guiding diagnosis and management in patients with known or suspected cardiac sarcoidosis. J Nucl Cardiol 2013;20(2):297–306.

125. Birnie DH, Sauer WH, Bogun F, et al. HRS expert consensus statement on the diagnosis and management of arrhythmias associated with cardiac sarcoidosis. Heart Rhythm 2014;11(7):1305–23.

Identifying Novel Biomarkers in Sarcoidosis Using Genome-Based Approaches

Nancy Casanova, MD[a,b,1], Tong Zhou, PhD[a,c,1],
Kenneth S. Knox, MD[a,d], Joe G.N. Garcia, MD[a,e],*

KEYWORDS

- Sarcoidosis • Biomarkers • Molecular signature • GWAS • Microarray • Sequencing

KEY POINTS

- The use of biomarkers to support diagnosis and predict disease activity remains a focal point in routine clinical care of sarcoidosis.
- Monitoring subclinical disease activity and likelihood of progression or remission in a longitudinal fashion remains a challenge.
- Genome-wide gene expression signature strategies and genetic variation data represent a new venue to generate useful biomarkers in sarcoidosis.
- Recent advances in genome-wide expression profiling techniques, such as gene expression microarray and RNA sequencing in blood provide a highly useful, non-invasive method to assess inflammatory activities in sarcoidosis.

SARCOIDOSIS: OVERVIEW AND NEED FOR BIOMARKERS

Sarcoidosis is a systemic heterogeneous inflammatory disease characterized by the presence of noncaseating epithelioid granulomas in one or multiple organs, with the lung affected in ~90% of cases. Lung involvement is commonly manifested as bilateral hilar lymphadenopathy (BHL) and pulmonary infiltration with more severe cases developing pulmonary fibrosis. Ocular and skin lesions may become sight threatening or disfiguring, requiring aggressive treatment. Cardiac and neurologic involvement may cause morbidity and death.[1,2] Löfgren syndrome, an acute presentation of sarcoidosis, is characterized by erythema nodosum, BHL, and polyarthralgia and is associated with spontaneous regression.[3,4] In addition, more

Disclosures: The authors have nothing to disclose.
Funding Source: This work was supported by National Institutes of Health U01 HL112696 (J.G.N. Garcia).
[a] Department of Medicine, Arizona Respiratory Center, University of Arizona Health Sciences Center, University of Arizona, Tucson, AZ 78721, USA; [b] Department of Medicine, Arizona Health Sciences Center, University of Arizona, Medical Research Building, Room 412, 1656 East Mabel Street, Tucson, AZ 85721, USA; [c] Department of Medicine, Arizona Health Sciences Center, University of Arizona, Medical Research Building, Room 410, 1656 East Mabel Street, Tucson, AZ 85721, USA; [d] Pulmonary Division, Department of Medicine, Arizona Health Sciences Center, University of Arizona, 1501 North Campbell, Tucson, AZ 85721, USA; [e] Department of Medicine, Arizona Health Sciences Center, University of Arizona, Drachman Hall, Room B-207, 1295 North Martin Avenue, Tucson, AZ 85721, USA
[1] These authors contributed equally to this work.
* Corresponding author. Department of Medicine, Arizona Health Sciences Center, University of Arizona, Drachman Hall, Room B-207, 1295 North Martin Avenue, Tucson, AZ 85721.
E-mail address: skipgarcia@email.arizona.edu

Clin Chest Med 36 (2015) 621–630
http://dx.doi.org/10.1016/j.ccm.2015.08.005
0272-5231/15/$ – see front matter © 2015 Elsevier Inc. All rights reserved.

than 50% of sarcoidosis patients will experience remission within 3 years after diagnosis, with more than 66% of patients experiencing remission within 10 years.[5,6] It is clear that although certain disease phenotypes and chest radiograph stages portend a good prognosis, a large proportion of patients would benefit from technological advances in biomarker development.

The need to develop useful biomarkers in the diagnosis and prognosis of subjects with sarcoidosis has long been recognized because sarcoidosis is a diagnosis of exclusion and may mimic multiple other rheumatologic illnesses.[7,8] Furthermore, a significant percentage of patients with sarcoidosis (about one-third) develop complications with granulomatous involvement of vital organs with progressive disease. Thus, monitoring subclinical disease activity and likelihood of progression or remission in a longitudinal fashion remains a challenge. Finally, significant racial and gender differences in disease development and prognosis have been reported in African American,[9] Irish, Scandinavian, and Hispanic populations. Again, these differences represent a compelling need for racial and ethnic-selective biomarkers to assess disease progression and response to therapy in diverse populations. In this article, traditional biomarkers in sarcoidosis as well as biomarkers emerging from technology-driven strategies are reviewed. Discussed are the integration of genome-wide gene expression signature strategies and genetic variation data as additional opportunities to generate useful biomarkers in sarcoidosis, particularly in assessment of personal risk for developing complicated sarcoidosis.

Traditional Biomarkers in Sarcoidosis

Despite limitations, the use of biomarkers to support diagnosis and predict disease activity remains a focal point in routine clinical care. Multiple methodologies have been applied to detect biomarkers in serum, lung tissue, bronchoalveolar lavage fluid (BALF), and exhaled breath condensate (EBC) using enzyme-linked immunosorbent assays, proteomic analysis, and mass spectrometry.[10] Traditionally, clinical biomarkers measured in sarcoidosis were limited to soluble factors measured in blood, bronchoalveolar lavage (BAL), or cerebral spinal fluid (Table 1). Data remain inconsistent regarding the validity of EBC biomarkers.[11] As technology improves, biomarker panels generated from array data will continue to emerge.

SOLUBLE BIOMARKERS ASSOCIATED WITH MONOCYTE-MACROPHAGE ACTIVATION

Although specific biomarkers have been suggested as useful tools in sarcoidosis, reduced specificity has been a major limitation with angiotensin-converting enzyme (ACE), the most commonly used biomarker in sarcoidosis. ACE is derived from activated macrophages in granulomatous pulmonary remodeling[12] and is useful in supporting a diagnosis and monitoring disease activity in some patients.[12,13] ACE levels are increased in approximately two-thirds of patients with sarcoidosis with elevated levels reported in neurosarcoidosis.[14] However, elevated ACE levels are not specific for sarcoidosis and are observed in granulomatous diseases such as tuberculosis,

Table 1
Conventional sarcoidosis biomarkers and their clinical association

Biomarker	Origin and Clinical Association
ACE	Monocyte-macrophage origin; acute stage, levels influenced by polymorphisms
sIL-2R	Lymphocyte associated; disease severity, extrapulmonary organ involvement
SAA	Monocyte-macrophage origin; higher level in tissue and serum in sarcoidosis
α-1-antitrypsin (BALF)	Cytokine associated; downregulated only in patients without LS; associated with spontaneous resolution
Protocadherin-2 precursor (BALF)	Cell adhesion; upregulated in sarcoidosis across all studied phenotypes
Chitotriosidase	Monocyte-macrophage origin; disease progression
Tenascin-C (BALF)	Fibrosis and ECM associated; levels correlated with infiltrates on chest radiographs in sarcoidosis
IL-17RC	Lymphocyte associated; elevated expression in retinal tissues
TGF-β1	Fibrosis and ECM related; associated with pulmonary fibrosis

Abbreviations: ECM, extracellular matrix; LS, Lofgren syndrome.

fungal infections, and Gaucher disease.[12,15,16] Moreover, there is no evidence that ACE levels significantly differ between active and inactive sarcoidosis[13] and do not reliably correlate with the severity of disease.[17] Serum concentrations at diagnosis were noted to be significantly lower in acute sarcoidosis and in Löfgren syndrome.[18] In addition, ACE concentration and activity are influenced by genetic polymorphisms with enzymatic activity significantly higher in individuals with the DD genotype than in individuals with the II genotype.[16,19,20] The utility of ACE as a biomarker in the diagnosis of sarcoidosis remains limited, although future studies using conformational fingerprinting of ACE may yield better specificity.[21] Although ACE is the prototypic sarcoid biomarker, similar conclusions are made regarding other soluble biomarkers outlined in later discussion.

Serum Amyloid A

Serum amyloid A (SAA) is an acute phase protein produced in the liver and upregulated by monocyte- and macrophage-derived cytokines.[22] SAA levels were significantly higher in sarcoidosis patients than in healthy controls[10,23,24] and significantly higher in sarcoidosis patients with active disease.[13] However, similar to ACE, this biomarker suffers from low specificity, although SAA levels may be more useful during follow-up because SAA levels are less sensitive to immunosuppressive drugs, such as corticosteroids. Cytokines such as tumor necrosis factor (TNF-α, TNF-β) play a major role in granuloma formation and are released in greater quantities from alveolar macrophages obtained from sarcoidosis patients.[25]

Lysozyme

Lysozyme is an enzyme produced by macrophages to degrade bacteria and is elevated in numerous inflammatory conditions, including sarcoidosis. Lysozyme historically has been associated with extrapulmonary sarcoidosis, particularly uveitis,[26] and in a recent study was more sensitive than ACE.[27] Serum chitotriosidase concentrations were significantly higher in advanced (stage 3) sarcoidosis compared with healthy controls, directly correlated with ACE levels, and were highest in those with persistent disease on therapy.[27]

SOLUBLE BIOMARKERS ASSOCIATED WITH LYMPHOCYTE ORIGIN
Soluble Interleukin-2 Receptor

Soluble interleukin-2 receptor (sIL-2R) levels shed from lymphocytes are increased in active sarcoidosis and, similar to ACE levels, may predict response to therapy.[16] Elevated levels have been correlated with parenchymal infiltration and lung function.[28,29] Similarly, persistently elevated sIL-2R may suggest extrapulmonary manifestations of sarcoidosis.[13,25,30] Interleukin-17 (IL-17), an interleukin important in mucosal immunity and autoimmunity, is increased in patients with ocular sarcoidosis[31] and in the BAL fluid of patients with Lofgren syndrome.

BIOMARKERS ASSOCIATED WITH FIBROSIS AND EXTRACELLULAR MATRIX
Tenascin-C

Tenascin-C, an extracellular matrix molecule expressed during wound healing in various tissues, is increased in granulomatous sarcoidosis[30] and in BALF in patients with parenchymal infiltration on chest radiographs.[31] Transforming growth factor (TGF-β1) is associated with tissue healing and recruits fibroblasts and myofibroblasts to the matrix, and overexpression of TGF-β1 fibrosis can occur. Significantly higher levels of TGF-β1 and ACE were reported in sarcoidosis patients.[12]

Measurement of biomarkers to diagnose and predict remitting or progressive disease remains promissory and relevant in the management of sarcoidosis. Despite a rich history and intense study, however, it is clear that no single soluble biomarker has proven to be sufficiently sensitive and specific to be recommended for widespread clinical use.

EMERGING STRATEGIES FOR BIOMARKER DEVELOPMENT

Recent advances in genome-wide expression profiling techniques, such as gene expression microarray and RNA sequencing, provide opportunities to discover novel disease mechanisms. These high-throughput approaches have been applied to diseases of unknown cause to help understand disease pathogenesis,[32–34] including identification of disease-associated candidate genes with diagnostic and prognostic applications.[35–38]

SARCOIDOSIS BIOMARKERS IDENTIFIED BY EXPRESSION PROFILING IN LUNG TISSUES

In a targeted approach using primers to well-established sarcoid inflammatory pathways, Christophi and coworkers[39] isolated RNA from paraffin-embedded samples and compared sarcoid granulomas (mostly lymph nodes) of gene expression to granulomas of other causes (fungal granulomas from lung and foreign body granulomas from skin). Interestingly, T-bet mRNA expression was the only marker significantly greater in sarcoid granulomas than both suture granulomas and fungal granulomas. Expression of cyclo-oxygenase-2, interferon-γ, and interferon regulatory factor-1 was significantly higher in sarcoid granulomas than suture granulomas. IL-13 was more highly expressed in fungal granulomas than in suture granulomas, but not significantly different from sarcoid granulomas. In a more comprehensive study to identify the genes contributing to inflammation and lung remodeling in patients with pulmonary sarcoidosis, Crouser and colleagues[40] compared the gene expression pattern between normal lung tissues (n = 6) and tissues obtained from untreated patients with pulmonary sarcoidosis (n = 6), using Affymetrix Human Genome U133 Plus 2.0 Array (Gene Expression Omnibus [GEO] Accession Number: GSE16538). This whole-transcriptome expression analysis of lung tissue identified interacting gene networks that engage in the maintenance of granulomatous inflammation of the lung and associated lung damage.[40] As expected, many of the genes identified in the most overrepresented network are associated with Th1-type immune responses, such as STAT1, CCL5, IL7, and IL15.[40] Furthermore, the expression of 2 genes regulating macrophage-derived proteases, matrix metallopeptidase 12 (MMP12) and ADAM-like, decysin 1 (ADAMDEC1), was dramatically upregulated in sarcoidosis lung tissues.[40] These findings were validated in an independent series of patients with sarcoidosis, wherein MMP12 and ADAMDEC1 gene/protein expression in BALF correlated with disease severity.[40] Therefore, Crouser and colleagues[40] suggested that MMP12 and ADAMDEC1 are potential mediators of lung damage or remodeling and may serve as biomarkers of pulmonary sarcoidosis.

Most patients with pulmonary sarcoidosis recover spontaneously, whereas a significant number of patients exhibit progressive disease leading to varying degrees of pulmonary fibrosis.[1,41,42] To understand the molecular basis of fibrotic progression in pulmonary sarcoidosis, Lockstone and colleagues[43] examined the gene expression pattern in transbronchial biopsies of granulomatous areas in lung of patients with self-limiting sarcoidosis and patients with progressive-fibrotic sarcoidosis, using Affymetrix Human Gene 1.0 ST Array (GEO Accession Number: GSE19976). In total, 334 genes were found to be differentially expressed between self-limiting and progressive-fibrotic sarcoidosis. Gene Set Enrichment Analysis showed that the gene upregulated in lung samples obtained from patients with progressive-fibrotic sarcoidosis comprised predominantly the genes involved in host defense and immune responses.[43] In addition, genes overexpressed in patients exhibiting progressive-fibrotic sarcoidosis are also significantly enriched for genes upregulated in hypersensitivity pneumonitis, another granulomatous lung disease.[43] Lockstone and colleagues[43] suggested that the gene expression profiling in transbronchial lung biopsy samples can be used for prognostic purposes in pulmonary sarcoidosis.

GENE SIGNATURES IN BLOOD SERVE AS POTENTIAL DIAGNOSTIC TOOL FOR SARCOIDOSIS

The above-cited studies suggest that gene expression profiling in lung tissues displays potential diagnostic and prognostic power in sarcoidosis. However, development of less-invasive biomarkers that predict clinical course or sarcoidosis disease status remains an urgent need.[44] To determine whether gene expression profiling of blood elements reflects inflammatory pathways in the lung of sarcoidosis patients, Koth and colleagues[45] analyzed the transcriptomic gene expression data from whole blood of sarcoidosis patients enrolled at University of California, San Francisco (UCSF cohort), using Affymetrix Human Genome U133 Plus 2.0 Array (GEO Accession Number: GSE19314) and built a machine-learning algorithm-based classifier using the UCSF microarray data, which distinguished sarcoidosis patients from healthy controls in an external validation cohort with 92% sensitivity and 92% specificity.[45] To understand how whole blood gene expression patterns relate to lung granulomatous tissues, differentially expressed genes of sarcoidosis in blood (USCF dataset) were compared with lung tissue (dataset generated by Crouser and colleagues[40]). Gene expression profiles induced in blood were found to significantly overlap with those in lung biopsies[45] with concordantly dysregulated genes identified as critical transcriptional regulators in interferon signaling pathways.[45] These investigators conclude that the gene expression signature identified in blood provides a highly useful, noninvasive method to assess inflammatory activities in sarcoidosis.

Recently, the authors analyzed genome-wide gene expression in peripheral blood mononuclear cells (PBMCs) in sarcoidosis patients enrolled from the Chicago area (Chicago cohort), using Affymetrix Human Exon 1.0 ST Array (GEO Accession Number: GSE37912).[46] A 20-gene signature was identified that distinguishes uncomplicated sarcoidosis from complicated sarcoidosis defined as progressive lung sarcoidosis with fibrosis, or extrapulmonary manifestations such as cardiac sarcoidosis and neurosarcoidosis. The expression levels of the genes within 20-gene signature showed a pattern of an additive model between uncomplicated and complicated sarcoidosis, that is, when the signature gene is upregulated, patients with complicated sarcoidosis exhibited higher expression levels than patients with uncomplicated sarcoidosis. Conversely, complicated sarcoidosis cases exhibit lower expression levels than patients with uncomplicated sarcoidosis when the signature gene is downregulated.[46] This gene signature exhibited a substantial predictive accuracy when classifying sarcoidosis patients from healthy controls in 2 independent external cohorts. Additional validation strategies included significant genetic association of single-nucleotide polymorphisms (SNPs) in signature genes with sarcoidosis susceptibility and severity.[46]

The authors have evaluated the performance of their blood gene signature (Zhou and colleagues, Chicago signature), the signature developed by Koth and colleagues[45] (UCSF signature), and an independent validation dataset from Oregon Health Sciences University (Oregon cohort; GEO Accession Number: GSE18781),[47] in which genome-wide gene expression data in PBMC are available for 25 healthy controls and 12 sarcoidosis patients. The predictive power of the top 20 discriminative genes proposed by Koth and colleagues was compared with that of the 20-gene signature proposed by Zhou and colleagues (**Table 2**). Despite the absence of genes shared by these 2 gene sets, the principal component analysis (PCA) indicated that both the Chicago and the UCSF signatures significantly distinguish patients with sarcoidosis from healthy controls in the Oregon cohort (**Fig. 1**A, B). In order to systematically compare these 2 signatures, a classification score was assigned to each subject based on the first principal component of the given signature.[48] The authors found that the classification score based on both signatures distinguishes sarcoidosis patients from healthy controls with good accuracy: the areas under the receiver operating characteristic (ROC) curve (AUC) were 0.957 and 0.963 for the Chicago and UCSF signature, respectively (see **Fig. 1**C). Significant differences between the AUCs of both signatures were not detected (DeLong's Test: $P = .843$).

A controversial computational study[48] suggested that most published gene signatures failed to perform significantly better than gene sets of identical size that were randomly selected from human genome. To address this issue in the

authors' study, they conducted a resampling test and obtained 10,000 random gene signatures by randomly selecting 20 genes from human genome (the same size as the Chicago and UCSF signatures) and calculated the AUC for each random gene signature. The alternative hypothesis was that the AUCs of the Chicago and UCSF signatures should be more positive than expected by chance if the predictive power of both signatures was significantly better than the random gene sets. The authors' analysis indicates that for both signatures, the null hypothesis that the predictive power is by chance could be rejected. The AUC of both signatures is significantly larger than that of random gene signatures (right-tailed: $P = .0005$ for the Chicago signature; $P = .0003$ for the UCSF signature) (see **Fig. 1**D). However, it should also be noted that the AUC is larger than 0.8 for most random gene signatures (see **Fig. 1**D). Therefore, the performance of a signature to identify gene signatures for a given disease cannot be measured by the prediction accuracy (eg, AUC) as many randomly generated gene signatures could also classify subjects with a fairly low error rate (indicated in **Fig. 1**D). In light of this finding, the authors suggest that the resampling test should be a standard procedure when generating biomarkers or molecular signatures for specific human disease. Prediction accuracy or nominal P values does not address the appropriate statistical question as to whether a given set of genes is related to disease and more related to disease than random gene sets.[48]

DISTINGUISHING PULMONARY SARCOIDOSIS FROM TUBERCULOSIS BY BLOOD GENE EXPRESSION PROFILING

Although the cause of sarcoidosis remains unclear, there has long been an implicated linkage to mycobacterial and propionibacterial organisms,[49–54] although a consensus on the nature of a microbial pathogenesis in sarcoidosis and environmental factors (eg, mold/mildew exposure)[15] has not yet been reached. Koth and colleagues[45] pointed out the significant overlap in gene expression profiles between sarcoidosis and tuberculosis due to the histologic similarities (eg, interferon signaling-related genes). Similar observations were reported by 2 independent groups.[55,56] However, blood transcriptional heterogeneity between sarcoidosis and tuberculosis has been explored. For example, Maertzdorf and colleagues[55] analyzed the difference in PBMC gene expression between sarcoidosis and tuberculosis, using Agilent-014850 Whole Human Genome Microarray

Table 2
The Chicago and University of California, San Francisco signatures

Cohort	Gene Symbol	Gene Title	D
Chicago	HBEGF	Heparin-binding EGF-like growth factor	↑
	SAP30	Sin3A-associated protein, 30 kDa	↑
	APOBEC3D	Apolipoprotein B mRNA editing enzyme, catalytic polypeptide-like 3D	↓
	CRIP1	Cysteine-rich protein 1 (intestinal)	↓
	CX3CR1	Chemokine (C-X3-C motif) receptor 1	↓
	FITM2	Fat storage–inducing transmembrane protein 2	↓
	FKBP1A	FK506 binding protein 1A, 12 kDa	↓
	KIAA1147	KIAA1147	↓
	KLRB1	Killer cell lectin-like receptor subfamily B, member 1	↓
	LOC100132356	Hypothetical protein LOC100132356	↓
	LOC100287290	Cytokine receptor CRL2	↓
	MEI1	Meiosis inhibitor 1	↓
	NOG	Noggin	↓
	RBM12B	RNA binding motif protein 12B	↓
	SERTAD1	SERTA domain containing 1	↓
	SESN3	Sestrin 3	↓
	TSHZ2	Teashirt zinc finger homeobox 2	↓
	ZNF540	Zinc finger protein 540	↓
	ZNF614	Zinc finger protein 614	↓
	ZNF671	Zinc finger protein 671	↓
UCSF	ATF3	Activating transcription factor 3	↑
	CEACAM1	Carcinoembryonic antigen-related cell adhesion molecule 1	↑
	DHRS9	Dehydrogenase/reductase member 9	↑
	GBP2	Guanylate binding protein 2, interferon-inducible	↑
	IRF1	Interferon regulatory factor 1	↑
	STX11	Syntaxin 11	↑
	TAP1	Transporter 1, ATP-binding cassette, subfamily B (MDR/TAP)	↑
	CD27	CD27 molecule	↓
	CD3G	CD3g molecule, γ (CD3-TCR complex)	↓
	CHIC1	Cysteine-rich hydrophobic domain 1	↓
	GIMAP5	GTPase, IMAP family member 5	↓
	IL7R	Interleukin 7 receptor	↓
	KCNA3	Potassium voltage-gated channel, shaker-related subfamily, member 3	↓
	LRRN3	Leucine-rich repeat neuronal 3	↓
	PAQR8	Progestin and adipoQ receptor family member VIII	↓
	TTC3	Tetratricopeptide repeat domain 3	↓
	XPO4	Exportin 4	↓
	ZNF512	Zinc finger protein 512	↓
	ZNF662	Zinc finger protein 662	↓
	ZNF709	Zinc finger protein 709	↓

Note: "D" stands for the direction of dysregulation. "↑" indicates upregulation in sarcoidosis, whereas "↓" means downregulation in sarcoidosis.

and found that the gene expression profiles of sarcoidosis showed an enrichment of downregulated genes involved in mitochondrial oxidative phosphorylation and translational activity compared with tuberculosis patients. Furthermore, sarcoidosis patients displayed significantly lower expression levels of genes related to antimicrobial defense responses.[55] Bloom and colleagues[56] compared the transcriptional profiles in whole blood between sarcoidosis and tuberculosis, using Illumina HumanHT-12 V4.0 expression BeadChip and identified a gene signature consisting of 144 transcripts that showed good sensitivity and specificity in all 3 independent cohorts from their own study (training, test, and validation sets)[56] and an external cohort from the study by Maertzdorf and colleagues.[55] However, few overlapping transcripts existed between the studies of Bloom and colleagues[56] and Maertzdorf and colleagues.

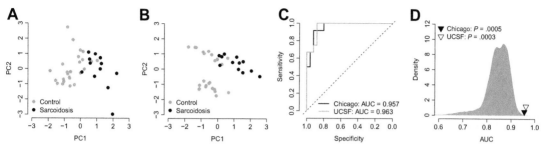

Fig. 1. Performance comparison between the Chicago and UCSF gene signatures in the Oregon cohort. (*A*) PCA on the expression of the Chicago signature. PC1: the first principal component; PC2: the second principal component. (*B*) PCA on the expression of the UCSF signature. PC1: the first principal component; PC2: the second principal component. (*C*) The ROC curves of the Chicago and UCSF signatures in classifying the subjects in the Oregon cohorts. (*D*) Superior predictive power of the 17-gene signature compared with random gene set. The gray area shows the distribution of the AUC for the 10,000 resampled gene signatures (with the identical size as the Chicago and UCSF signatures) randomly picked up from human genome. The solid triangle stands for the AUC of the Chicago signature and the empty triangle denotes the AUC of the UCSF signature. Right-tailed *P* values of the sampling distribution were calculated.

HIGH-THROUGHPUT GENETIC STUDIES TO IDENTIFY NOVEL CANDIDATE GENES OF SARCOIDOSIS

Complex diseases such as sarcoidosis are likely influenced by multiple environmental factors and genetic variation. Previous studies based on a priori assumptions from clinical observations have suggested that the susceptibility to sarcoidosis is partially affected by the genetic variation in the genes and pathways related to granuloma formation and immune response, such as HLA class I and class II genes,[1,2,57,58] *IL1A* (interleukin 1α),[59] *IFNG* (interferon γ),[60] *NRAMP1* (natural resistance associated macrophage protein),[61] *IL18* (interleukin 18),[58] and *CFTR* (cystic fibrosis transmembrane regulator).[62,63] The heterogeneity of sarcoidosis in clinical course and development of organ involvement[1,2] suggest that an individual patient's genetic makeup may interact with various genetic and nongenetic factors to present certain clinical manifestations. High-throughput techniques such as whole-genome genotyping array and next-generation sequencing technologies allow for interrogation of the entire human genome with a high resolution for common genetic variants associated with sarcoidosis patients as well as for those genetic markers potentially associated with complicated sarcoidosis by carefully defining the sarcoidosis subphenotypes. These high-throughput techniques significantly expand the coverage and resolution of the human genome compared with several previously published genetic studies using microsatellite markers for identifying sarcoidosis susceptibility loci.[64,65] More importantly,

whole-genome screening for genetic variants associated with sarcoidosis will aid identification of novel candidate genes implicated in sarcoidosis pathology, which potentially serve as biomarkers in this disease.[66]

The first genome-wide association study (GWAS) in sarcoidosis was conducted by Hofmann and colleagues,[67] using Affymetrix Genome-Wide Human SNP Array 5.0 in a predominant German population. This study identified a nonsynonymous SNP, rs1049550, residing in the first of 4 annexin core domains within the gene *ANXA11* (annexin A11), which was associated with sarcoidosis susceptibility,[67] a finding confirmed in an independent case-control study in Czech patients[68] and in African and European Americans.[69,70] In a separate GWAS conducted by Hofmann and colleagues,[70] a nonsynonymous SNP, rs1040461, in gene *RAB23* (RAB23, member RAS oncogene family), was associated with sarcoidosis in a German population with this association replicated in African Americans but not in European Americans. More recently, a sarcoidosis GWAS in both African and European Americans, using Illumina HumanOmni1-Quad array,[70] identified a novel sarcoidosis-associated SNP, rs715299, within the introduction region of the gene *NOTCH4* (notch 4) in African Americans but not in European Americans.[70] The locus of this SNP is close to several MHC class II genes known to be associated with sarcoidosis[71,72] and within the region of high-linkage disequilibrium.[73] Using stepwise conditional association analyses, it was confirmed that the observed signal within *NOTCH4* is independent of the SNPs within the MHC class II genes.[70]

SUMMARY

Sarcoidosis is a challenging disease of undefined cause and heterogeneous clinical course. Although there has been significant progress over the past years, significant and vexing questions remain unsolved. Relevant and promissory approaches have been developed to identify potential blood transcripts and genomic signatures to facilitate diagnosis and predict disease course. Better understanding of environmental factors and molecular approaches such as profiling whole genome gene expression could provide an opportunity to explore genome-based biomarkers associated with sarcoidosis and advance precision medicine into clinical practice.

REFERENCES

1. Iannuzzi MC, Rybicki BA, Teirstein AS. Sarcoidosis. N Engl J Med 2007;357(21):2153–65.
2. Newman LS, Rose CS, Maier LA. Sarcoidosis. N Engl J Med 1997;336(17):1224–34.
3. Byun CW, Yang SN, Yoon JS, et al. Lofgren's syndrome-acute onset sarcoidosis and polyarthralgia: a case report. Ann Rehabil Med 2013;37(2): 295–9.
4. Statement on sarcoidosis. Joint Statement of the American Thoracic Society (ATS), the European Respiratory Society (ERS) and the World Association of Sarcoidosis and Other Granulomatous disorders (WASOG) adopted by the ATS Board of Directors and by the ERS Executive Committee, February 1999. Am J Respir Crit Care Med 1999; 160(2):736–55.
5. Nunes H, Bouvry D, Soler P, et al. Sarcoidosis. Orphanet J Rare Dis 2007;2:46.
6. What is sarcoidosis? Available at: https://www.nhlbi. nih.gov/health/health-topics/topics/sarc/. Accessed April 3, 2015.
7. Sweiss NJ, Patterson K, Sawaqed R, et al. Rheumatologic manifestations of sarcoidosis. Semin Respir Crit Care Med 2010;31(4):463–73.
8. Drent M, Cremers JP, Jansen TL. Pulmonology meets rheumatology in sarcoidosis: a review on the therapeutic approach. Curr Opin Rheumatol 2014;26(3):276–84.
9. Rybicki BA, Major M, Popovich J Jr, et al. Racial differences in sarcoidosis incidence: a 5-year study in a health maintenance organization. Am J Epidemiol 1997;145(3):234–41.
10. Bons JA, Drent M, Bouwman FG, et al. Potential biomarkers for diagnosis of sarcoidosis using proteomics in serum. Respir Med 2007;101:1687–95.
11. Rozy A, Czerniawska J, Stepniewska A, et al. Inflammatory markers in the exhaled breath condensate of patients with pulmonary sarcoidosis. J Physiol Pharmacol 2006;57(Suppl 4):335–40.
12. Ahmadzai H, Cameron B, Chui J, et al. Measurement of neopterin, TGF-beta(1) and ACE in the exhaled breath condensate of patients with sarcoidosis. J Breath Res 2013;7(4):046003.
13. Gungor S, Ozseker F, Yalcinsoy M, et al. Conventional markers in determination of activity of sarcoidosis. Int Immunopharmacol 2015;25(1):174–9.
14. Tahmoush AJ, Amir MS, Connor WW, et al. CSF-ACE activity in probable CNS neurosarcoidosis. Sarcoidosis Vasc Diffuse Lung Dis 2002;19(3):191–7.
15. Beneteau-Burnat B, Baudin B. Angiotensin-converting enzyme: clinical applications and laboratory investigations on serum and other biological fluids. Crit Rev Clin Lab Sci 1991;28(5–6):337–56.
16. Baughman R, editor. Sarcoidosis, vol. 210. New York: Taylor and Francis Group; 2006.
17. Baudin B. Angiotensin I-converting enzyme (ACE) for sarcoidosis diagnosis. Pathol Biol (Paris) 2005; 53(3):183–8 [in French].
18. Alia P, Mana J, Capdevila O, et al. Association between ACE gene I/D polymorphism and clinical presentation and prognosis of sarcoidosis. Scand J Clin Lab Invest 2005;65:691–7.
19. Floe A, Hoffmann HJ, Nissen PH, et al. Genotyping increases the yield of angiotensin-converting enzyme in sarcoidosis–a systematic review. Dan Med J 2014;61:A4815.
20. Pietinalho A, Furuya K, Yamaguchi E, et al. The angiotensin-converting enzyme DD gene is associated with poor prognosis in Finnish sarcoidosis patients. Eur Respir J 1999;13(4):723–6.
21. Danilov SM, Balyasnikova IV, Danilova AS, et al. Conformational fingerprinting of the angiotensin I-converting enzyme (ACE). Application in sarcoidosis. J Proteome Res 2010;9(11):5782–93.
22. Salazar A, Pinto X, Mana J. Serum amyloid A and high-density lipoprotein cholesterol: serum markers of inflammation in sarcoidosis and other systemic disorders. Eur J Clin Invest 2001;31(12):1070–7.
23. Bargagli E, Bennett D, Maggiorelli C, et al. Human chitotriosidase: a sensitive biomarker of sarcoidosis. J Clin Immunol 2013;33(1):264–70.
24. Zhang Y, Chen X, Hu Y, et al. Preliminary characterizations of a serum biomarker for sarcoidosis by comparative proteomic approach with tandem-mass spectrometry in ethnic Han Chinese patients. Respir Res 2013;14:18.
25. Bargagli E, Mazzi A, Rottoli P. Markers of inflammation in sarcoidosis: blood, urine, BAL, sputum, and exhaled gas. Clin Chest Med 2008;29(3):445–58.
26. Herbort CP, Rao NA, Mochizuki M. International criteria for the diagnosis of ocular sarcoidosis: results of the first International Workshop on ocular Sarcoidosis (IWOS). Ocul Immunol Inflamm 2009; 17(3):160–9.

27. Febvay C, Kodjikian L, Maucort-Boulch D, et al. Clinical features and diagnostic evaluation of 83 biopsy-proven sarcoid uveitis cases. Br J Ophthalmol 2015. [Epub ahead of print].

28. Miyoshi S, Hamada H, Kadowaki T, et al. Comparative evaluation of serum markers in pulmonary sarcoidosis. Chest 2010;137(6):1391–7.

29. Vorselaars AD, van Moorsel CH, Zanen P, et al. ACE and sIL-2R correlate with lung function improvement in sarcoidosis during methotrexate therapy. Respir Med 2015;109(2):279–85.

30. Grutters JC, Fellrath JM, Mulder L, et al. Serum soluble interleukin-2 receptor measurement in patients with sarcoidosis: a clinical evaluation. Chest 2003; 124(1):186–95.

31. Wu W, Jin M, Wang Y, et al. Overexpression of IL-17RC associated with ocular sarcoidosis. J Transl Med 2014;12:152.

32. Calvano SE, Xiao W, Richards DR, et al. A network-based analysis of systemic inflammation in humans. Nature 2005;437(7061):1032–7.

33. Rolph MS, Sisavanh M, Liu SM, et al. Clues to asthma pathogenesis from microarray expression studies. Pharmacol Ther 2006;109(1–2):284–94.

34. Selman M, Pardo A, Kaminski N. Idiopathic pulmonary fibrosis: aberrant recapitulation of developmental programs? PLoS Med 2008;5(3):e62.

35. Herazo-Maya JD, Noth I, Duncan SR, et al. Peripheral blood mononuclear cell gene expression profiles predict poor outcome in idiopathic pulmonary fibrosis. Sci Transl Med 2013;5(205):205ra136.

36. Zhou T, Wang T, Garcia JG. Expression of nicotinamide phosphoribosyltransferase-influenced genes predicts recurrence-free survival in lung and breast cancers. Sci Rep 2014;4:6107.

37. Desai AA, Zhou T, Ahmad H, et al. A novel molecular signature for elevated tricuspid regurgitation velocity in sickle cell disease. Am J Respir Crit Care Med 2012;186(4):359–68.

38. Pitroda SP, Zhou T, Sweis RF, et al. Tumor endothelial inflammation predicts clinical outcome in diverse human cancers. PLoS One 2012;7(10):e46104.

39. Christophi GP, Caza T, Curtiss C, et al. Gene expression profiles in granuloma tissue reveal novel diagnostic markers in sarcoidosis. Exp Mol Pathol 2014;96(3):393–9.

40. Crouser ED, Culver DA, Knox KS, et al. Gene expression profiling identifies MMP-12 and ADAM-DEC1 as potential pathogenic mediators of pulmonary sarcoidosis. Am J Respir Crit Care Med 2009; 179(10):929–38.

41. Neville E, Walker AN, James DG. Prognostic factors predicting the outcome of sarcoidosis: an analysis of 818 patients. QJM 1983;52(208):525–33.

42. Hillerdal G, Nou E, Osterman K, et al. Sarcoidosis: epidemiology and prognosis. A 15-year European study. Am Rev Respir Dis 1984;130(1):29–32.

43. Lockstone HE, Sanderson S, Kulakova N, et al. Gene set analysis of lung samples provides insight into pathogenesis of progressive, fibrotic pulmonary sarcoidosis. Am J Respir Crit Care Med 2010; 181(12):1367–75.

44. Su R, Li MM, Bhakta NR, et al. Longitudinal analysis of sarcoidosis blood transcriptomic signatures and disease outcomes. Eur Respir J 2014;44(4): 985–93.

45. Koth LL, Solberg OD, Peng JC, et al. Sarcoidosis blood transcriptome reflects lung inflammation and overlaps with tuberculosis. Am J Respir Crit Care Med 2011;184(10):1153–63.

46. Zhou T, Zhang W, Sweiss NJ, et al. Peripheral blood gene expression as a novel genomic biomarker in complicated sarcoidosis. PLoS One 2012;7(9): e44818.

47. Sharma SM, Choi D, Planck SR, et al. Insights in to the pathogenesis of axial spondyloarthropathy based on gene expression profiles. Arthritis Res Ther 2009;11(6):R168.

48. Venet D, Dumont JE, Detours V. Most random gene expression signatures are significantly associated with breast cancer outcome. PLoS Comput Biol 2011;7(10):e1002240.

49. Song Z, Marzilli L, Greenlee BM, et al. Mycobacterial catalase-peroxidase is a tissue antigen and target of the adaptive immune response in systemic sarcoidosis. J Exp Med 2005;201(5):755–67.

50. Gupta D, Agarwal R, Aggarwal AN, et al. Molecular evidence for the role of mycobacteria in sarcoidosis: a meta-analysis. Eur Respir J 2007;30(3):508–16.

51. Drake WP, Dhason MS, Nadaf M, et al. Cellular recognition of Mycobacterium tuberculosis ESAT-6 and KatG peptides in systemic sarcoidosis. Infect Immun 2007;75(1):527–30.

52. Oswald-Richter KA, Beachboard DC, Seeley EH, et al. Dual analysis for mycobacteria and propionibacteria in sarcoidosis BAL. J Clin Immunol 2012; 32(5):1129–40.

53. Ishige I, Usui Y, Takemura T, et al. Quantitative PCR of mycobacterial and propionibacterial DNA in lymph nodes of Japanese patients with sarcoidosis. Lancet 1999;354(9173):120–3.

54. Chen ES, Moller DR. Etiologic role of infectious agents. Semin Respir Crit Care Med 2014;35(3):285–95.

55. Maertzdorf J, Weiner J 3rd, Mollenkopf HJ, et al. Common patterns and disease-related signatures in tuberculosis and sarcoidosis. Proc Natl Acad Sci U S A 2012;109(20):7853–8.

56. Bloom CI, Graham CM, Berry MP, et al. Transcriptional blood signatures distinguish pulmonary tuberculosis, pulmonary sarcoidosis, pneumonias and lung cancers. PLoS One 2013;8(8):e70630.

57. Iannuzzi MC, Rybicki BA. Genetics of sarcoidosis: candidate genes and genome scans. Proc Am Thorac Soc 2007;4(1):108–16.

58. Kelly DM, Greene CM, Meachery G, et al. Endotoxin up-regulates interleukin-18: potential role for gram-negative colonization in sarcoidosis. Am J Respir Crit Care Med 2005;172(10):1299–307.

59. Hutyrova B, Pantelidis P, Drabek J, et al. Interleukin-1 gene cluster polymorphisms in sarcoidosis and idiopathic pulmonary fibrosis. Am J Respir Crit Care Med 2002;165(2):148–51.

60. Akahoshi M, Ishihara M, Remus N, et al. Association between IFNA genotype and the risk of sarcoidosis. Hum Genet 2004;114(5):503–9.

61. Maliarik MJ, Chen KM, Sheffer RG, et al. The natural resistance-associated macrophage protein gene in African Americans with sarcoidosis. Am J Respir Cell Mol Biol 2000;22(6):672–5.

62. Bombieri C, Luisetti M, Belpinati F, et al. Increased frequency of CFTR gene mutations in sarcoidosis: a case/control association study. Eur J Hum Genet 2000;8(9):717–20.

63. Schurmann M, Albrecht M, Schwinger E, et al. CFTR gene mutations in sarcoidosis. Eur J Hum Genet 2002;10(11):729–32.

64. Iannuzzi MC, Iyengar SK, Gray-McGuire C, et al. Genome-wide search for sarcoidosis susceptibility genes in African Americans. Genes Immun 2005;6(6):509–18.

65. Schurmann M, Reichel P, Muller-Myhsok B, et al. Results from a genome-wide search for predisposing genes in sarcoidosis. Am J Respir Crit Care Med 2001;164(5):840–6.

66. Rybicki BA, Sinha R, Iyengar S, et al. Genetic linkage analysis of sarcoidosis phenotypes: the sarcoidosis genetic analysis (SAGA) study. Genes Immun 2007;8(5):379–86.

67. Hofmann S, Franke A, Fischer A, et al. Genome-wide association study identifies ANXA11 as a new susceptibility locus for sarcoidosis. Nat Genet 2008;40(9):1103–6.

68. Mrazek F, Stahelova A, Kriegova E, et al. Functional variant ANXA11 R230C: true marker of protection and candidate disease modifier in sarcoidosis. Genes Immun 2011;12(6):490–4.

69. Levin AM, Iannuzzi MC, Montgomery CG, et al. Association of ANXA11 genetic variation with sarcoidosis in African Americans and European Americans. Genes Immun 2013;14(1):13–8.

70. Adrianto I, Lin CP, Hale JJ, et al. Genome-wide association study of African and European Americans implicates multiple shared and ethnic specific loci in sarcoidosis susceptibility. PLoS One 2012;7(8):e43907.

71. Rossman MD, Thompson B, Frederick M, et al. HLA-DRB1*1101: a significant risk factor for sarcoidosis in blacks and whites. Am J Hum Genet 2003;73(4):720–35.

72. Grunewald J, Eklund A, Olerup O. Human leukocyte antigen class I alleles and the disease course in sarcoidosis patients. Am J Respir Crit Care Med 2004;169(6):696–702.

73. Miretti MM, Walsh EC, Ke X, et al. A high-resolution linkage-disequilibrium map of the human major histocompatibility complex and first generation of tag single-nucleotide polymorphisms. Am J Hum Genet 2005;76(4):634–46.

Pulmonary Sarcoidosis

Dominique Valeyre, MD[a,b],*, Jean-François Bernaudin, MD, PhD[c],
Florence Jeny, MD[a,b], Boris Duchemann, MD[b], Olivia Freynet, MD[b], Carole Planès, MD, PhD[a,d],
Marianne Kambouchner, MD[e], Hilario Nunes, MD, PhD[a,b]

KEYWORDS

- Sarcoidosis • Lung • Pathology • Pulmonary function • Evolution

KEY POINTS

- Modes of onset of pulmonary sarcoidosis are various and often unspecific, leading to diagnosis delay.
- Noncaseating granulomas are shown at a high rate through bronchial flexible endoscopy and represent an important element for confirming diagnosis in the context of typical clinical-radiographic presentation with bilateral hilar lymphadenopathy or micronodular lesions with typical distribution along lymphatic vessels.
- Monitoring evolution has to be scheduled every 3 to 6 months with clinical evaluation, chest radiography, and pulmonary function tests.
- The evolution of pulmonary sarcoidosis may be variable, with different evolution patterns from rapid spontaneous recovery to progressive inexorable respiratory insufficiency that is insensitive to treatments.

INTRODUCTION

Sarcoidosis is a systemic disease affecting the lung in almost all cases.[1–3] Whatever the various revealing symptoms, the evidence of abnormal chest radiography is usually a key step for considering diagnosis.[4,5] Bronchial flexible endoscopy allows typical granulomas to be obtained at a high rate.[6–10] The lung is investigated through imaging; pulmonary function; and, when required, 6-minute walk test (6MWT), cardiopulmonary exercise testing, or right heart catheterization.[5,10–13] The impact of pulmonary sarcoidosis may be benign or severe. The evolution of pulmonary sarcoidosis may be variable from rapid spontaneous recovery to progressive inexorable respiratory insufficiency insensitive to treatments.[14,15]

This article focuses on lung disorders, modes of onset, some investigations (especially lung function and bronchoalveolar lavage [BAL]), the prognosis, and the evolution. It does not address pathogenesis, diagnosis of sarcoidosis, chest imaging, severe manifestations, pulmonary hypertension, or treatment, which are also discussed in this issue.

PATHOLOGY

Pulmonary sarcoidosis is a granulomatous interstitial pneumonia, a group of diseases that includes a variety of infectious and noninfectious settings.[16] Observation of the characteristic noncaseating granuloma is essential for the diagnosis of sarcoidosis. Sarcoid granulomas are well formed and

Disclosures: None.
[a] EA2363, University Paris 13, COMUE Sorbonne-Paris-Cité, 74 rue Marcel Cachin, Bobigny 93009, France; [b] Assistance Publique Hôpitaux de Paris, Pulmonary Department, Avicenne University Hospital, 125 rue de Stalingrad, Bobigny 93009, France; [c] Assistance Publique Hôpitaux de Paris, Pathology Department, Tenon University Hospital, 4 rue de la Chine, Paris 75020, France; [d] Assistance Publique Hôpitaux de Paris, Physiology Department, Avicenne University Hospital, 125 rue de Stalingrad, Bobigny 93009, France; [e] Assistance Publique Hôpitaux de Paris, Pathology Department, Avicenne University Hospital, 125 rue de Stalingrad, Bobigny 93009, France
* Corresponding author. Service de Pneumologie, Hôpital Avicenne, 125 rue de Stalingrad, Bobigny 93009, France.
E-mail address: dominique.valeyre@avc.aphp.fr

consist of a compact core of macrophages/mononuclear phagocytes converted into epithelioid cells and giant cells[17,18] (**Fig. 1**A, B). Epithelioid cells are metabolically active cells, particularly in the synthesis of angiotensin-converting enzyme and 1α-25(OH)$_2$ vitamin D (calcitriol).[19–21] Epithelioid cells are closely associated with CD4$^+$ T lymphocytes, whereas CD8 lymphocytes, CD4$^+$ FOXP3$^+$ T$_{reg}$, Th17 cells, B lymphocytes, as well as immunoglobulin (Ig) A–producing plasma cells are present in the peripheral area.[22–24] In contrast with other granulomatous interstitial pneumonias, sarcoidosis shows a particularly florid proliferation of granulomas with a trend to coalesce.[18] Sarcoid granulomas occasionally show a focal central coagulative necrosis. Collections of granulomas

may form macroscopically small white nodules (micronodules) or large masses (macronodules) with the lung in between relatively spared.[25] The topographic predilection of granulomas for lymphatic routes (collecting lymphatics in pleural interstitium, interlobular septa, and bronchovascular interstitium, as well as intralobular lymphatics) provides a valuable histopathologic diagnostic criterion for pulmonary sarcoidosis[18,26] (see **Fig. 1**B, C). Such a distribution suggests a critical role of lymphatics in the emergence of these lesions, reinforcing a putative role of airborne particles in the pathogenesis of pulmonary sarcoidosis.[26] In addition to granulomas close to small airways, a peribronchiolitis with a narrowing of the bronchiolar lumen is common (see **Fig. 1**D).

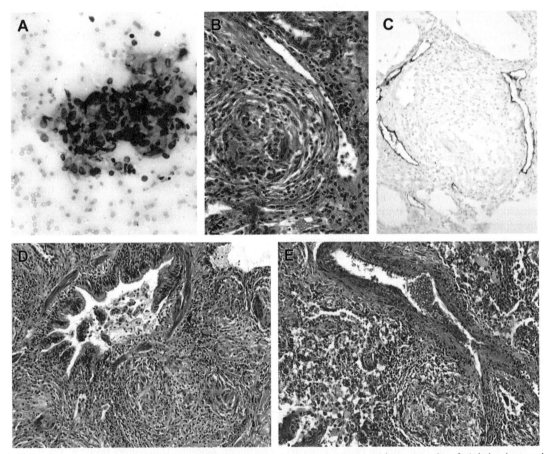

Fig. 1. Examples of the characteristic well-circumscribed noncaseating granulomas made of tightly clustered histiocytes, epithelioid cells, and lymphocytes observed in various situations in pulmonary sarcoidosis. (*A*) A granuloma obtained by fine-needle aspiration using endobronchial ultrasonography of a mediastinal lymph node (May-Grünwald-Giemsa, original magnification × 200). (*B–E*) Images obtained from paraffin-embedded surgical lung biopsies. (*B, C*) The characteristic proximity of granulomas and lymphatics observed in pulmonary sarcoidosis (*B*); lymphatic lumen is observed above rhe granuloma (hematoxylin-eosin-saffron [HES], original magnification × 100). (*C*) The lymphatics wrapping a granuloma appear brown after incubation with the lymphatic marker antipodoplanin D2-40 antibody, original magnification × 100). (*D*) The bronchiolar involvement by granulomas (HES, original magnification × 100). (*E*) The vascular involvement by a granuloma in the wall of a pulmonary artery (HES, original magnification × 100). (*Courtesy of* [*A*] Dr J. Fleury-Feith, APHP, Paris.)

Furthermore a vascular involvement observed in areas of granulomatous inflammation is found in more than half of the patients after open-lung biopsy or autopsy studies.[27–29] Vasculitis is observed at all levels from large elastic pulmonary arteries to venules, and venous involvement is more prominent than arterial involvement[28,30] (see **Fig. 1**E). Necrotizing sarcoid granulomatosis is characterized by an extensive noncaseating granulomatous inflammation with areas of parenchymal necrosis in addition to a marked vasculitis.[17,18] Pleural involvement is less frequent.

Bronchial mucosa is another predilection site for granulomas, thus when macroscopically mucosal abnormalities are noticed, granulomas are observed in 54% to 90% of the biopsies.[31] Bronchi may be typically affected, as in the classic endobronchial sarcoidosis characterized by waxy yellow mucosal nodules with 2-mm to 4-mm diameter. They are more profuse in the lobar and the segmental bronchi and their coalescence may occlude the bronchial lumen, mimicking a malignant mass.[32,33]

The mediastinal lymph nodes' involvement is a key feature of stages I and II sarcoidosis. The nodes show various-sized noncaseating epithelioid granulomas. In the early phase, small epithelioid cell nodules appear in the cortex, thereafter well-demarcated granulomas are observed throughout the lymph node and they may coalesce. In the late phase, they result in fibrosis and hyalinization.[34] However, pathologists must be aware that epithelioid granulomas may be associated with a nonsarcoidosis underlying disease; the so-called sarcoidlike reaction.[34] Needle aspiration of intrathoracic lymph nodes under ultrasonographic guidance, either from the airways (transbronchial needle aspiration) or from the esophagus (transesophageal needle aspiration), is currently the method of choice for mediastinal node sampling in patients with presumed radiographic stages I and II sarcoidosis[8,34–36] (see **Fig. 1**A).

The dynamics of pulmonary lesions in sarcoidosis and their mechanisms are still largely unknown. There is evidence that alveolitis is an early event preceding granulomatous modifications.[37–39] Such a sequence is in keeping with the concept that granulomas result from the presence of activated Th1 cells and macrophages in the context of a lower respiratory tract compartmentalization of an exaggerated immune reaction.[40,41] Thereafter, according to BAL results from stage I to III sarcoidosis, the initial lymphocytic alveolitis with a high CD4/CD8 ratio, does shift to a normalization of the alveolar lymphocytosis.[42] Granulomas either resolve or leave behind fibrotic changes. In addition, a progressive pulmonary fibrosis by interstitial thickening with hyalinized fibrous tissue may be responsible for parenchymal fibrosis and for honeycombing of the lung leading to end-stage sarcoidosis.[18,43,44] After reviewing the charts and lung samples from explants of patients with sarcoidosis who underwent lung transplantation, persistence of granulomas was reported. In addition, evidence of associated interstitial pneumonitis was also frequently observed.[43,44] Patients without interstitial pneumonitis had sarcoidosis for a longer time before transplantation.[43] Moreover, findings consistent with a usual interstitial pneumonia (UIP) pattern (patchy distribution of lesions, honeycombing, fibroblastic foci) were reported by Shigemitsu and colleagues[43] but not by Xu and colleagues,[44] who observed that the honeycombing was predominantly central without the subpleural predominance of UIP. The chronic interstitial pneumonitis observed in end-stage explant lungs of patients with sarcoidosis suggests that chronic inflammation may be a key factor in progressive fibrotic changes in sarcoidosis, as already suggested by gene set analysis of transbronchial biopsies.[45]

EPIDEMIOLOGY

Sarcoidosis is a global disease but with significant variations according to age, gender, race, and geography. In almost all series, the lung is involved in 90% to 95% of cases.[1–3]

Pulmonary sarcoidosis is the disease with the highest incidence and prevalence among chronic interstitial lung diseases (ILDs), representing 23% to 38%, more than idiopathic interstitial pneumonias and ILDs of an identified cause. Figures of incidence and prevalence are variable from study to study because of methodological or epidemiologic factors.[46] Most consistent studies give an incidence between 3.5 and 10.9 per 100,000 person-years in white people. The disease incidence and prevalence are higher in African Americans and in northern Europe populations, whereas they are lower for the Japanese. Both incidence and prevalence are highest in people between 25 and 45 years old, with a possible second peak in women after 50 years of age.[47,48] At presentation, Scadding radiographic stages I and II are frankly predominant before 45 years of age, whereas stages 0, III, and IV are common after 45 years of age.[48] There is an overrepresentation of women compared with men, with an female/male ratio from 1.12 to 1.75.[1,2]

Sarcoidosis is most often sporadic but may be familial in 3.6% to 9% of cases, with an increased risk in siblings of index cases (4-fold to 6-fold)[49] and with a far higher risk (80-fold) in homozygotic twins of index cases.[50] Environmental factors like exposure to musty odors, insecticides, or metal processing industries have been associated with an increased risk of sarcoidosis, whereas being a smoker could decrease this risk.[51] Altogether, these epidemiologic findings suggest the combined influence of genetic and environmental factors in sarcoidosis.

MODES OF ONSET

The modes of onset of pulmonary sarcoidosis are multiple. Pulmonary symptoms (persistent cough, gradually developed dyspnea at exercise, or chest pain) are revealing symptoms in half of all cases; isolated symptoms or symptoms associated with extrapulmonary symptoms are both found in one-quarter of cases (**Table 1**).[2,52,53] In some patients of African American or African ancestry, dyspnea may develop more rapidly to a disabling level. Other initial manifestations include Löfgren syndrome or frequent specific extrapulmonary manifestations (skin or eye symptoms or peripheral lymphadenopathy). Manifestations of Löfgren syndrome may differ between men and women, with erythema nodosum found predominantly in women, whereas ankle periarticular inflammation or arthritis is seen preferentially in men. General symptoms, particularly fatigue (sometimes very severe), may be isolated or not, and in this latter situation may be at the forefront of manifestations. Less frequent extrapulmonary revealing symptoms may also be encountered: splenomegaly; parotitis; diabetes insipidus; or clinical consequences of nervous system, cardiac, renal,

nasosinusal, epididymal, or other localizations. Also, multiple other circumstances may lead to consideration of pulmonary sarcoidosis: symptoms caused by hypercalcemia, nephrolithiasis, hemoptysis, cor pulmonale, or incidental discovery of abnormal blood tests (eg, abnormal liver biologic tests or the fortuitous evidence on a surgical specimen of noncaseating granulomas).

Besides skin or eye manifestations, which lead to a rapid diagnosis, most symptoms, particularly general and pulmonary symptoms, often result at first in misdiagnoses like asthma or bronchitis. Unexplained persistent symptoms do not prompt enough chest radiography, despite its value for guiding the diagnosis.

Patients often have their sarcoidosis diagnosed more than 3 months after their first symptoms and their first visit to a physician, 1 out 4 being diagnosed after 6 months.[52] When there are only pulmonary symptoms, the diagnosis is even more delayed[52] and the intervention of several physicians is required before diagnosis is considered.

In around one-third of patients, the disease is asymptomatic and may be discovered through a fortuitous chest radiograph indicated for any reason. This figure is lower than in earlier series because of the withdrawal of mass radiography.[47,52]

PULMONARY CLINICAL SIGNS AND INVESTIGATIONS

Clinical and radiological findings are extremely variable (**Table 2**).

Physical Examination

Pulmonary physical examination is usually normal. Crackles are heard at presentation in only 4% of

Table 1
Modes of onset of pulmonary sarcoidosis

Modes of Onset	Description	Incidence (%)	References
Pulmonary	Cough, dyspnea, chest pain, wheezing	50 (25 isolated; 25 associated)	2,52
Erythema nodosum/ankle arthritis	—	4–43	1–3,47
Frequent extrapulmonary localizations	Skin/eye/superficial lymphadenopathy	3–37/3–50/2.3–33	1,2
General symptoms	Fatigue, weight loss, fever, night sweats	50–70	2
Rare pulmonary initial manifestations	Hemoptysis	1	2
Fortuitous chest radiography discovery	Trend to decrease because of withdrawal of mass radiography	20–60	2,3,47,53,89

Table 2
Pulmonary investigation at presentation work-up, follow-up visits, or events: computed tomography (CT)

Investigations	Work-up at Presentation	Follow-up Visits	Events
Clinical evaluation	Always	Always	Always
Chest radiography	Always	Always	Always
Thoracic CT	Only in difficult diagnosis or severe pulmonary sarcoidosis	No	When progression is of unclear origin
18FDG-PET	Very rarely	No	Very rarely
Bronchial endoscopy	Most often	No, except for control of severe bronchial lesions under treatment	When progression is of unclear origin
Pulmonary function tests	Always	Always	Always
6MWT	When required	When required	Often
Cardiopulmonary exercise testing	When required	No	Sometimes
Right heart catheterization	Rarely (when pulmonary hypertension is suspected)	For evaluation of therapy	When pulmonary hypertension is suspected or before transplantation listing

Abbreviation: FDG, fluorodeoxyglucose.

cases[2] but among the patients with advanced pulmonary disease about one-quarter present crackles.[54] Finger clubbing is rarely observed at diagnosis (2% of cases).[2] Wheezing may be heard, particularly in severe bronchial involvement.[32] Ankle edema and vena cava syndrome are very uncommon at presentation.

Imaging is discussed in an article by Keijsers, Veltkamp and Grutters,[55] as is bronchoscopy, which is also discussed later in this article.

Besides obtaining granulomas, bronchial flexible endoscopy allows the identification of macroscopic lesions like inflammation; loss of normal angular contours of spurs at the level of bifurcation caused by mucosal thickening; waxy yellow mucosal nodules from 2 to 4 mm in diameter; localized bronchial stenoses, sometimes with a malignant mass appearance, most often at the lobar or segmental level; extrinsic compression caused by lymphadenopathy; or distortion and narrowing secondary to lung fibrosis.[32,56,57]

Bronchoalveolar Lavage

BAL is a safe, minimally invasive procedure, widely performed for 30 years but its relevance for diagnosis of diffuse ILDs is still discussed.[58,59] If its value in diagnosis and follow-up of patients with sarcoidosis is still debated, BAL has to its credit the identification of the CD4+ T-cell lymphocytic alveolitis, which has been a major breakthrough in the approach to the disease pathogenesis.[40,60] Even if alveolar lymphocytosis is not specific, a lymphocytic count greater than 25% after exclusion of infectious causes strongly suggests sarcoidosis, as well as hypersensitivity pneumonitis or drug toxicity (other ILDs that may be associated with an alveolar lymphocytosis include cellular nonspecific pneumonitis, lymphoid interstitial pneumonia, and cryptogenic organized pneumonia).[59] Characteristically, BAL in sarcoidosis displays a moderate (20%–50%) lymphocytosis in 80% of cases and a T-lymphocyte CD4/CD8 ratio higher than 3.5 in 50% of cases.[61] The diagnostic relevance of the CD4/CD8 ratio is controversial and in practice it should be considered if higher than 3.5 (with a specificity of 93%–96% but a sensitivity of 53%–59%). In contrast, a CD4/CD8 ratio in the normal range may suggest an inactive disease.[61] Other parameters of T-lymphocyte analysis, such as a decreased CD103 integrin expression, combining the CD103+ CD4+/CD4+ and the CD4+/CD8+ ratios, have been proposed to add to the specificity but have not been confirmed.[62–64]

In addition, integrated differential analyses of BAL cells have been proposed using either a computer program based on a logistic model[65] or a bayesian analysis,[66] and more recently the integration of HLA-DR(+), CD8+ T cells, and natural killer T cells.[67] However, these methods have not yet been applied in routine practice. Furthermore, an increased neutrophil count in advanced sarcoidosis may denote the presence of pulmonary fibrosis and thus indicate an unfavorable prognosis.[58,61] However, even if BAL is not diagnostically decisive, it still plays a major role in research investigation in sarcoidosis. Recently the proteomic profiling of noncellular components, particularly the intra-alveolar IgG repertoire using protein microarrays, revealed autoimmune targets that may function as autoantigens in sarcoidosis.[68]

Pulmonary Function

Pulmonary function tests are part of the systematic diagnosis work-up at presentation. Reduction of volumes, particularly forced vital capacity (FVC), is the most common finding at spirometry and tends to be more frequent and marked from radiographic stage I to stage IV but with significant overlaps at an individual level. FVC is the simplest and most accurate parameter to reflect the impact of pulmonary sarcoidosis.[13] Airflow obstruction occurs in variable figures according to criteria used. Frank airflow obstruction is mainly observed in stage IV[69,70] or for diverse other conditions from diffuse macroscopic involvement or multiple endobronchial stenosis mainly caused by profuse granulomas, whereas extrinsic bronchial stenosis caused by lymphadenopathy compression is rarely observed.[32,56,57,71] Some degree of bronchial hyperreactivity may also be encountered. Often several mechanisms are combined at the origin of airflow obstruction in the same patient.[56]

Reduction of the diffusing capacity for carbon monoxide (DL_{CO}), and particularly its membrane component, is the most frequent respiratory impairment at function tests and best predicts a widened alveolar-arterial gradient with exercise.[72]

In cases of lung fibrosis, the pulmonary function profile is linked to the computed tomography (CT) pattern, with more airflow reduction in cases of airways distortion and more reduction of volumes and DL_{CO} in patients with honeycombing.[70]

Six-minute Walk Test

The 6MWT is a useful test to assess the functional status of patients with sarcoidosis.[11] Multiple patients from a referral center had reduced 6MWT. Reduced 6MWT is multifactorial and predictive of oxygen desaturation at exercise. Patients with pulmonary hypertension tend to have a lower 6MWT distance but other parameters are also associated with low 6MWT distance, such as St George Respiratory Questionnaire (SGRQ) activity component, reduced FVC, and the fatigue assessment scale.

Cardiopulmonary Exercise Testing

Cardiopulmonary exercise testing[73–75] may be particularly useful to detect impaired gas exchange during exercise in patients with unexplained disabling symptoms despite normal pulmonary function and absence of echocardiographic abnormality. It also helps to decipher dyspnea mechanisms of unclear origin and helps recognize its respiratory, cardiac, or other origin. It remains an excellent tool for assessing the overall disease impact.

PROGNOSTIC FACTORS

Despite a poor interobserver agreement,[76] Scadding radiographic classification remains useful for predicting evolution with a high rate of rapid spontaneous resolution for stages I and II and more chronicity, treatment need, and events for stages III and IV.[77] Some findings are associated with an increased mortality risk, like pulmonary hypertension,[12,30,78] pulmonary fibrosis,[54] and frankly altered pulmonary function.[79,80] Recently a reliable prognosis algorithm based on the composite physiologic index, the main pulmonary diameter/ascending aorta diameter ratio, and the extent of fibrosis at CT has been shown to accurately predict mortality.[81]

EVOLUTION
Modes of Evolution

The evolution is variable, from rapidly self-resolving disease in less than 24 months to long-standing disease with an inexorable progression (**Fig. 2**). Nine evolution patterns have been described in the World Association for Sarcoidosis and Other Granulomatous Disorders Task Force clinical outcome status,[14] whereas 6 have been proposed by Prasse and colleagues.[15] This article schematizes most of the encountered patterns, taking into account the duration of the disease, the need and duration of treatments and the response to them, and the inflammatory and fibrotic components of the disease (see **Fig. 2**). The proportion of patients with each of the evolution patterns depends primarily on the mode of recruitment: primary care setting or referral center.[2,14,47,82]

In primary care settings, most patients are asymptomatic or present few symptoms; are at radiographic stage I or II; and have a disease that spontaneously resolves in less than 5 years without any treatment, most often in less than 2 to 3 years

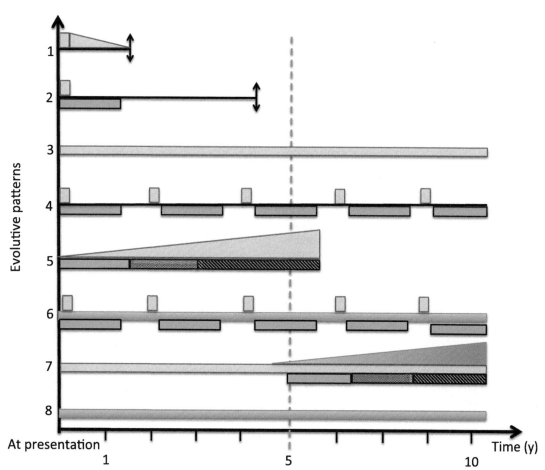

Fig. 2. Various evolution patterns in pulmonary sarcoidosis. Recovery (↕); granulomatous inflammatory lesions (*yellow*); fibrotic lung lesions (*blue*); first-line, second-line, and third-line treatments (*green*). Rapidly spontaneous recovery, evolution pattern 1; rapid recovery after a 1-year course of treatment, evolution pattern 2; light stable disease without a trend to fibrosis and not treated, evolution pattern 3; persistent disease needing prolonged treatment (in 1 or several courses) but without a trend toward any fibrosis, evolution pattern 4; progressive active multidrug-resistant disease, evolution pattern 5; both fibrotic and active lung disease with response of active lesions and without progression of fibrotic lesions under therapy, evolution pattern 6; slowly progressive lung fibrosis insensitive to therapy, evolution pattern 7. Only fibrotic lung disease with no activity, no need for treatment, and further viability, evolution pattern 8.

(see **Fig. 2**: evolutive pattern 1).[2,82] Only a small number of patients progress from one radiographic stage to another.[2] Some patients need a short course of treatment (1 year) and recover before 5 years (see **Fig. 2**: evolutive pattern 2).

By contrast, in referral centers highly specialized in sarcoidosis, many patients present a symptomatic disease with iterative relapses during dose reduction or after withdrawal of treatment (see **Fig. 2**: evolutive pattern 4 or 6 according to the absence or presence of pulmonary fibrosis). In some cases, the disease resists 1 or several treatments (see **Fig. 2**: evolutive pattern 5). Some patients have inexorably progressive fibrosis despite treatment (see **Fig. 2**: evolutive pattern 7). Sometimes, patients have a diagnosis at

a fibrotic stage with no more activity (see **Fig. 2**: evolutive pattern 8).

In most cases, when indicated, a treatment is most often initiated at diagnosis. However, it is sometimes delayed because of a progression of the disease.

Follow-up and Events

The follow-up is scheduled every 3 to 6 months and sometimes quickened by an event; it includes a clinical, radiographic (extent of pulmonary disease), and pulmonary function evaluation including measures of FVC, forced expiratory volume in 1 second, and DL_{CO} (see **Table 2**). The evolution (progression, improvement, or stability) is easy to determine when symptoms, pulmonary involvement, extent at chest radiography, and pulmonary function follow a consistent route. For difficult situations, spirometry might be the most accurate parameter.[13] However, for advanced pulmonary fibrosis with bronchiectasis, respiratory suprainfections may be an alternative explanation for acute worsening in one-half of cases.[83]

An important point is to think of pulmonary hypertension in patients with no clear explanation for dyspnea; a discordant decrease in DL_{CO} far more significant than expected, taking into account pulmonary infiltration extent at radiography; and FVC decrease, an abnormal 6MWT, or suspect echocardiography. In such a context, right heart catheterization confirms pulmonary hypertension and determines whether pulmonary hypertension is secondary to left ventricular dysfunction.[12]

Another potentially severe event is the occurrence of cavitary lesions[84] that predispose to chronic pulmonary aspergillosis,[85] which is a cause of massive hemoptysis.

The occurrence of atypical clinical or radiological signs may prompt the search for an associated disease like pulmonary embolism, lymphoma, or lung carcinoma.[86]

Mortality

In North America and western Europe, pulmonary sarcoidosis is associated with an increased mortality.[87,88] Severe manifestations, particularly pulmonary hypertension, represent a significant underlying cause, especially in African Americans.[78]

SUMMARY

Pulmonary manifestations of sarcoidosis are important because of their high prevalence, their role in guiding and confirming diagnosis, and their impact on the evolution and the treatment of the disease.

REFERENCES

1. Baughman RP, Teirstein AS, Judson MA, et al. Clinical characteristics of patients in a case control study of sarcoidosis. Am J Respir Crit Care Med 2001;164:1885–9.
2. Chappell AG, Cheung WY, Hutchings HA. Sarcoidosis: a long-term follow up study. Sarcoidosis Vasc Diffuse Lung Dis 2000;17:167–73.
3. Siltzbach LE, James DG, Neville E, et al. Course and prognosis of sarcoidosis around the world. Am J Med 1974;57:847–52.
4. Bein ME, Putman CE, McLoud TC, et al. A reevaluation of intrathoracic lymphadenopathy in sarcoidosis. AJR Am J Roentgenol 1978;131:409–15.
5. Nunes H, Uzunhan Y, Gille T, et al. Imaging of sarcoidosis of the airways and lung parenchyma and correlation with lung function. Eur Respir J 2012;40:750–65.
6. Baughman RP, Culver DA, Judson MA. A concise review of pulmonary sarcoidosis. Am J Respir Crit Care Med 2011;183:573–81.
7. Valeyre D, Prasse A, Nunes H, et al. Sarcoidosis. Lancet 2014;383:1155–67.
8. Von Bartheld MB, Dekkers OM, Szlubowski A, et al. Endosonography vs conventional bronchoscopy for the diagnosis of sarcoidosis: the GRANULOMA randomized clinical trial. JAMA 2013;309:2457–64.
9. Plit ML, Havryk AP, Hodgson A, et al. Rapid cytological analysis of endobronchial ultrasound-guided aspirates in sarcoidosis. Eur Respir J 2013;42:1302–8.
10. Valeyre D, Bernaudin J-F, Uzunhan Y, et al. Clinical presentation of sarcoidosis and diagnostic workup. Semin Respir Crit Care Med 2014;35:336–51.
11. Baughman RP, Sparkman BK, Lower EE. Six-minute walk test and health status assessment in sarcoidosis. Chest 2007;132:207–13.
12. Baughman RP, Engel PJ, Taylor L, et al. Survival in sarcoidosis-associated pulmonary hypertension: the importance of hemodynamic evaluation. Chest 2010;138:1078–85.
13. Zappala CJ, Desai SR, Copley SJ, et al. Accuracy of individual variables in the monitoring of long-term change in pulmonary sarcoidosis as judged by serial high-resolution CT scan data. Chest 2014; 145:101–7.
14. Baughman RP, Nagai S, Balter M, et al. Defining the clinical outcome status (COS) in sarcoidosis: results of WASOG Task Force. Sarcoidosis Vasc Diffuse Lung Dis 2011;28:56–64.
15. Prasse A, Katic C, Germann M, et al. Phenotyping sarcoidosis from a pulmonary perspective. Am J Respir Crit Care Med 2008;177:330–6.
16. Cheung OY, Muhm JR, Helmers RA, et al. Surgical pathology of granulomatous interstitial pneumonia. Ann Diagn Pathol 2003;7:127–38.
17. Myers JL, Tazelaar HD. Challenges in pulmonary fibrosis: 6–Problematic granulomatous lung disease. Thorax 2008;63:78–84.
18. Travis W, Colby T, Koss M, et al. Non-neoplastic disorders of the lower respiratory tract. Washington, DC: American Registry of Pathology and the Armed Forces Institute of Pathology; 2002.
19. Soler P, Basset F, Bernaudin JF, et al. Morphology and distribution of the cells of a sarcoid granuloma: ultrastructural study of serial sections. Ann N Y Acad Sci 1976;278:147–60.
20. Silverstein E, Pertschuk LP, Friedland J. Immunofluorescent localization of angiotensin converting enzyme

in epithelioid and giant cells of sarcoidosis granulomas. Proc Natl Acad Sci U S A 1979;76:6646–8.

21. Okabe T, Ishizuka S, Fujisawa M, et al. Sarcoid granulomas metabolize 25-hydroxyvitamin D3 in vitro. Biochem Biophys Res Commun 1984;123:822–30.

22. Miyara M, Amoura Z, Parizot C, et al. The immune paradox of sarcoidosis and regulatory T cells. J Exp Med 2006;203:359–70.

23. Facco M, Cabrelle A, Teramo A, et al. Sarcoidosis is a Th1/Th17 multisystem disorder. Thorax 2011;66: 144–50.

24. Kamphuis LS, van Zelm MC, Lam KH, et al. Perigranuloma localization and abnormal maturation of B cells: emerging key players in sarcoidosis? Am J Respir Crit Care Med 2013;187:406–16.

25. Criado E, Sánchez M, Ramírez J, et al. Pulmonary sarcoidosis: typical and atypical manifestations at high-resolution CT with pathologic correlation. Radiographics 2010;30:1567–86.

26. Kambouchner M, Pirici D, Uhl J-F, et al. Lymphatic and blood microvasculature organisation in pulmonary sarcoid granulomas. Eur Respir J 2011;37: 835–40.

27. Carrington CB. Structure and function in sarcoidosis. Ann N Y Acad Sci 1976;278:265–83.

28. Takemura T, Matsui Y, Saiki S, et al. Pulmonary vascular involvement in sarcoidosis: a report of 40 autopsy cases. Hum Pathol 1992;23:1216–23.

29. Corte TJ, Wells AU, Nicholson AG, et al. Pulmonary hypertension in sarcoidosis: a review. Respirology 2011;16:69–77.

30. Nunes H, Humbert M, Capron F, et al. Pulmonary hypertension associated with sarcoidosis: mechanisms, haemodynamics and prognosis. Thorax 2006;61:68–74.

31. Chapman JT, Mehta AC. Bronchoscopy in sarcoidosis: diagnostic and therapeutic interventions. Curr Opin Pulm Med 2003;9:402–7.

32. Chambellan A, Turbie P, Nunes H, et al. Endoluminal stenosis of proximal bronchi in sarcoidosis: bronchoscopy, function, and evolution. Chest 2005;127: 472–81.

33. Polychronopoulos VS, Prakash UBS. Airway involvement in sarcoidosis. Chest 2009;136:1371–80.

34. Asano S. Granulomatous lymphadenitis. J Clin Exp Hematop 2012;52:1–16.

35. Garwood S, Judson MA, Silvestri G, et al. Endobronchial ultrasound for the diagnosis of pulmonary sarcoidosis. Chest 2007;132:1298–304.

36. Oki M, Saka H, Kitagawa C, et al. Prospective study of endobronchial ultrasound-guided transbronchial needle aspiration of lymph nodes versus transbronchial lung biopsy of lung tissue for diagnosis of sarcoidosis. J Thorac Cardiovasc Surg 2012;143: 1324–9.

37. Keogh BA, Crystal RG. Alveolitis: the key to the interstitial lung disorders. Thorax 1982;37:1–10.

38. Rosen Y, Athanassiades TJ, Moon S, et al. Nongranulomatous interstitial pneumonitis in sarcoidosis. Relationship to development of epithelioid granulomas. Chest 1978;74:122–5.

39. Lacronique J, Bernaudin J-F, Soler P, et al. Alveolitis and granulomas: sequential course in pulmonary sarcoidosis. In: Chretien J, Marsac J, Saltiel JC, editors. Sarcoidosis. Paris: Pergamon Press; 1983. p. 36–42.

40. Crystal RG, Bitterman PB, Rennard SI, et al. Interstitial lung diseases of unknown cause. Disorders characterized by chronic inflammation of the lower respiratory tract (first of two parts). N Engl J Med 1984;310:154–66.

41. Müller-Quernheim J, Prasse A, Zissel G. Pathogenesis of sarcoidosis. Presse Med 2012;41:e275–87.

42. Capelli A, Di Stefano A, Lusuardi M, et al. Increased macrophage inflammatory protein-1alpha and macrophage inflammatory protein-1beta levels in bronchoalveolar lavage fluid of patients affected by different stages of pulmonary sarcoidosis. Am J Respir Crit Care Med 2002;165:236–41.

43. Shigemitsu H, Oblad JM, Sharma OP, et al. Chronic interstitial pneumonitis in end-stage sarcoidosis. Eur Respir J 2010;35:695–7.

44. Xu L, Kligerman S, Burke A. End-stage sarcoid lung disease is distinct from usual interstitial pneumonia. Am J Surg Pathol 2013;37:593–600.

45. Lockstone HE, Sanderson S, Kulakova N, et al. Gene set analysis of lung samples provides insight into pathogenesis of progressive, fibrotic pulmonary sarcoidosis. Am J Respir Crit Care Med 2010;181:1367–75.

46. Reich JM. A critical analysis of sarcoidosis incidence assessment. Multidiscip Respir Med 2013;8:57.

47. Hillerdal G, Nöu E, Osterman K, et al. Sarcoidosis: epidemiology and prognosis. A 15-year European study. Am Rev Respir Dis 1984;130:29–32.

48. Sawahata M, Sugiyama Y, Nakamura Y, et al. Age-related differences in chest radiographic staging of sarcoidosis in Japan. Eur Respir J 2014;43:1810–2.

49. Rybicki BA, Iannuzzi MC, Frederick MM, et al. Familial aggregation of sarcoidosis. A Case-control Etiologic Study of Sarcoidosis (ACCESS). Am J Respir Crit Care Med 2001;164:2085–91.

50. Sverrild A, Backer V, Kyvik KO, et al. Heredity in sarcoidosis: a registry-based twin study. Thorax 2008;63:894–6.

51. Newman LS, Rose CS, Bresnitz EA, et al. A case control etiologic study of sarcoidosis: environmental and occupational risk factors. Am J Respir Crit Care Med 2004;170:1324–30.

52. Judson MA, Thompson BW, Rabin DL, et al. The diagnostic pathway to sarcoidosis. Chest 2003; 123:406–12.

53. Lynch JP, Kazerooni EA, Gay SE. Pulmonary sarcoidosis. Clin Chest Med 1997;18:755–85.

54. Nardi A, Brillet P-Y, Letoumelin P, et al. Stage IV sarcoidosis: comparison of survival with the general

population and causes of death. Eur Respir J 2011; 38:1368–73.

55. Ruth G, Keijsers RG, Veltkamp M, et al. Chest Imaging. Clin Chest Med 2015, in press.

56. Naccache J-M, Lavolé A, Nunes H, et al. High-resolution computed tomographic imaging of airways in sarcoidosis patients with airflow obstruction. J Comput Assist Tomogr 2008;32:905–12.

57. Baughman RP, Lower EE, Tami T. Upper airway. 4: sarcoidosis of the upper respiratory tract (SURT). Thorax 2010;65:181–6.

58. Wells AU. The clinical utility of bronchoalveolar lavage in diffuse parenchymal lung disease. Eur Respir Rev 2010;19:237–41.

59. Meyer KC, Raghu G. Bronchoalveolar lavage for the evaluation of interstitial lung disease: is it clinically useful? Eur Respir J 2011;38:761–9.

60. Grunewald J, Eklund A. Role of CD4+ T cells in sarcoidosis. Proc Am Thorac Soc 2007;4:461–4.

61. Costabel U, Bonella F, Ohshimo S, et al. Diagnostic modalities in sarcoidosis: BAL, EBUS, and PET. Semin Respir Crit Care Med 2010;31:404–8.

62. Kolopp-Sarda MN, Kohler C, De March AK, et al. Discriminative immunophenotype of bronchoalveolar lavage CD4 lymphocytes in sarcoidosis. Lab Invest 2000;80:1065–9.

63. Heron M, Slieker WAT, Zanen P, et al. Evaluation of CD103 as a cellular marker for the diagnosis of pulmonary sarcoidosis. Clin Immunol 2008;126: 338–44.

64. Hyldgaard C, Kaae S, Riddervold M, et al. Value of s-ACE, BAL lymphocytosis, and CD4+/CD8+ and CD103+CD4+/CD4+ T-cell ratios in diagnosis of sarcoidosis. Eur Respir J 2012;39:1037–9.

65. Drent M, van Nierop MA, Gerritsen FA, et al. A computer program using BALF-analysis results as a diagnostic tool in interstitial lung diseases. Am J Respir Crit Care Med 1996;153:736–41.

66. Welker L, Jörres RA, Costabel U, et al. Predictive value of BAL cell differentials in the diagnosis of interstitial lung diseases. Eur Respir J 2004;24: 1000–6.

67. Tøndell A, Rø AD, Åsberg A, et al. Activated CD8(+) T cells and NKT cells in BAL fluid improve diagnostic accuracy in sarcoidosis. Lung 2014;192:133–40.

68. Häggmark A, Hamsten C, Wiklundh E, et al. Proteomic profiling reveals autoimmune targets in sarcoidosis. Am J Respir Crit Care Med 2015;191: 574–83.

69. Hansell DM, Milne DG, Wilsher ML, et al. Pulmonary sarcoidosis: morphologic associations of airflow obstruction at thin-section CT. Radiology 1998;209: 697–704.

70. Abehsera M, Valeyre D, Grenier P, et al. Sarcoidosis with pulmonary fibrosis: CT patterns and correlation with pulmonary function. AJR Am J Roentgenol 2000;174:1751–7.

71. Lavergne F, Clerici C, Sadoun D, et al. Airway obstruction in bronchial sarcoidosis: outcome with treatment. Chest 1999;116:1194–9.

72. Lamberto C, Nunes H, Le Toumelin P, et al. Membrane and capillary blood components of diffusion capacity of the lung for carbon monoxide in pulmonary sarcoidosis: relation to exercise gas exchange. Chest 2004;125:2061–8.

73. Delobbe A, Perrault H, Maitre J, et al. Impaired exercise response in sarcoid patients with normal pulmonary functio. Sarcoidosis Vasc Diffuse Lung Dis 2002;19:148–53.

74. Wallaert B, Talleu C, Wemeau-Stervinou L, et al. Reduction of maximal oxygen uptake in sarcoidosis: relationship with disease severity. Respiration 2011; 82:501–8.

75. Marcellis RGJ, Lenssen AF, de Vries GJ, et al. Is there an added value of cardiopulmonary exercise testing in sarcoidosis patients? Lung 2013;191: 43–52.

76. Baughman RP, Shipley R, Desai S, et al. Changes in chest roentgenogram of sarcoidosis patients during a clinical trial of infliximab therapy: comparison of different methods of evaluation. Chest 2009;136: 526–35.

77. Scadding JG. Prognosis of intrathoracic sarcoidosis in England. A review of 136 cases after five years' observation. Br Med J 1961;2:1165–72.

78. Mirsaeidi M, Machado RF, Schraufnagel D, et al. Racial difference in sarcoidosis mortality in the United States. Chest 2015;147:438–49.

79. Baughman RP, Winget DB, Bowen EH, et al. Predicting respiratory failure in sarcoidosis patients. Sarcoidosis Vasc Diffuse Lung 1997;14:154–8.

80. Viskum K, Vestbo J. Vital prognosis in intrathoracic sarcoidosis with special reference to pulmonary function and radiological stage. Eur Respir J 1993; 6:349–53.

81. Walsh SL, Wells AU, Sverzellati N, et al. An integrated clinicoradiological staging system for pulmonary sarcoidosis: a case-cohort study. Lancet Respir Med 2014;2:123–30.

82. Reich JM, Johnson RE. Course and prognosis of sarcoidosis in a nonreferral setting. Analysis of 86 patients observed for 10 years. Am J Med 1985; 78:61–7.

83. Baughman RP, Lower EE. Frequency of acute worsening events in fibrotic pulmonary sarcoidosis patients. Respir Med 2013;107:2009–13.

84. Hours S, Nunes H, Kambouchner M, et al. Pulmonary cavitary sarcoidosis: clinico-radiologic characteristics and natural history of a rare form of sarcoidosis. Medicine (Baltimore) 2008;87:142–51.

85. Denning DW, Pleuvry A, Cole DC. Global burden of allergic bronchopulmonary aspergillosis with asthma and its complication chronic pulmonary aspergillosis in adults. Med Mycol 2013;51:361–70.

86. Bonifazi M, Bravi F, Gasparini S, et al. Sarcoidosis and cancer risk: systematic review and meta-analysis of observational studies. Chest 2015;147: 778–91.

87. Gribbin J, Hubbard RB, Le Jeune I, et al. Incidence and mortality of idiopathic pulmonary fibrosis and sarcoidosis in the UK. Thorax 2006;61:980–5.

88. Swigris JJ, Olson AL, Huie TJ, et al. Sarcoidosis-related mortality in the United States from 1988 to 2007. Am J Respir Crit Care Med 2011;183:1524–30.

89. Reich JM. Mortality of intrathoracic sarcoidosis in referral vs population-based settings: influence of stage, ethnicity, and corticosteroid therapy. Chest 2002;121:32.

Neurosarcoidosis

Jinny O. Tavee, MD[a],*, Barney J. Stern, MD[b]

KEYWORDS

- Neurosarcoidosis • Meningitis • Cranial neuropathy • Sarcoidosis • Myelopathy

KEY POINTS

- Although the clinical presentation of neurosarcoidosis greatly varies, cranial neuropathy, particularly facial nerve palsy, and aseptic meningitis are the most common manifestations.
- Characteristic gadolinium-enhanced MRI patterns include nodular leptomeningeal enhancement, preferential basilar involvement of the brain, and patchy noncontiguous lesions of the spinal cord spanning ≥3 segments.
- Corticosteroids are the mainstay of treatment of neurosarcoidosis, although other immunosuppressive drugs and biologic agents, such as TNF-α antagonists, are effective in treating severe cases affecting the brain and spinal cord.

INTRODUCTION

Sarcoidosis is a multisystemic granulomatous disorder of unknown cause that leads to neurologic complications in 5% to 10% of cases.[1–4] The actual prevalence may be higher as evidence of subclinical neurologic involvement has been seen in up to 27% of sarcoidosis patients postmortem.[5] Because any portion of the nervous system may be affected, neurosarcoidosis encompasses a broad range of clinical manifestations and is difficult to distinguish from other diseases. However, classic presentations, such as facial nerve palsy, and characteristic diagnostic findings can help guide the clinician toward establishing the diagnosis of neurosarcoidosis and initiating the appropriate treatment regimen.

EPIDEMIOLOGY AND PATHOLOGY

Although less common than thoracic, skin, and lymph node involvement, the neurologic manifestations of sarcoidosis are the presenting symptom in 50% to 70% of neurosarcoidosis cases and often develop within 2 years of systemic disease onset.[6] Sarcoidosis itself has been reported in all ethnic groups, and is most common in northern Europeans and African Americans with an estimated incidence of 15 to 20 and 35 to 80 cases per 100,000, respectively.[7] Most cases present between the third and fifth decades, and there is a 30% increased risk in women.[7] Similarly, neurosarcoidosis is more common in women and African Americans between the ages of 20 and 40.[1,3,8]

The primary histopathologic finding in sarcoidosis is the nonnecrotizing granuloma, an organized cluster of epithelioid and multinucleated giant cells that is surrounded by a rim of T lymphocytes. Although the inciting pathogen is still unknown, epidemiologic studies have demonstrated an increased incidence of sarcoidosis with various environmental exposures that include infections, such as mycobacterium and *Proprionibacterium*

Disclosure Statement: J.O. Tavee receives research support from Mallinckrodt Inc and Araim Pharmaceuticals, Inc. B.J. Stern has served as an expert witness, editor of *The Neurologist*, and serves on the Data and Safety Monitoring Board and as a medical safety monitor at the National Institute of Neurologic Disorders and Stroke. B.J. Stern receives research support from the National Institute of Neurologic Disorders and Stroke and Remedy Pharmaceuticals.

[a] Cleveland Clinic Foundation, Neuromuscular Center, 9500 Euclid Avenue S90, Cleveland OH 44195, USA;
[b] Department of Neurology, University of Maryland School of Medicine, 16 S Eutaw Street #500, Baltimore, MD 21201, USA
* Corresponding author.
E-mail address: taveej2@ccf.org

Clin Chest Med 36 (2015) 643–656
http://dx.doi.org/10.1016/j.ccm.2015.08.007
0272-5231/15/$ – see front matter © 2015 Elsevier Inc. All rights reserved.

chestmed.theclinics.com

acnes; pesticides; mold; fire-fighting; metal dusts; and naval ship-service.[7,9–13] Many other factors seem to be important in the development of sarcoidosis, such as race, genetic polymorphisms, host immune status, and geography.[14,15]

Granulomatous inflammation most commonly affects the leptomeninges and has been shown in pathologic and radiographic studies to invade the brain and spinal cord parenchyma via Virchow-Robin spaces.[16–18] These cerebrospinal fluid (CSF)-filled perivascular channels communicate with the cervical lymphatics and may represent the interface between the immune system and the brain.[16] In addition, the greater size of the Virchow-Robin spaces at the base of the brain in combination with CSF flow dynamics may account for the preferential involvement of the basal meninges, cranial nerves, and midline neuroendocrine structures seen in neurosarcoidosis.[17,18]

CLINICAL PRESENTATION

Patients with neurosarcoidosis may present with various symptoms depending on which part of the neurologic axis is affected, and up to half have more than one manifestation (**Fig. 1**).[6] The most common presentation is cranial neuropathy, followed by basal meningitis, hypothalamic-pituitary dysfunction, encephalopathy, and other symptoms related to intraparenchymal brain involvement.

Cranial Nerve

Neurosarcoidosis affecting the central nervous system (CNS) was first reported in 1909 by Heerfordt[19] who described a series of patients presenting with facial palsy in the setting of uveitis and parotid gland enlargement. Although direct granulomatous infiltration or compression may affect any of the cranial nerves, facial neuropathy is the most common manifestation and is seen in up to 50% of all neurosarcoidosis cases.[1] Weakness is usually unilateral, but a third of cases may be bilateral. Most patients respond favorably to corticosteroids with little to no residual deficits, and some may even resolve spontaneously.

The second most commonly reported manifestation is optic neuropathy, which presents with blurred or loss of vision that can be in one or both eyes and is sometimes accompanied by pain (**Fig. 2**). Reduced visual acuity with color desaturation, pale optic disks, and papilledema may be seen on ophthalmologic examination. Patients with unilateral lesions tend to have a more favorable outcome, whereas those with bilateral involvement are often left with severe visual defects.[20]

The next most common presentation is hearing loss, which is usually bilateral and caused by cochlear nerve involvement that may be related to direct nerve involvement or more diffuse meningeal disease. In the authors' experience, significant hearing loss often remains permanent despite aggressive treatment. Dizziness can also occur if the vestibular component of the eighth cranial nerve is involved in the inflammatory process. Focal deficits of the remaining cranial nerves may occur in isolation or in combination with meningitis or other neurologic manifestations.

Meningeal

Leptomeningeal involvement of the brain with or without parenchymal disease presents as a

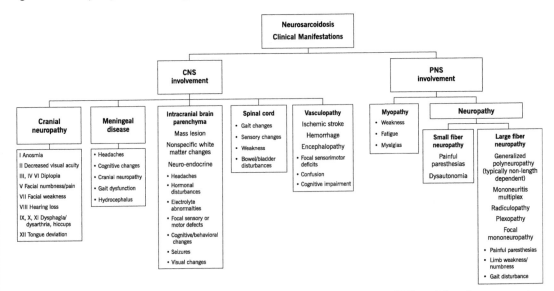

Fig. 1. Clinical manifestations of neurosarcoidosis. CNS, central nervous system; PNS, peripheral nervous system.

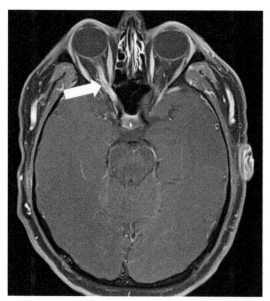

Fig. 2. Optic nerve enhancement (*arrow*) is seen on the right in a 34-year-old man with sarcoidosis presenting with visual loss and headaches.

chronic or subacute aseptic meningitis and has been reported to be the most common clinical manifestation by some authors, accounting for up to 78% of neurosarcoidosis cases in one series.[2,21] Most patients present with headache, and may also demonstrate concomitant cranial neuropathies or evidence of neuroendocrine dysfunction with focal involvement of the basilar meninges. With more diffuse leptomeningeal disease, the headache may be accompanied by gait dysfunction, cognitive changes, and/or seizures, suggesting involvement of the brain parenchyma. Patients presenting acutely with this complex of symptoms should be evaluated urgently for hydrocephalus, which can often complicate severe cases of leptomeningeal inflammation and is considered a neurologic emergency.

Intracranial Parenchyma

Headache, seizures, and focal neurologic deficits related to the location of a space-occupying lesion may occur with intraparenchymal brain involvement presenting as a mass lesion. Nonspecific white matter changes related to neurosarcoidosis are often asymptomatic, although they may be associated with memory loss and other cognitive disturbances in cases where there are numerous periventricular or subcortical lesions. Involvement of the hypothalamus and/or pituitary gland may result in polydipsia, which may be seen with diabetes insipidus, or the syndrome of inappropriate antidiuretic hormone. The resultant sodium derangements (both hyponatremia and hypernatremia) may result in episodes of confusion and hallucinations. Galactorrhea, amenorrhea, and other signs of hormonal dysfunction may also be seen with pituitary or hypothalamic involvement.

Spinal Cord

The presentation of patients with spinal cord sarcoidosis is often disproportionate to the degree of disease seen on MRI. Despite extensive cord lesions involving multiple vertebral segments, patients often report a vague sense of imbalance, difficulty walking, and leg numbness. There may also be increased bladder urgency or sexual dysfunction, but this information is usually not volunteered and must be obtained through direct questioning. Furthermore, examination typically demonstrates only minimal deficits with patchy nondermatomal sensory changes and/or a mildly unsteady gait. More definitive myelopathic signs and symptoms (hyperreflexia, weakness, a clear sensory level, and bowel/bladder incontinence) may also be seen, but their absence does not exclude the possibility of spinal cord involvement.

Neurovascular

Stroke related to neurosarcoidosis is rare and may be caused by granulomatous infiltration of the vessel walls with resultant stenosis or occlusion, usually in the setting of severe meningeal inflammation. Necrotizing granulomatous angiitis, embolic infarction related to cardiac sarcoidosis, transient ischemic attack, and intracerebral hemorrhage have also been reported.[22,23] Of note, sarcoidosis vasculitis more commonly results in a slowly progressive encephalopathy rather than a discrete ischemic infarct as demonstrated in a neuropathologic review of 19 cases with histologically proved vasculitic changes.[22] Of these cases, 14 were clinically manifested as encephalopathy, whereas only five had presented with a stroke or transient ischemic attack.[22]

Neuromuscular

Sarcoidosis myopathy often presents with myalgias, fatigue, and generalized weakness. It may also be asymptomatic because granulomatous muscle involvement has been seen in up to 50% of sarcoidosis cases at autopsy.[24] In some patients with sarcoidosis myopathy, intramuscular nodules can be palpated under the skin, a finding that is more common in men. Large-fiber nerve involvement typically presents with a painful, non-length-dependent axon loss polyneuropathy caused by granulomatous compression or infiltration of the nerve fibers and vasculitis.[25] The asymmetric distribution of findings as opposed to a distal stocking-glove pattern can help distinguish sarcoidosis-related neuropathy from those caused by diabetes and other more common etiologies. A subacute demyelinating polyneuropathy mimicking Guillain-Barré syndrome or more chronic form similar to chronic inflammatory demyelinating polyneuropathy has also been reported in a handful of cases.[26] Small-fiber neuropathy associated with sarcoidosis is discussed elsewhere in this issue.

Other

Fatigue, memory loss, difficulty concentrating, intermittent speech disturbances, mood disorders, and other cognitive-behavioral changes are often reported by patients with systemic sarcoidosis. Known by patients and clinicians as a "sarcoidosis fog," these symptoms do not correlate with specific structural changes within the CNS and are likely caused by multiple factors, which include sarcoidosis-associated systemic inflammation, medication side effects, exacerbation of underlying depression, and sleep disturbances among other conditions.[18]

DIAGNOSTIC TESTING
Tissue Biopsy

Definitive diagnosis of neurosarcoidosis is established when biopsy of the affected neural tissue reveals evidence of nonnecrotizing granulomas. However, accessing parenchymal tissue or elegant structures within the nervous system may result in chronic neurologic deficits that are worse than the presenting symptoms. Thus, in suspected cases of neurosarcoidosis with no history of systemic disease, the focus should be on confirming the presence of neurologic involvement and evaluating for an extraneural source of biopsy or other supportive evidence of sarcoidosis (**Fig. 3**).

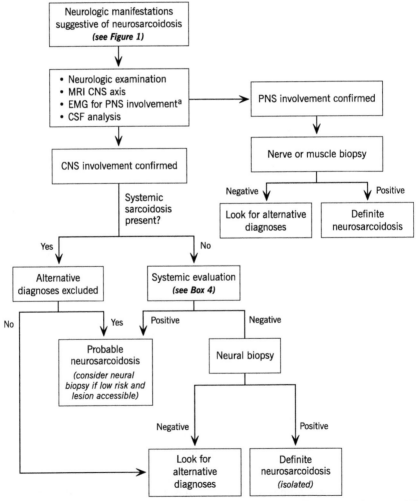

Fig. 3. Diagnostic algorithm for neurosarcoidosis. CNS, central nervous system; CSF, cerebrospinal fluid; PNS, peripheral nervous system. [a] Small fiber neuropathy evaluation is discussed elsewhere.

The most widely used diagnostic criteria is the modified Zajicek's criteria, which is divided into three categories: (1) "definite" when there is histologic confirmation of neurologic tissue, (2) "probable" when there is evidence of neurologic involvement and tissue confirmation of systemic sarcoidosis, and (3) "possible" when characteristic neurologic involvement is seen in the absence of any tissue diagnosis of sarcoidosis (**Box 1**).[27] For patients with a known history of systemic sarcoidosis, the exclusion of malignancy, infection, and other potential etiologies is key (**Box 2**).

MRI

MRI with gadolinium is the initial test of choice for patients with suspected CNS neurosarcoidosis. Although the diverse MRI findings of neurosarcoidosis often mimic other disorders, certain abnormalities or predilections for specific structures may be more characteristic of the disease.

- The most common radiographic abnormality seen in up to 40% of cases is leptomeningeal thickening and enhancement, which may be diffuse or focal along the basal surface of the brain affecting cranial nerves and neuroendocrine structures.[28] The pattern of enhancement may be smooth or nodular in appearance. In extensive cases, the leptomeningeal abnormalities may involve the entire length of the CNS axis in a patchy distribution along with exiting nerve roots at multiple levels and the cauda equina (**Fig. 4**).
- Dural thickening is also common and can be diffuse, mimicking idiopathic hypertrophic pachymeningitis and lymphoma, or focal, appearing similar to a meningioma (**Fig. 5**).
- Hydrocephalus may be seen in severe cases of meningeal inflammation, and can be communicating or noncommunicating (**Fig. 6**).
- Intraparenchymal brain involvement may present as a focal mass lesion, nonenhancing white matter changes, dense infiltration, or areas of patchy enhancement. In some patients with neuroendocrine dysfunction, thickening and enhancement of the hypothalamic-pituitary structures may be seen (**Figs. 7** and **8**).
- Intramedullary spinal cord lesions often affect multiple (≥ 3) segments in a noncontiguous, patchy distribution and are accompanied by meningeal enhancement in about half of the cases.[29] Concomitant intracerebral lesions have also been found to occur with a similar frequency.[29,30] Acute lesions may demonstrate focal cord expansion, whereas more chronic cases result in cord atrophy (**Fig. 9**).
- Vasculitic sarcoidosis can arise from leptomeningeal infiltration of the perivascular space or granulomatous formation in vessel walls. These can appear as ischemic lesions in specific vascular distributions, cerebral hemorrhage, or more commonly nonspecific white matter changes (**Fig. 10**). These latter lesions may be unrelated to the sarcoidosis and can occur because of hypertension, diabetes, smoking, and other inflammatory or infectious disorders.

MRI abnormalities may not have a clinical correlate, especially in the setting of cranial nerve,

---

Box 1
Diagnostic criteria for neurosarcoidosis

In patients with a clinical presentation suggestive of neurosarcoidosis and exclusion of other diagnoses, classification is as follows:

Definite

- Histologic confirmation of affected neural tissue

Probable

- Evidence of CNS inflammation on MRI or CSF (elevated protein, cells, IgG index, or presence of oligoclonal bands) compatible with neurosarcoidosis AND
- Evidence of systemic sarcoidosis with histologic confirmation and/or at least two of the following indirect indicators: fluorodeoxyglucose PET, gallium scan, chest imaging, serum angiotensin-converting enzyme

Possible

- Above criteria not met

Adapted from Zajicek JP, Scolding NJ, Foster O, et al. Central nervous system sarcoidosis-diagnosis and management. QJM 1999;92:104.

Box 2
Differential diagnosis of neurosarcoidosis

Infection

- Progressive multifocal leukoencephalopathy (JC virus)
- Cryptococcus
- Histoplasmosis
- Tuberculosis
- HIV
- Varicella zoster virus
- Neurosyphilis
- Listeria
- Borrelia (Lyme disease)
- Cytomegalovirus
- Toxoplasmosis
- Whipple disease

Immune-mediated

- IgG4-related meningeal disease
- CNS vasculitis
- Wegener granulomatosis
- Common variable immunodeficiency syndrome
- Sjögren syndrome
- Behçet syndrome
- Systemic lupus erythematosus
- Vogt-Koyanagi-Harada syndrome
- Lymphocytic hypophysitis
- Rosai-Dorfman disease
- Chronic lymphocytic infiltration with pontine perivascular enhancement responsive to steroids

Malignancy

- CNS lymphoma
- Carcinomatous meningitis
- Leptomeningeal or dural metastases
- Meningioma
- Glioma
- Germ cell tumors

Demyelinating

- Multiple sclerosis
- Neuromyelitis optica (Devic disease)
- Acute demyelinating encephalomyelitis
- Transverse myelitis

spinal cord, and nonenhancing white matter lesions. Conversely, reported symptoms may not be explained by radiographic findings. However, one retrospective case series found that pituitary and gadolinium-enhancing white matter lesions did correlate clinically in most cases.[30] Finally, MRI should always be done with gadolinium (if there is no allergy and renal function allows) to evaluate for the presence of leptomeningeal involvement, active inflammation, or infiltrative lesions that would otherwise go undetected in a nonenhanced scan. However, not all cases of active CNS inflammation demonstrate gadolinium-enhanced lesions.

Cerebrospinal Fluid

CSF analysis should be performed in all patients with suspected neurosarcoidosis to help confirm the presence of inflammation and exclude the possibilities of infection and malignancy. The CSF demonstrates abnormalities of one or more routine parameters in 70% to 95% of neurosarcoidosis cases (**Box 3**).[31,32]

- In a literature review that included more than 700 neurosarcoidosis patients from multiple case series, elevated CSF protein (64% of cases) and cell count (54% of cases) were the most commonly reported abnormalities.[31] Although these findings are nonspecific for neurosarcoidosis, they may indicate the presence of inflammation as abnormal CSF protein levels greater than or equal to 200 mg/dL, and cell count greater than or equal to 50 cells/μL has been found to correlate with diffuse leptomeningeal enhancement on MRI and clinically active disease.[31]
- Hypoglycorrhachia (low CSF glucose) is seen in up to a third of cases caused by disruption of the CSF glucose transport system, and in combination with abnormal CSF protein or pleocytosis can help point toward neurosarcoidosis as compared with other inflammatory diseases, although infection and carcinomatous meningitis also share this feature.
- An elevated IgG index and the presence of oligoclonal bands have been reported in 43% and 34% of combined neurosarcoidosis cases, respectively.[31] Increased CSF lactate and other markers of inflammation may also be seen.
- In one recent study, elevated CSF-soluble interleukin-2 receptor levels over 150 pg/mL detected untreated neurosarcoidosis patients with a 61% sensitivity and 93% specificity in comparison with healthy control subjects

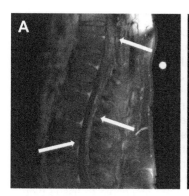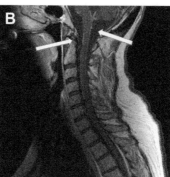

Fig. 4. (*A*) Patchy leptomeningeal enhancement (*arrow*) of the thoracic cord and cauda equina is seen in a 44-year-old man with neurosarcoidosis. (*B*) Extensive leptomeningeal enhancement (*arrow*) of the brainstem and cervical spinal cord in a 34-year-old man with sexual dysfunction and gait disturbance.

and other inflammatory diseases, such as multiple sclerosis and CNS vasculitis, although there was no significant difference when compared with infection.[33] Levels were found to change accordingly with disease activity and treatment status in serial measurements of patients with neurosarcoidosis.

- Although serum angiotensin-converting enzyme (ACE) is still widely used in evaluating systemic disease, CSF ACE is less helpful in the diagnosis of neurosarcoidosis given its low sensitivity (13%–25%) and has been absent even in the setting of a positive brain biopsy.[33,34]

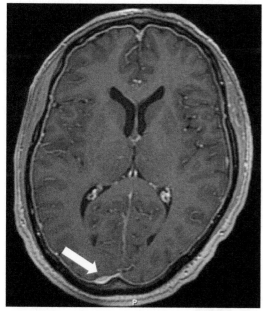

Fig. 5. Diffuse dural enhancement (*arrow*) is seen with a small area of focal thickening in the right occipital region in a 62-year-old man with cognitive impairment and hallucinations.

- Cytology, flow cytometry, and cultures (fungal, bacterial, and viral) should be obtained in all patients with suspected neurosarcoidosis because malignancy and infectious meningitis may demonstrate very similar MRI and CSF findings, including hypoglycorrhachia. In known sarcoidosis patients who are chronically immunosuppressed, progressive multifocal leukoencephalopathy should be excluded with polymerase chain reaction studies for JC virus DNA.

Peripheral Nervous System Testing

Electromyogram is the primary study to evaluate patients with evidence of neuromuscular involvement (eg, myalgias, large-fiber neuropathy, mononeuritis multiplex) and can help determine localization, demyelinating versus axon loss pathophysiology, degree of severity, and chronicity of the lesion. MRI of the musculoskeletal system may also demonstrate nodular lesions within the muscle suggestive of sarcoidosis involvement. Histologic confirmation may be obtained via nerve or muscle biopsy, which is less invasive than CNS biopsy and can demonstrate the characteristic nonnecrotizing granulomatous lesions needed for definite diagnosis.

For patients presenting with a painful small-fiber neuropathy or dysautonomia, specialized testing including skin biopsy with quantitative nerve fiber analysis, autonomic studies, and confocal corneal microscopy may objectively confirm small nerve fiber loss or dysfunction (discussed elsewhere in this issue).

Other Testing

Various presentations require more focused testing. Electroencephalogram should be obtained in patients presenting with seizures. Neuroendocrine evaluation with cortisol, vasopressin, and other hormonal levels may be needed in

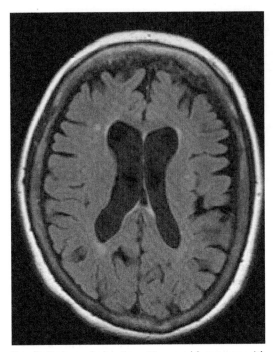

Fig. 6. Hydrocephalus in a 68-year-old woman with meningeal neurosarcoidosis who presented with gait imbalance and urinary incontinence.

patients presenting with symptoms of hypothalamic-pituitary dysfunction. Cardiac evaluation, computed tomography or MR angiography, or even conventional angiography may be considered in patients with sarcoidosis and stroke.

Systemic Evaluation

The search for systemic disease in patients with suspected neurosarcoidosis typically begins with serologic and pulmonary evaluation (**Box 4**). Although the serum ACE level is still part of the diagnostic criteria, it may be affected by genetic polymorphisms, is of insufficient sensitivity

(57%), and does not correlate well with disease activity.[35,36] In contrast, the soluble interleukin-2 receptor protein, which like ACE is also secreted by granulomas, has been found to correlate with the presence of active disease and is increasingly being used in the setting of sarcoidosis. However, elevated levels may also be seen in lymphoma, systemic lupus erythematosus, and other inflammatory disorders.[37]

Additional testing should include computed tomography imaging studies of the chest, abdomen, and pelvis to evaluate for lymphadenopathy or other lesions that are amenable to tissue biopsy or that are supportive of the diagnosis. If no evidence of extraneural disease is seen, fluorodeoxyglucose PET and 67-gallium scanning may be considered because both increase the sensitivity of detecting subclinical systemic involvement, but are significantly more expensive.[38] However, fluorodeoxyglucose PET is more sensitive in detecting inflammation than gallium scanning and is the preferred imaging modality.

Conjunctival Biopsy

Conjunctival biopsy has been described as a potentially useful and minimally invasive study that demonstrates findings consistent with sarcoidosis in up to 55% cases even in the absence of conjunctival lesions.[39,40] Bilateral biopsy is recommended because abnormalities can often be seen only on one side. However, a more recent retrospective study evaluating the use of conjunctival biopsy in 440 suspected cases of neurosarcoidosis (the diagnosis had to be included as a surgical indication or in the neurology clinic notes) reported only a 3% (13 of 440) rate of abnormalities consistent with ocular sarcoidosis, of which 1% (4 of 440) was ultimately found to have another cause for the neurologic symptoms.[41] Although the authors concluded that the yield was insufficient to recommend

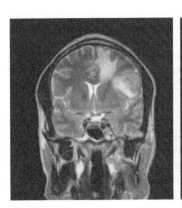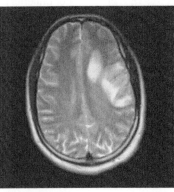

Fig. 7. Increased signal intensity in left frontal lobe of 42-year-old man presenting with seizures. Biopsy of the underlying mass demonstrated nonnecrotizing granulomas.

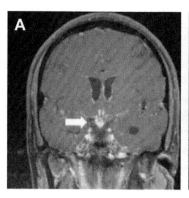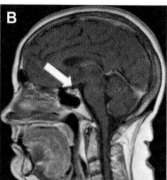

Fig. 8. (A) Hypothalamus, basal meninges, and frontal horns of lateral ventricles demonstrate post–gadolinium enhancement in a patient with severe neurosarcoidosis and the syndrome of inappropriate antidiuretic hormone secretion. (B) Gadolinium-enhancing pituitary gland in a patient with neurosarcoidosis and diabetes insipidus.

routinely in the setting of neurosarcoidosis, further studies are needed.

Isolated Neurosarcoidosis

In patients in which no evidence of systemic disease is found despite a comprehensive investigation, proceeding with CNS biopsy may be necessary because the lack of a firm diagnosis should be considered cautionary for the prescription of any immunosuppressive agents outside of corticosteroids because of the risks and side effect profiles of these medications. Fortunately, isolated neurosarcoidosis is rare and seen in only 10% to 17% of all cases.[2,34] In the largest series of isolated neurosarcoidosis to date, which included a total of 10 patients, intraparenchymal brain involvement was the most common manifestation (7 of 10) followed by leptomeningeal disease (6 of 10).[34] For patients with isolated neurosarcoidosis, continued surveillance for systemic disease or latent findings suggestive of an alternative diagnosis should be maintained.

TREATMENT

Although up to 40% of sarcoidosis patients are managed without pharmacologic therapy,

neurosarcoidosis often requires immunosuppressive treatment especially in the setting of brain or spinal cord involvement (**Box 5**).[3] Given the lack of controlled clinical trials, treatment guidelines are largely based on anecdotal evidence and small case series. Factors to consider in choosing a specific therapy include length of anticipated treatment, and severity of clinical manifestation, which may be loosely categorized as mild (facial palsy), moderate (cranial neuropathies involving II or VIII, myopathy, neuropathy, dural meningeal involvement), and severe disabling disease (brain and spinal cord lesions, leptomeningeal involvement, hydrocephalus). An algorithmic approach to treatment based on these categories is provided in **Fig. 11**.[42]

Corticosteroids

The first-line therapy for all manifestations of neurosarcoidosis requiring treatment is corticosteroids. For mild to moderate cases, an oral dose of 20 to 40 mg/day may be initiated. In severe cases, particularly those of recent onset, pulse dose intravenous methylprednisolone at 500 to 1000 mg/day for 3 to 5 days is usually considered followed by an oral maintenance dose of 0.5 to 1 mg/kg or about 60 mg daily. During the next 6

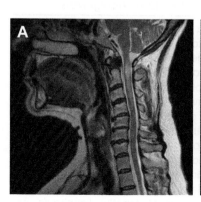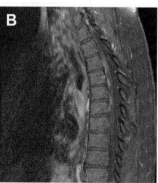

Fig. 9. (A) Focal cord expansion with increased signal intensity is seen within the cervical cord down to C4 in a patient with biopsy-confirmed neurosarcoidosis. (B) Patchy gadolinium enhancement throughout the anterior thoracic cord in a patient with sarcoidosis presenting with paraparesis bowel/bladder disturbances.

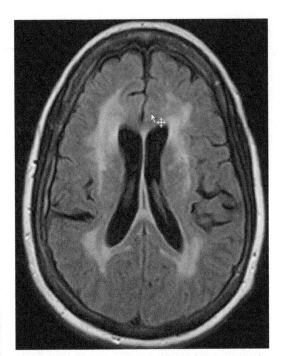

Fig. 10. Confluent periventricular white matter lesions in a 60-year-old woman with neurosarcoidosis presenting with progressive memory loss with episodic confusion.

to 12 months, the dose may be slowly tapered with careful monitoring for exacerbation or recurrence of disease, although many patients ultimately require low doses of 5 to 10 mg daily for at least 2 years. For mild to moderate cases, monotherapy with corticosteroids is usually sufficient. However,

Box 3
Cerebrospinal fluid abnormalities in neurosarcoidosis

Routine analysis

- Pleocytosis (lymphocytic or neutrophilic predominance may be seen)
- Elevated protein
- Reduced glucose
- All parameters may be normal in up to 30% of cases

Inflammatory markers

- Elevated IgG index
- Presence of oligoclonal bands
- Elevated angiotensin-converting enzyme
- Elevated soluble interleukin-2 receptor level
- Elevated lactic acid

Box 4
Systemic evaluation

First Tier

- Serologic studies
  - Comprehensive metabolic profile with liver function testing
  - Complete blood count
  - Angiotensin-converting enzyme
  - Soluble interleukin-2 receptor level
- Chest radiograph
- Pulmonary function testing
- Ophthalmologic evaluation with slit-lamp
- Skin survey
- Purified protein derivative or interferon-γ assay for mycobacterium tuberculosis
- Electrocardiogram

Second Tier

- Computed tomography of body with biopsy of abnormal tissue suggestive of sarcoidosis
- Bronchoscopy or endobronchial ultrasound-guided transbronchial needle aspiration

Third Tier

- Fluorodeoxyglucose PET
- 67-Gallium scanning
- Conjunctival biopsy

in those with refractory or severe disabling disease, combination therapy with a second immunosuppressive agent should be considered. Corticosteroids are effective in reducing inflammation and repairing the blood-brain barrier, but may result in significant dose-related side effects that should be monitored for in all patients requiring chronic treatment (see **Box 5**).

Tumor Necrosis Factor-α Antagonists

Infliximab is a monoclonal antibody against tumor necrosis factor (TNF)-α that has emerged as a promising agent in treating CNS and refractory neurosarcoidosis.[43] Early in the course, it may be used in combination with oral corticosteroids but is also effective as maintenance monotherapy. In the authors' experience, infliximab is especially helpful in patients with severe leptomeningeal, brain, and spinal cord disease. Another TNF-α antagonist, adalimumab, has also been found to be beneficial in corticosteroid-refractory neurosarcoidosis.[44] Major side effects include progressive multifocal leukoencephalopathy, lymphoma, and

Box 5
Therapies for neurosarcoidosis

Drug	Dosage	Adverse Effects	Monitoring
Prednisone	5–40 mg daily	Diabetes, hypertension, weight gain, cataracts, glaucoma steroid myopathy	Blood pressure, weight, glucose if clinically indicated, osteoporosis and bone density checks
Hydroxychloroquine	200–400 mg daily	Ocular, hepatic, cutaneous	Eye examination every 6–12 mo
Methotrexate	5–20 mg weekly	Hematologic, hepatoxic	CBC, hepatic every 1–3 mo
Azathioprine	50–200 mg daily	Hematologic, gastrointestinal	CBC, hepatic every 1–3 mo
Mycophenylate	500–1500 mg daily twice daily	Hematologic, gastrointestinal	CBC, hepatic every 1–3 mo
Infliximab	3–5 mg/kg initially, 2 wk later, then every 4–8 wk	Allergic reactions, increased risk for infections, especially tuberculosis, worsening congestive heart failure, possible increased risk for malignancy, PML	PPD before initiating therapy, hold drug in face of active infection
Adalimumab	40–80 mg SQ every 1–2 wk	Allergic reactions, increased risk for infections, especially tuberculosis, worsening congestive heart failure, possible increased risk for malignancy, PML	PPD before initiating therapy, hold drug in face of active infection
Rituximab	1000 mg IV, 2 doses, 2 wk apart	Hematologic, allergic reactions increased risk for infections, especially HBV, PML, renal	HBV screening before initiating therapy, hold drug in face of active infection, CBC, renal function every 1–3 mo

Abbreviations: CBC, complete blood count; HBV, hepatitis B virus; IV, intravenous; PML, progressive multifocal leukoencephalopathy; PPD, purified protein derivative, skin test to diagnose tuberculosis; SQ, subcutaneous.

Adapted from Stern B. Sarcoidosis treatment guidelines. Chicago, IL: Foundation for Sarcoidosis Research; 2015. Available at: http://www.stopsarcoidosis.org/wp-content/uploads/2013/03/FSR-Physicians-Protocol1.pdf. Accessed March 27, 2015; with permission.

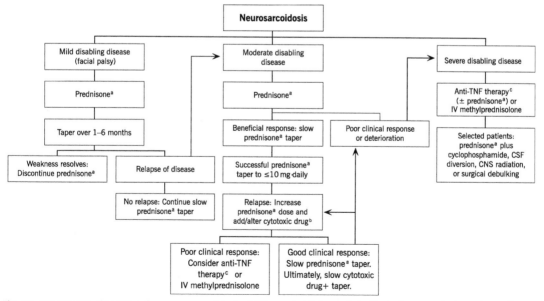

Fig. 11. Treatment algorithm for neurosarcoidosis. [a] Where prednisone is indicated, an equivalent dose of corticosteroids (ie, methylprednisolone) could also be used. See text for dosing recommendations. [b] Cytotoxic drugs include methotrexate, azathioprine, and mycophenolate. [c] Anti-TNF therapy includes infliximab and adalimumab. IV, intravenous; TNF, tumor necrosis factor. (*Adapted from* Stern B. Sarcoidosis treatment guidelines. Chicago, IL: Foundation for Sarcoidosis Research; 2015. Available at: http://www.stopsarcoidosis.org/wp-content/uploads/2013/03/FSR-Physicians-Protocol1.pdf. Accessed March 27, 2015; with permission.)

reactivation of tuberculosis, all of which should be considered in sarcoidosis patients who develop new neurologic findings while on TNF-α antagonists.

Box 6
Therapy for specific complications of neurosarcoidosis

- Hydrocephalus
  - Ventriculostomy and drainage with subsequent shunt placement
- Seizures
  - Antiepileptic medications
  - Seizure precautions (eg, no driving as per state law)
- Hypothalamic-pituitary dysfunction
  - Endocrine consultation
  - Electrolyte monitoring
  - Fluid management
  - Hormone-replacement therapy
- Peripheral neuropathy, trigeminal neuralgia
  - Antidepressants
  - Antiepileptics
  - Opioid or opioid agonists
  - Topical medications
  - Pain management consultation
  - Intravenous immune globulin for large and small-fiber neuropathy[a]
  - ARA-290 (experimental erythropoietin agonist for small-fiber neuropathy)[a]
- Neurovascular complications
  - Antiplatelet medications or anticoagulants if indicated
  - Statins and other medications targeting stroke risk factors
- Fatigue and weight gain
  - Physical therapy
  - Exercise
  - Nutrition consultation
- Depression and cognitive changes
  - Counseling
  - Psychiatry consultation
  - Neuropsychology or behavioral health referral

[a] Small-fiber neuropathy treatment is discussed elsewhere in this issue.

Other Corticosteroid-Sparing Agents

For patients with severe disease who are not candidates for TNF-α antagonists because of medical contraindications or cost, azathioprine is an effective alternative. Thiopurine methyltransferase genotype testing should be obtained before initiation of treatment to identify patients at risk for hematologic toxicity. Cyclophosphamide may also be considered for severe disease, but is limited by significant adverse effects. Methotrexate and hydroxychloroquine may be used in combination with corticosteroids or other agents for treating neurosarcoidosis, but are typically insufficient as monotherapy. In contrast, mycophenylate mofetil is helpful in some cases of CNS involvement, and can be used in conjunction with infliximab for severe disease. Recently, rituximab has demonstrated benefit in severely ill patients. Whole-brain radiation therapy is another potential option for refractory CNS cases, although most reports were published before the use of TNF-α antagonists in neurosarcoidosis.[45] Finally, treatment of specific complications, such as shunt placement for hydrocephalus, is shown in **Box 6**.

SUMMARY

Although involvement of the nervous system is relatively rare compared with other organs, neurosarcoidosis often results in serious deficits that can significantly impact quality of life. Early recognition and aggressive treatment can stop worsening of disease and in some cases help restore neurologic function.

REFERENCES

1. Stern BJ, Krumholz A, Johns C, et al. Sarcoidosis and its neurological manifestations. Arch Neurol 1985;42:909.
2. Chapelon C, Ziza JM, Piette JC, et al. Neurosarcoidosis: signs, course and treatment in 35 confirmed cases. Medicine 1990;69:261–76.
3. Judson MA, Boan AD, Lackland DT. The clinical course of sarcoidosis: presentation, diagnosis, and treatment in a large white and black cohort in the United States. Sarcoidosis Vasc Diffuse Lung Dis 2012;29:119–27.
4. Maycock RL, Bertrand P, Morrison LE, et al. Manifestations of sarcoidosis. Am J Med 1963;35:67–89.
5. Manz HJ. Pathobiology of neurosarcoidosis and clinicopathologic correlation. Can J Neurol Sci 1983;10:50–5.
6. Krumholz A, Stern BJ. Neurologic manifestations of sarcoidosis. Handb Clin Neurol 2014;119:305–33.

7. Rybicki BA, Iannuzzi MC. Epidemiology of sarcoidosis: recent advances and future prospects. Semin Respir Crit Care Med 2007;28:22–35.

8. Baughman RP, Teirstein AS, Judson MA, et al. Clinical characteristics of patients in a case control study of sarcoidosis. Am J Respir Crit Care Med 2001;164:1885–9.

9. Ishige I, Usui Y, Takemura T, et al. Quantitative PCR of mycobacterial and propionibacterial DNA in lymph nodes of Japanese patients with sarcoidosis. Lancet 1999;354:120–3.

10. Prezant DJ, Dhala A, Goldstein A. The incidence, prevalence, and severity of sarcoidosis in New York City firefighters. Chest 1999;116:1183–93.

11. Kucera GP, Rybicki BA, Kirkey KL, et al. Occupational risk factors for sarcoidosis in African-American siblings. Chest 2003;123:1526–35.

12. Newman LS, Rose CS, Bresnitz EA, et al. A case control etiologic study of sarcoidosis: environmental and occupational risk factors. Am J Respir Crit Care Med 2004;170:1324–30.

13. Gorham ED, Garland CF, Garland FC, et al. Trends and occupational associations in incidence of hospitalized pulmonary sarcoidosis and other lung diseases in Navy personnel: a 27-year historical prospective study, 1975–2001. Chest 2004;126:1431–8.

14. Culver DA. Sarcoidosis. Immunol Allergy Clin N Am 2012;32:487–511.

15. Iannuzzi MC, Rybicki BA, Teirstein AS. Sarcoidosis. N Engl J Med 2007;357:2153–65.

16. Mirfakhraee M, Crofford MJ, Guinto FC, et al. Virchow-Robin space: a path of spread in neurosarcoidosis. Radiology 1986;158:715–20.

17. Nowak DA, Widenka DC. Neurosarcoidosis: a review of its intracranial manifestation. J Neurol 2001;248:363–72.

18. Tavee J, Stern B. Neurosarcoidosis. Continuum (Minneap Minn) 2014;20:545–59.

19. Heerfordt CF. Über eine "Febris uveo-parotidea subchronica" an der Glandula parotis und der Uvea des Auges lokalisiert und häufug mit Paresen cerebrospinaler Nerven kompliziert. Albrecht von Grafes Archiv für Ophthalmologie 1909;70:254–73.

20. Pawate S, Moses H, Sriram S. Presentations and outcomes of neurosarcoidosis: a study of 54 cases. QJM 2009;102:449–60.

21. Aksamit A. Neurosarcoidosis. Continuum Lifelong Learn Neurol 2008;14:181–96.

22. Brown MM, Thompson AJ, Wedzicha JA, et al. Sarcoidosis presenting with stroke. Stroke 1989;20:400–5.

23. Herring AB, Urich H. Sarcoidosis of the central nervous system. J Neurol Sci 1969;9:405–22.

24. Iwai K, Tachibana T, Takemura T, et al. Pathological studies on sarcoidosis autopsy. I. Epidemiological features of 320 cases in Japan. Pathol Int 1993;43:372–6.

25. Burns TM, Dyck PJB, Aksamit AJ, et al. The natural history and long-term outcome of 57 limb sarcoidosis neuropathy cases. J Neurol Sci 2006;244:77–87.

26. Said G, Lacroix C, Planté-Bordeneuve V, et al. Nerve granulomas and vasculitis in sarcoid peripheral neuropathy: a clinicopathological study of 11 patients. Brain 2002;125:264–75.

27. Zajicek JP, Scolding NJ, Foster O, et al. Central nervous system sarcoidosis-diagnosis and management. QJM 1999;92:103–17.

28. Smith JK, Matheus MG, Castillo M. Imaging manifestations of neurosarcoidosis. AJR Am J Roentgenol 2004;182:289–95.

29. Sohn M, Culver DA, Judson MA, et al. Spinal cord neurosarcoidosis. Am J Med Sci 2013;347:195–8.

30. Shah R, Roberson GH, Curé JK. Correlation of MR imaging findings and clinical manifestations in neurosarcoidosis. AJNR Am J Neuroradiol 2009;20:953–61.

31. Wengert O, Rothenfusser-Korber E, Vollrath B, et al. Neurosarcoidosis: correlation of cerebrospinal fluid findings with diffuse leptomeningeal gadolinium enhancement on MRI and clinical disease activity. J Neurol Sci 2013;335:124–30.

32. Oksanen V. Neurosarcoidosis: clinical presentations and course in 50 patients. Acta Neurol Scand 1986;73:283–90.

33. Petereit HF, Reske D, Tumani H, et al. Soluble CSF interleukin 2 receptor as indicator of neurosarcoidosis. J Neurol 2010;247:1855–63.

34. Nozaki K, Scott TF, Sohn M, et al. Isolated neurosarcoidosis: case series in 2 sarcoidosis centers. Neurologist 2012;18:373–7.

35. Tomita H, Ina Y, Sugiura Y, et al. Polymorphism in the angiotensin-converting enzyme (ACE) gene and sarcoidosis. Am J Respir Crit Care Med 1997;156:255–9.

36. Studdy PR, James DG. The specificity and sensitivity of serum angiotensin-converting enzyme in sarcoidosis and other diseases. In: Chretien J, Marsac J, Saltiel JC, editors. Sarcoidosis. Paris: Pergamon Press; 1983. p. 332–44.

37. Keicho N, Kitamura K, Takaku F, et al. Serum concentration of soluble interleukin-2 receptor as a sensitive parameter of disease activity in sarcoidosis. Chest 1990;98:1125–9.

38. Mañá J, Gámez C. Molecular imaging in sarcoidosis. Curr Opin Pulm Med 2011;17:325–31.

39. Leavitt JA, Campbell RJ. Cost-effectiveness in the diagnosis of sarcoidosis: the conjunctival biopsy. Eye 1998;12:959–62.

40. Nichols DW, Eagle RC Jr, Yanoff M, et al. Conjunctival biopsy as an aid in the evaluation of the patient with suspected sarcoidosis. Ophthalmology 1980;87:287–91.

41. Pichler MR, Flanagan EP, Aksamit AJ, et al. Conjunctival biopsy to diagnose neurosarcoidosis in patients with inflammatory nervous system disease of unknown etiology. Neurolog Clin Pract 2015;10:2012.

42. Stern B. Sarcoidosis treatment guidelines. Chicago, IL: Foundation for Sarcoidosis Research; 2015. Available at: http://www.stopsarcoidosis.org/wp-content/uploads/2013/03/FSR-Physicians-Protocol1.pdf. Accessed March 27, 2015.

43. Moravan M, Segal BM. Treatment of CNS sarcoidosis with infliximab and mycophenolate mofetil. Neurology 2009;72:337–40.

44. Marnane M, Lynch T, Scott J, et al. Steroid-unresponsive neurosarcoidosis successfully treated with adalimumab. J Neurol 2009;256:139–40.

45. Motta M, Alongi F, Bolognesi A, et al. Remission of refractory neurosarcoidosis treated with brain radiotherapy: a case report and a literature review. Neurologist 2008;14:120–4.

Cardiac Sarcoidosis

David Birnie, MD, MB ChB[a],*, Andrew C.T. Ha, MD[b], Lorne J. Gula, MD, MSc[c],
Santabhanu Chakrabarti, MBBS, MD[d], Rob S.B. Beanlands, MD[a], Pablo Nery, MD[a]

KEYWORDS

- Cardiac sarcoidosis • Clinically silent • Clinically manifest • Atrioventricular block
- Ventricular arrhythmias • Heart failure • Sudden cardiac death

KEY POINTS

- Studies have suggested that clinically manifest cardiac involvement occurs in perhaps 5% of patients with pulmonary/systemic sarcoidosis.
- The 3 principal manifestations of cardiac sarcoidosis (CS) are conduction abnormalities, ventricular arrhythmias, and heart failure.
- An estimated 20% to 25% of patients with pulmonary/systemic sarcoidosis have asymptomatic cardiac involvement (clinically silent cardiac involvement).
- The prognosis of clinically manifest disease primarily relates to the extent of left ventricular (LV) dysfunction.
- Recently a consensus document detailed recommendations on the management of most aspects of CS.

EPIDEMIOLOGY AND CLINICAL MANIFESTATIONS

Studies have suggested that clinically manifest cardiac involvement occurs in perhaps 5% of patients with pulmonary/systemic sarcoidosis. Clinical features of CS depend on the location, extent, and activity of the disease.[1,2] The 3 principal manifestations of CS are (1) conduction abnormalities,[3–8] (2) ventricular arrhythmias,[9] and (3) heart failure.[2] Other data indicate that many patients with pulmonary/systemic sarcoidosis have asymptomatic cardiac involvement (clinically silent disease). For example, autopsy studies have estimated the prevalence of cardiac involvement to be at least 25% of patients with sarcoidosis in North America.[10–12] These incidence data from autopsy series are very consistent with recent data using

modern late gadolinium enhancement–cardiac magnetic resonance (LGE-CMR) technology. These LGE-CMR studies in patients with extracardiac sarcoidosis found clinically silent cardiac involvement in 13%,[13] 25.5%[14] and 25.9%[15] of cases respectively.

DIAGNOSIS

In 2014, an international guideline for the diagnosis of CS was published (**Box 1**).[16] The international expert consensus statement was written by experts in the field who were chosen by the Heart Rhythm Society in collaboration with multiple other societies. Before this consensus document, the only published diagnostic guidelines were the Japanese Ministry of Health and Welfare criteria[17] and the National Institutes of Health's A Case

Disclosure statement: The authors have nothing to disclose.
[a] Division of Cardiology, University of Ottawa Heart Institute, 40 Ruskin Street, Ottawa, Ontario K1Y 4 W7, Canada; [b] Department of Medicine, Peter Munk Cardiac Centre, University Health Network, University of Toronto, GW 3-558A, 200 Elizabeth Street, Toronto, Ontario M5G 2C4, Canada; [c] Division of Cardiology, London Health Sciences Centre, 339 Windermere Road, c6-110, London, Ontario N6A 5A5, Canada; [d] Division of Cardiology, Department of Medicine, University of British Columbia, 211 1033, Davie Street, Vancouver, British Columbia V6E 1M7, Canada
* Corresponding author.
E-mail address: dbirnie@ottawaheart.ca

chestmed.theclinics.com

Box 1
Expert consensus recommendations on criteria for diagnosis of cardiac sarcoidosis

There are 2 pathways to a diagnosis of CS:

1. Histologic diagnosis from myocardial tissue

    CS is diagnosed in the presence of noncaseating granuloma on histologic examination of myocardial tissue with no alternative cause identified (including negative organismal stains if applicable)

2. Clinical diagnosis from invasive and noninvasive studies

    It is probable[a] that there is CS if

    a. There is a histologic diagnosis of extracardiac sarcoidosis and

    b. One or more of following is present

        i. Steroid +/− immunosuppressant responsive cardiomyopathy or heart block

        ii. Unexplained reduced left ventricular ejection fraction (<40%)

        iii. Unexplained sustained (spontaneous or induced) ventricular tachycardia

        iv. Mobitz type II second-degree heart block or third-degree heart block

        v. Patchy uptake on dedicated cardiac PET (in a pattern consistent with CS)

        vi. LGE on CMR (in a pattern consistent with CS)

        vii. Positive gallium uptake (in a pattern consistent with CS)

        Plus

    c. Other causes for the cardiac manifestations have been reasonably excluded

[a] In general, probable involvement is considered adequate to establish a clinical diagnosis of CS.[24]
From Birnie DH, Sauer WH, Bogun F, et al. HRS expert consensus statement on the diagnosis and management of arrhythmias associated with cardiac sarcoidosis. Heart Rhythm 2014;11(7):1306; with permission.

Control Etiology of Sarcoidosis Study (ACCESS) set of criteria published in 1999.[18]

Role of Endomyocardial Biopsy in the Diagnosis of Cardiac Sarcoidosis

In patients with extracardiac sarcoidosis, lymph node or lung biopsy is typically targeted first due to the higher diagnostic yield and lower procedural risk. In cases of isolated CS or negative extracardiac biopsy, endomyocardial biopsy (EMB) may be required to confirm the diagnosis. However, EMB has low sensitivity due to the focal nature of the disease, revealing noncaseating granulomas in less than 25% of patients with CS.[19,20] To increase the sensitivity of the procedure, electrophysiological (electroanatomic mapping)[21] or image-guided (PET or CMR)[22] biopsy procedures have been described. Consensus guidelines recommend that EMB for investigation of a possible diagnosis of CS should always be guided.[16,23]

Screening for Cardiac Involvement in Patients with Biopsy-Proven Extracardiac Sarcoidosis

There are few data comparing the sensitivity and specificity of various screening tests for cardiac involvement in patients with sarcoidosis. Mehta and colleagues[25] studied 62 subjects with sarcoidosis. Those with symptoms (significant palpitations, syncope, or presyncope) or abnormal results (electrocardiogram [ECG], Holter monitoring, and echocardiography) were studied with CMR or PET scanning. The diagnosis of CS was based on abnormalities detected by PET or CMR. Subjects with CS had more cardiac symptoms than those without CS (46% vs 5%); and they were more likely to have abnormal Holter monitor findings (50% vs 3%, respectively) and trans-thoracic echocardiography findings (25% vs 5%).[25] It should be noted that the presence of 1 abnormal screening variable had a sensitivity of 100% and a specificity of 87% for the diagnosis of CS.[25] There are no data on whether interval rescreening is necessary in patients with an initial negative work-up.[16]

It is clear that larger studies are required to define the sensitivity and specificity (and cost-effectiveness) of various screening strategies/tests to detect clinically silent cardiac involvement. Also, research is required to look at other proposed screening tests or potential risk markers, including signal-averaged ECG and fragmented QRS.[26,27] Recent consensus guidelines have made recommendations for screening (**Box 2** and **3, Fig. 1**).

Box 2
Expert consensus recommendations on screening for cardiac involvement in patients with biopsy-proven extracardiac sarcoidosis

Class I recommendations

It is recommended that patients with biopsy-proven extracardiac sarcoidosis should be asked about unexplained syncope, presyncope, or significant palpitations.[a]

It is recommended that patients with biopsy-proven extracardiac sarcoidosis should be screened for cardiac involvement with a 12-lead ECG.

Class IIa recommendations

Screening for cardiac involvement with an echocardiogram can be useful in patients with biopsy-proven extracardiac sarcoidosis.[b]

Advanced cardiac imaging, CMR, or FDG–PET, at a center with experience in CS imaging protocols can be useful in patients with 1 or more abnormalities detected on initial screening by symptoms, ECG, or echocardiogram.

Class III recommendation

Advanced cardiac imaging, CMR, or FDG–PET, is not recommended for patients without abnormalities on initial screening by symptoms, ECG, or echocardiogram.

   [a] Palpitations are defined as "a prominent patient complaint lasting greater than 2 weeks."[25]
   [b] Echocardiographic findings suggestive of cardiac involvement include ventricular dysfunction, wall motion abnormalities, aneurysms, or basal septal thinning.
   From Birnie DH, Sauer WH, Bogun F, et al. HRS expert consensus statement on the diagnosis and management of arrhythmias associated with cardiac sarcoidosis. Heart Rhythm 2014;11(7):1307; with permission.

PROGNOSIS

Patients with CS have a poorer prognosis than patients without cardiac involvement.[34] In Japan, CS is reported to be responsible for as many as 85% of deaths from sarcoidosis.[35] Cardiac death is due to either heart failure or sudden cardiac death (SCD). Sadek and colleagues[36] recently published a systematic review of mortality data in patients with clinically manifest CS. The extent of left ventricular (LV) dysfunction seems to be the most important predictor of survival.[36] For example, Yazaki and colleagues[8] reported that 89% of patients with normal LV ejection fraction (LVEF) were alive at 10 years; patients with depressed LVEF had a 10-year survival rate of 27%. Similarly, Chiu and colleagues[37] found that all patients with normal LVEF were alive at 10 years; in patients with severe dysfunction (LVEF <30%), the survival rate was 91% after 1 year, 57% after 5 years, and 19% after 10 years. However, these data were published in 2001[8] and 2005.[37] Contemporary outcomes are likely to be better with modern heart failure therapies and broader use of implantable cardioverter-defibrillators (ICDs) for SCD prevention.

Seven studies looked at the prognosis of clinically silent CS. Five studies, including a total of 286 subjects, found that subjects with clinically silent CS have a completely benign course (no cardiac events for an average of 23 months).[7,13,25,38,39] Two studies, however, reported starkly contrasting findings.[14,15] Patel and colleagues[15] followed 81 subjects with biopsy-proven extracardiac sarcoidosis and detected clinically silent myocardial involvement in 21 out of 81 (26%) subjects. Subjects were followed for 21 months; there were 4 out of 21 (19%) cardiac deaths in subjects with clinically

---

Box 3
Screening for cardiac sarcoidosis in patients with specific cardiac presentations

There are several situations in which cardiac presentations can be the first and/or an unrecognized manifestation of sarcoidosis:

1. Idiopathic advanced conduction system disease in younger patients (age <60 years)[28,29]

2. Sustained monomorphic ventricular tachycardia of unknown cause[30]

3. Arrhythmogenic right ventricular cardiomyopathy.[21,31–33]

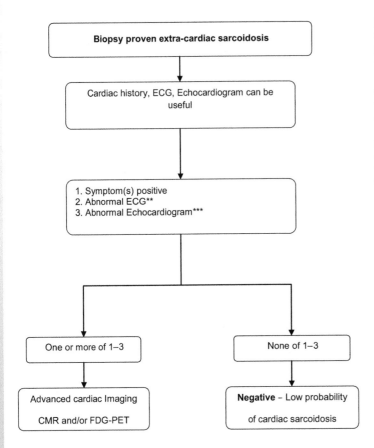

Fig. 1. Suggested algorithm of investigation for patients with biopsy-proven extracardiac sarcoidosis. ** abnormal ECG defined as complete left or right bundle branch block and/or presence of unexplained pathological Q waves in 2 or more leads and/or sustained 2 or 3 degree AV block and/or sustained or non-sustained VT; *** abnormal echocardiogram defined as RWMA and/or wall aneurysm and/or basal septum thinning and/or LVEF < 40%. (*From* Birnie DH, Sauer WH, Bogun F, et al. HRS expert consensus statement on the diagnosis and management of arrhythmias associated with cardiac sarcoidosis. Heart Rhythm 2014; 11(7):1309; with permission.)

silent CS. In 2014, Greulich and colleagues[14] reported on 155 consecutive subjects with systemic sarcoidosis diagnosed by biopsy and/or clinical criteria who underwent CMR. Primary endpoints were death, aborted SCD, and appropriate ICD therapy. The median follow-up time was 2.6 years. Clinically silent CS was found in 39 subjects (25.5%) and 11 of 39 (28.2%) had a primary endpoint (all cardiac) in follow-up.[14] Hence, there is considerable controversy in the literature about the prognosis of patients with clinically silent CS. The prognosis of clinically silent CS is a key clinical question with very important relevance to large numbers of patients. This question can only be answered by a multicenter prospective study with excellent epidemiologic methodology and such studies are ongoing (NCT01477359).

CLINICAL MANAGEMENT: ROLE OF IMMUNOSUPPRESSION

Sadek and colleagues[36] recently published a systematic review of corticosteroids in the treatment of CS. Only 10 articles met the inclusion criteria; there were no randomized trials and all publications were of poor to fair quality. In the 10 reports,

257 subjects received corticosteroids and 42 subjects did not. Eight articles had data on atrioventricular (AV) block, 4 reported on LV function recovery; 2 reported on ventricular arrhythmia burden; and 9 reported on mortality. Twenty-seven of 57 subjects (47.4%) with corticosteroids had improvements in AV conduction. In contrast, 16 subjects were not treated with corticosteroids and 0 of 16 improved.[36] Overall, the data quality was too limited to draw clear conclusions for any outcome. Despite the paucity of data immunosuppression (primarily with corticosteroids), therapy has been advocated for the treatment of CS by most experts for many years.[1,2,40] However, the optimal doses of corticosteroids and how best to assess response to therapy is not known. Also, it is unknown whether all patients with CS should be treated or only those with clinically manifest disease.

Role of FDG-PET Imaging to Guide Immunosuppression

FDG-PET is a glucose analog that is useful in differentiating between normal and active inflammatory lesions in which the activated proinflammatory macrophages show a higher metabolic rate and glucose utilization.[41] Although no individual clinical finding is pathognomonic for the diagnosis, FDG–PET has gained interest in the functional imaging of inflammatory disease activity to assess fibrogranulomatous disease in the myocardium. Focal or focal-on-diffuse ^{18}F-FDG uptake patterns suggest active CS.[42–44] Also, FDG–PET may be able to identify ongoing active inflammation and potentially detect reversible stages of CS.[44] Furthermore, it has been suggested that PET might be useful as a disease activity marker to guide CS therapy.[2]

FDG–PET testing should be done at a center with experience in CS imaging protocols.[16] The suppression of physiologic ^{18}F-FDG uptake in the cardiac muscle is a key factor.[45] Various preparation and imaging protocols have been used.[45–48] Recently, the Japanese Society of Nuclear Medicine published a consensus guidelines.[45] **Fig. 2** shows serial FDG–PET scans with progressive decline in cardiac ^{18}F-FDG uptake after immunosuppression. **Fig. 3** shows fused FDG–PET and CMR images.

One study showed no significant difference in prognosis in subjects treated with greater than 40 mg or prednisone per day compared with those treated with 30 mg of prednisone or less.[8] Hence, most experts suggest an initial dose of 30 to 40 mg per day.[49] The response to treatment should be evaluated after 1 to 3 months. If there has been a response, the prednisone dose should be tapered to 5 to 15 mg per day, with treatment planned for an additional 9 to 12 months.[49] Other investigators have suggested an initial dose of 1 mg/kg/d.[50] Patients should followed for at least 3 years after discontinuing treatment to assess for relapse.[50]

For patients with clinically manifest disease, the lead author initially treats with 0.5 mg/kg/d (maximum dose 40 mg) and repeat FDG–PET scan after 2 to 3 months of treatment. If the 2 to 3 month FDG–PET is positive, increasing the steroid dose to 1 mg/kg/d or adding a second agent is considered. If the 2 to 3 month FDG–PET is negative, the steroids are tapered over 3 months to 0.2 mg/kg/d to continue for 9 months for a total of 12 months of treatment. LV function is followed at 6, 12, 18, and 36 months and repeating FDG–PET is considered if LVEF falls significantly. See **Fig. 4** for treatment algorithm (**Box 4**, **Table 1**).

MANAGEMENT OF LEFT VENTRICULAR DYSFUNCTION

The effect of corticosteroids on LV function has been reported in 4 studies.[37,51–53] The summary of the data[36] suggests that corticosteroid therapy is associated with

1. Maintenance of LV function in subjects with normal function at diagnosis
2. Improvement in LVEF in subjects with mild to moderate LV dysfunction
3. No improvement in subjects with severe LV dysfunction.

However, it is unclear whether the positive outcomes were secondary to corticosteroid therapy or simply the natural history of the disease.[36] Again, clearly much remains to be learned about the role of corticosteroids in improving or preserving LV function. However, many physicians use immunosuppression in patients with LV dysfunction and evidence of ongoing myocardial inflammation.

Patients with CS and LV dysfunction should also be treated with all standard heart failure medical and device therapies, including heart transplantation. Recurrent disease has been reported in the transplanted heart[54] but this is rare and long-term patient outcomes are similar to control groups.[55]

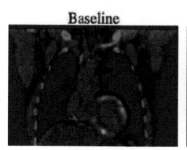
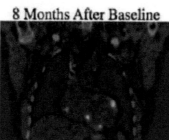
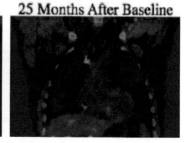

Baseline   **8 Months After Baseline**   **25 Months After Baseline**

Fig. 2. Serial FDG PET examinations showing change in inflammation. The results of the 3 serial studies over 25 months from a 46-year-old man treated with corticosteroids are shown. The color maps demonstrate the intensity of ^{18}F-FDG uptake in a coronal view. (*Adapted from* Osborne MT, Hulten EA, Singh A, et al. Reduction in F-fluorodeoxyglucose uptake on serial cardiac positron emission tomography is associated with improved left ventricular ejection fraction in patients with cardiac sarcoidosis. J Nucl Cardiol 2014;21(1):173; with permission.)

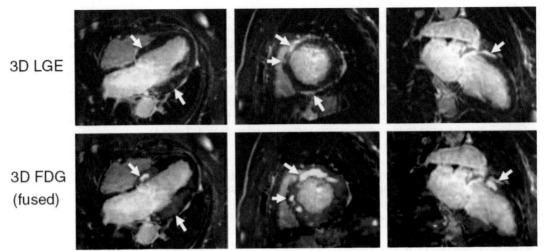

3D LGE

3D FDG
(fused)

Fig. 3. CMR images for respective 4-chamber, short-axis, and 2-chamber orientations showing 3-dimensional (3D) LGE scar imaging. White arrows indicate regions of abnormal LGE, consistent with mature scar. Bottom row shows 3D LGE images with fusion of FDG-PET signal suggestive of active inflammation surrounding regions of established scar.

MANAGEMENT OF CONDUCTION ABNORMALITIES

Advanced AV block is a common presentation of clinically manifest CS due to the involvement of the basal septum by scar tissue, granulomas, or the involvement of the nodal artery.[6] Furthermore, it can be the first manifestation of sarcoidosis in any organ. A recent study from Finland reported on 72 young subjects (age <55 years) with unexplained, new onset, significant conduction system disease. Biopsy-verified CS was found in 14 out of 72 (19%), probable CS in 4 out of 72 (6%), and giant cell myocarditis in 4 out of 72 (6%). Subjects with CS had significantly poorer prognoses

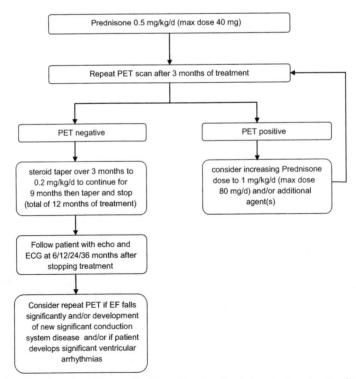

Fig. 4. Treatment algorithm for clinically manifest CS at lead author's institution. EF, ejection fraction.

Box 4
Clinical situations in which immunosuppression should be considered in patients with cardiac sarcoidosis

- In patients presenting with Mobitz II or third-degree heart block (see consensus recommendations)[16]
- In patients with frequent ventricular ectopy or nonsustained ventricular arrhythmias and evidence of myocardial inflammation (see consensus recommendations)[16]
- In patients with sustained ventricular arrhythmias and evidence of myocardial inflammation (see consensus recommendations)[16]
- In patients with LV dysfunction and evidence of myocardial inflammation.

---

compared with the subjects with idiopathic chronic heart block.[28] Nery and colleagues[56] presented similar data from a tertiary Canadian center. They prospectively evaluated patients aged 18 to 60 years who presented unexplained Mobitz II or third-degree AV block and no previous history of sarcoidosis. CS was diagnosed in 11 out of 32 (34%) patients. During an average follow-up of 21 plus or minus 9 months, major adverse cardiac events occurred in 3 patients with CS and none in subjects with idiopathic AV block (**Box 5**).[56]

MANAGEMENT OF VENTRICULAR ARRHYTHMIAS
Mechanisms of Ventricular Arrhythmias

Triggered activity and abnormal automaticity have been described secondary to myocardial inflammation in myocarditis.[59,60] These nonreentrant ventricular arrhythmias are also observed clinically in patients with CS presenting with frequent ventricular ectopy. Some of these patients had a reduction in arrhythmia burden following corticosteroids.[53,61] However, the most common mechanism is likely to be macroreentrant arrhythmias around areas of granulomatous scar.[61–63] Active inflammation may play a role in promoting monomorphic ventricular tachycardia (VT) due to reentry, either by triggering it with ventricular ectopy[61] or by slowing conduction in diseased tissue within granulomatous scar.[53,64]

The Role of Immunosuppression

Despite modest data, immunosuppression with corticosteroids is often used in patients with ventricular arrythmias.[36] Several studies have suggested a benefit of immunosuppression,[53,63,65] whereas others failed to show benefit.[66] Furthermore, a worsening of ventricular arrhythmias has also been reported with steroid therapy in a few patients.[67,68] The use of corticosteroids has also been linked to aneurysm formation.[6] Some data suggest that immunosuppression may be more beneficial for ventricular arrhythmias in the early disease phase, in the presence of preserved LV function.[51,53]

Ablation for Ventricular Arrhythmias

Jefic and colleagues[63] described the role of radiofrequency catheter ablation in 9 subjects with CS after immunosuppression failed to control VT. Most of the VTs were due to a reentrant mechanism and were mapped using entrainment mapping and pace mapping. Ablation outcomes in the study by Jefic and colleagues[63] were favorable, with either elimination of VT recurrences or reductions in the VT burden. In contrast, Koplan and colleagues[62] reported recurrences of VT in most subjects.

A stepwise approach has been described in a registry of 42 patients with CS and VT.[63] The steps were initial treatment with immunosuppression;

Table 1
Suggested use of advanced imaging modalities in various clinical scenarios

Clinical Scenario	Suggested Test
Screening younger patients (age <60 y) with acute presentation of idiopathic advanced conduction system disease	FDG–PET
Screening for cardiac involvement in patients with extracardiac sarcoidosis and 1 initially abnormal screening test	MRI
To follow response to steroids or immunosuppression	FDG–PET
To assess for active disease in patients with manifest CS and increased ventricular arrhythmia burden	FDG–PET

In patients with VT/ventricular fibrillation storm, it is suggested that initial treatment be a combination of antiarrhythmic medication (usually amiodarone) and immunosuppression (if there is evidence of active inflammation). If the clinical situation or setting does not permit an urgent FDG–PET scan, empiric immunosuppression should be given. If the ventricular arrhythmias cannot be adequately controlled with these measures, VT ablation should be considered, even if there is active inflammation.

RISK STRATIFICATION FOR SUDDEN CARDIAC DEATH

Patients with CS are at risk of sudden death and there are few data to help with risk stratification. **Fig. 5** from the recent consensus document[16] shows suggested approach to risk stratification and when to consider ICD implantation.

Left Ventricular Function

Perhaps because of its element of active granulomatous inflammation, and perhaps because of the variable involvement of the LV and/or the right ventricular, CS may not behave in the same fashion as do other types of nonischemic cardiomyopathy with regard to ventricular arrhythmias, LVEF, and sudden death risk. For example, CS patient cohorts seem to have more frequent ICD therapies than other populations. In the 3 large published series, annualized appropriate therapy rates were 8.6%, 13.2%, and 14.5%, respectively.[69–71] All 3 studies examined associations with appropriate ICD therapies. The only consistent finding was

followed by antiarrhythmic medication; and, finally, catheter ablation if VT persisted. Medical therapy with corticosteroids alone or in combination with antiarrhythmic therapy effectively suppressed ventricular arrhythmias in 33 out of 42 subjects. In the remaining 9 subjects, catheter ablation was performed and resulted in effective arrhythmia suppression in most.[63] Recent consensus document recommended this stepwise approach to ventricular arrhythmias (**Box 6**).

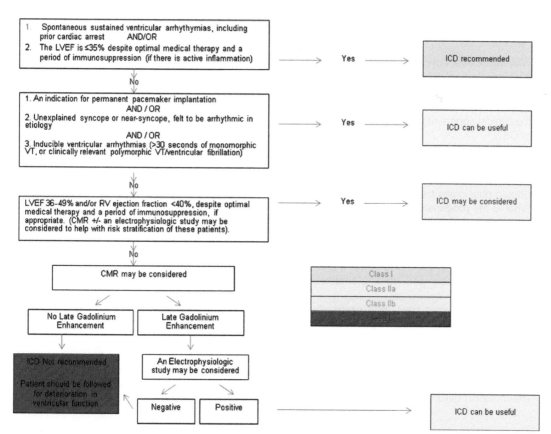

Fig. 5. Consensus recommendations for ICD implantations in patients diagnosed with CS. (*From* Birnie DH, Sauer WH, Bogun F, et al. HRS expert consensus statement on the diagnosis and management of arrhythmias associated with cardiac sarcoidosis. Heart Rhythm 2014;11(7):1318; with permission.)

that a lower LVEF was associated with appropriate ICD therapy. However, is should be noted that patients with mildly impaired LV function also had substantial risk of arrhythmia.[69–71]

Cardiac Magnetic Resonance

CMR is increasingly being used for the assessment of clinically silent CS in view of its ability to identify small regions of myocardial damage even in individuals with preserved LV systolic function (see **Fig. 3** for an example and previous discussion for more detail).[72]

MANAGEMENT OF ATRIAL ARRHYTHMIAS

The true frequency of atrial arrhythmias in CS is unknown.[6,73] It is also not clear whether atrial arrhythmias associated with CS are due to inflammation and/or scarring, or are secondary to LV dysfunction. An important clinical problem associated with atrial arrhythmias in CS is the risk of inappropriate ICD therapy.[69–71] Evidence regarding immunosuppression for the treatment of atrial arrhythmias in sarcoidosis patients is

limited to case reports.[74,75] There are no data on the risk of thromboembolism in sarcoidosis patients with atrial fibrillation or the effect of anticoagulation in this group. Hence it is suggested to apply guidelines for thromboprophylaxis in nonvalvular atrial fibrillation.[16] There are no specific data to guide antiarrhythmic drug selection in patients with CS. Beta blocker, calcium-channel blockers, sotalol, dofetilide, and amiodarone can be used. Class I agents are not recommended because patients with CS usually have myocardial scarring. Data on catheter ablation of atrial arrhythmias in CS are too scarce to guide reccommendations.[75]

SUMMARY AND FUTURE DIRECTIONS

Much remains to be learned about how to best diagnose and manage patients with CS. The recent expert consensus concluded with, "in this document we attempted to summarize the few things we currently know and to make the best possible recommendations. Equally importantly the document highlights the many knowledge gaps that still exist."[16]

Key unresolved questions include, but are not limited to[16]

1. What is the effect of corticosteroid treatment on the clinical course of the various manifestations of CS?
2. What is the effect of other immunotherapy on the clinical course of the various manifestations of CS?
3. What is the best, most cost-effective method to screen for CS? How frequently should patients be screened?
4. Should physicians treat clinically silent CS?
5. What is the prognosis of clinically silent CS?
6. How can physicians prevent SCD in CS? How should physicians stratify the risk for SCD? Who should receive ICDs?
7. What is the role of advanced imaging (PET and CMR) in diagnosis and guiding treatment of CS?
8. How can physicians best treat ventricular arrhythmias in CS? Should physicians treat ongoing inflammation before or after catheter ablation?
9. How can physicians best treat atrial arrhythmias in CS? Should physicians treat ongoing inflammation before or after catheter ablation?

REFERENCES

1. Ayyala US, Nair AP, Padilla ML. Cardiac sarcoidosis. Clin Chest Med 2008;29(3):493–508, ix.
2. Dubrey SW, Falk RH. Diagnosis and management of cardiac sarcoidosis. Prog Cardiovasc Dis 2010; 52(4):336–46.
3. Chapelon-Abric C, de ZD, Duhaut P, et al. Cardiac sarcoidosis: a retrospective study of 41 cases. Medicine (Baltimore) 2004;83(6):315–34.
4. Fleming HA, McMahon JN, McCarthy CF, et al. Sarcoid heart disease. Br Heart J 1983;50(5):498.
5. Matsui Y, Iwai K, Tachibana T, et al. Clinicopathological study of fatal myocardial sarcoidosis. Ann N Y Acad Sci 1976;278:455–69.
6. Roberts WC, McAllister HA Jr, Ferrans VJ. Sarcoidosis of the heart. A clinicopathologic study of 35 necropsy patients (group 1) and review of 78 previously described necropsy patients (group 11). Am J Med 1977;63(1):86–108.
7. Smedema JP, Snoep G, van Kroonenburgh MP, et al. Cardiac involvement in patients with pulmonary sarcoidosis assessed at two university medical centers in the Netherlands. Chest 2005; 128(1):30–5.
8. Yazaki Y, Isobe M, Hiroe M, et al. Prognostic determinants of long-term survival in Japanese patients with cardiac sarcoidosis treated with prednisone. Am J Cardiol 2001;88(9):1006–10.
9. Uusimaa P, Ylitalo K, Anttonen O, et al. Ventricular tachyarrhythmia as a primary presentation of sarcoidosis. Europace 2008;10(6):760–6.
10. Iwai K, Tachibana T, Takemura T, et al. Pathological studies on sarcoidosis autopsy. I. Epidemiological features of 320 cases in Japan. Acta Pathol Jpn 1993;43(7–8):372–6.
11. Iwai K, Takemura T, Kitaichi M, et al. Pathological studies on sarcoidosis autopsy. II. Early change, mode of progression and death pattern. Acta Pathol Jpn 1993;43(7–8):377–85.
12. Perry A, Vuitch F. Causes of death in patients with sarcoidosis. A morphologic study of 38 autopsies with clinicopathologic correlations. Arch Pathol Lab Med 1995;119(2):167–72.
13. Nagai T, Kohsaka S, Okuda S, et al. Incidence and prognostic significance of myocardial late gadolinium enhancement in patients with sarcoidosis without cardiac manifestation. Chest 2014;146(4):1064–72.
14. Greulich S, Deluigi CC, Gloekler S, et al. CMR imaging predicts death and other adverse events in suspected cardiac sarcoidosis. JACC Cardiovasc Imaging 2013;6(4):501–11.
15. Patel MR, Cawley PJ, Heitner JF, et al. Detection of myocardial damage in patients with sarcoidosis. Circulation 2009;120(20):1969–77.
16. Birnie DH, Sauer WH, Bogun F, et al. HRS expert consensus statement on the diagnosis and management of arrhythmias associated with cardiac sarcoidosis. Heart Rhythm 2014;11(7):1305–23.
17. Hiraga H, Hiroe M, Iwai K. Guideline for Diagnosis of Cardiac Sarcoidosis: Study Report on Diffuse Pulmonary Diseases. Tokyo, Japan: The Japanese Ministry of Health and Welfare; 1993. p. 23–4.
18. Judson MA, Baughman RP, Teirstein AS, et al. Defining organ involvement in sarcoidosis: the ACCESS proposed instrument. ACCESS Research Group. A case control etiologic study of sarcoidosis. Sarcoidosis Vasc Diffuse Lung Dis 1999;16(1):75–86.
19. Ardehali H, Howard DL, Hariri A, et al. A positive endomyocardial biopsy result for sarcoid is associated with poor prognosis in patients with initially unexplained cardiomyopathy. Am Heart J 2005;150(3):459–63.
20. Cooper LT, Baughman KL, Feldman AM, et al. The role of endomyocardial biopsy in the management of cardiovascular disease: a scientific statement from the American Heart Association, the American College of Cardiology, and the European Society of Cardiology. Circulation 2007;116(19):2216–33.
21. Nery PB, Keren A, Healey J, et al. Isolated cardiac sarcoidosis: establishing the diagnosis with electro-anatomic mapping- guided endomyocardial biopsy. Can J Cardiol 2013;29(8):1015.e1–3.
22. Kandolin R, Lehtonen J, Graner M, et al. Diagnosing isolated cardiac sarcoidosis. J Intern Med 2011; 270(5):461–8.

23. Leone O, Veinot JP, Angelini A, et al. 2011 consensus statement on endomyocardial biopsy from the Association for European Cardiovascular Pathology and the Society for Cardiovascular Pathology. Cardiovasc Pathol 2012;21(4):245–74.

24. Judson MA, Organ Assessment Instrument Investigators. The WASOG Sarcoidosis Organ Assessment Instrument: an update of a previous clinical tool. Sarcoidosis Vasc Diffuse Lung Dis 2014; 31(1):19–27.

25. Mehta D, Lubitz SA, Frankel Z, et al. Cardiac involvement in patients with sarcoidosis: diagnostic and prognostic value of outpatient testing. Chest 2008; 133(6):1426–35.

26. Schuller JL, Lowery CM, Zipse M, et al. Diagnostic utility of signal-averaged electrocardiography for detection of cardiac sarcoidosis. Ann Noninvasive Electrocardiol 2011;16(1):70–6.

27. Schuller JL, Olson MD, Zipse MM, et al. Electrocardiographic characteristics in patients with pulmonary sarcoidosis indicating cardiac involvement. J Cardiovasc Electrophysiol 2011;22(11):1243–8.

28. Kandolin R, Lehtonen J, Kupari M. Cardiac sarcoidosis and giant cell myocarditis as causes of atrioventricular block in young and middle-aged adults. Circ Arrhythm Electrophysiol 2011;4(3): 303–9.

29. Nery PB, Beanlands RS, Nair GM, et al. Atrioventricular block as the initial manifestation of cardiac sarcoidosis in middle-aged adults. J Cardiovasc Electrophysiol 2014;25(8):875–81.

30. Nery PB, Mc Ardle BA, Redpath CJ, et al. Prevalence of cardiac sarcoidosis in patients presenting with monomorphic ventricular tachycardia. Pacing Clin Electrophysiol 2014;37(3):364–74.

31. Santucci PA, Morton JB, Picken MM, et al. Electroanatomic mapping of the right ventricle in a patient with a giant epsilon wave, ventricular tachycardia, and cardiac sarcoidosis. J Cardiovasc Electrophysiol 2004;15(9):1091–4.

32. Vasaiwala SC, Finn C, Delpriore J, et al. Prospective study of cardiac sarcoid mimicking arrhythmogenic right ventricular dysplasia. J Cardiovasc Electrophysiol 2009;20(5):473–6.

33. Philips B, Madhavan S, James CA, et al. Arrhythmogenic right ventricular dysplasia/cardiomyopathy and cardiac sarcoidosis: distinguishing features when the diagnosis is unclear. Circ Arrhythm Electrophysiol 2014;7(2):230–6.

34. Kim JS, Judson MA, Donnino R, et al. Cardiac sarcoidosis. Am Heart J 2009;157(1):9–21.

35. Sekiguchi M, Numao Y, Imai M, et al. Clinical and histopathological profile of sarcoidosis of the heart and acute idiopathic myocarditis. Concepts through a study employing endomyocardial biopsy. I. Sarcoidosis. Jpn Circ J 1980;44(4): 249–63.

36. Sadek MM, Yung D, Birnie DH, et al. Corticosteroid therapy for cardiac sarcoidosis: a systematic review. Can J Cardiol 2013;29(9):1034–41.

37. Chiu CZ, Nakatani S, Zhang G, et al. Prevention of left ventricular remodeling by long-term corticosteroid therapy in patients with cardiac sarcoidosis. Am J Cardiol 2005;95(1):143–6.

38. Dhote R, Vignaux O, Blanche P, et al. Value of MRI for the diagnosis of cardiac involvement in sarcoidosis. Rev Med Interne 2003;24(3):151–7 [in French].

39. Vignaux O, Dhote R, Duboc D, et al. Detection of myocardial involvement in patients with sarcoidosis applying T2- weighted, contrast-enhanced, and cine magnetic resonance imaging: initial results of a prospective study. J Comput Assist Tomogr 2002;26(5):762–7.

40. Grutters JC, van den Bosch JM. Corticosteroid treatment in sarcoidosis. Eur Respir J 2006;28(3): 627–36.

41. Pellegrino D, Bonab AA, Dragotakes SC, et al. Inflammation and infection: imaging properties of 18F-FDG-labeled white blood cells versus 18F-FDG. J Nucl Med 2005;46(9):1522–30.

42. Okumura W, Iwasaki T, Toyama T, et al. Usefulness of fasting 18F-FDG PET in identification of cardiac sarcoidosis. J Nucl Med 2004;45(12):1989–98.

43. Langah R, Spicer K, Gebregziabher M, et al. Effectiveness of prolonged fasting 18f-FDG PET-CT in the detection of cardiac sarcoidosis. J Nucl Cardiol 2009;16(5):801–10.

44. Ishimaru S, Tsujino I, Takei T, et al. Focal uptake on 18F-fluoro-2- deoxyglucose positron emission tomography images indicates cardiac involvement of sarcoidosis. Eur Heart J 2005;26(15):1538–43.

45. Ishida Y, Yoshinaga K, Miyagawa M, et al. Recommendations for (18)F-fluorodeoxyglucose positron emission tomography imaging for cardiac sarcoidosis: Japanese Society of Nuclear Cardiology recommendations. Ann Nucl Med 2014;28(4): 393–403.

46. Mc Ardle BA, Birnie DH, Klein R, et al. Is there an association between clinical presentation and the location and extent of myocardial involvement of cardiac sarcoidosis as assessed by ^{18}F-fluorodeoxyglucose positron emission tomography? Circ Cardiovasc Imaging 2013;6(5):617–26.

47. Mc Ardle BA, Leung E, Ohira H, et al. The role of F(18)-fluorodeoxyglucose positron emission tomography in guiding diagnosis and management in patients with known or suspected cardiac sarcoidosis. J Nucl Cardiol 2013;20(2):297–306.

48. Osborne MT, Hulten EA, Singh A, et al. Reduction in ^{18}F-fluorodeoxyglucose uptake on serial cardiac positron emission tomography is associated with improved left ventricular ejection fraction in patients with cardiac sarcoidosis. J Nucl Cardiol 2014;21(1): 166–74.

49. Iannuzzi MC, Rybicki BA, Teirstein AS. Sarcoidosis. N Engl J Med 2007;357(21):2153–65.

50. Valeyre D, Prasse A, Nunes H, et al. Sarcoidosis. Lancet 2014;383(9923):1155–67.

51. Kato Y, Morimoto S, Uemura A, et al. Efficacy of corticosteroids in sarcoidosis presenting with atrioventricular block. Sarcoidosis Vasc Diffuse Lung Dis 2003;20(2):133–7.

52. Kudoh H, Fujiwara S, Shiotani H, et al. Myocardial washout of 99mTc-tetrofosmin and response to steroid therapy in patients with cardiac sarcoidosis. Ann Nucl Med 2010;24(5):379–85.

53. Yodogawa K, Seino Y, Ohara T, et al. Effect of corticosteroid therapy on ventricular arrhythmias in patients with cardiac sarcoidosis. Ann Noninvasive Electrocardiol 2011;16(2):140–7.

54. Luk A, Lee A, Ahn E, et al. Cardiac sarcoidosis: recurrent disease in a heart transplant patient following pulmonary tuberculosis infection. Can J Cardiol 2010;26(7):e273–5.

55. Zaidi AR, Zaidi A, Vaitkus PT. Outcome of heart transplantation in patients with sarcoid cardiomyopathy. J Heart Lung Transplant 2007;26(7):714–7.

56. Nery PB, Healey JS, Beanlands RS. Middle aged patients with new onset atrioventricular block should be investigated for cardiac sarcoidosis. Heart Rhythm 2013;10:S447.

57. Epstein AE, Dimarco JP, Ellenbogen KA, et al. 2012 ACCF/AHA/HRS focused update incorporated into the ACCF/AHA/HRS 2008 guidelines for device-based therapy of cardiac rhythm abnormalities: a report of the American College of Cardiology Foundation/American Heart Association Task Force on Practice Guidelines and the Heart Rhythm Society. Circulation 2013;127(3):e283–352.

58. Erdmann E. Angina pectoris, pathological stress EKG and a normal coronary angiogram. Internist (Berl) 1980;21(3):165–8 [in German].

59. Berte B, Eyskens B, Meyfroidt G, et al. Bidirectional ventricular tachycardia in fulminant myocarditis. Europace 2008;10(6):767–8.

60. Tai YT, Lau CP, Fong PC, et al. Incessant automatic ventricular tachycardia complicating acute coxsackie B myocarditis. Cardiology 1992;80(5–6): 339–44.

61. Stees CS, Khoo MS, Lowery CM, et al. Ventricular tachycardia storm successfully treated with immunosuppression and catheter ablation in a patient with cardiac sarcoidosis. J Cardiovasc Electrophysiol 2010;22(2):210–3.

62. Koplan BA, Soejima K, Baughman K, et al. Refractory ventricular tachycardia secondary to cardiac sarcoid: electrophysiologic characteristics, mapping, and ablation. Heart Rhythm 2006;3(8):924–9.

63. Jefic D, Joel B, Good E, et al. Role of radiofrequency catheter ablation of ventricular tachycardia in cardiac sarcoidosis: report from a multicenter registry. Heart Rhythm 2009;6(2):189–95.

64. Tselentakis EV, Woodford E, Chandy J, et al. Inflammation effects on the electrical properties of atrial tissue and inducibility of postoperative atrial fibrillation. J Surg Res 2006;135(1):68–75.

65. Futamatsu H, Suzuki J, Adachi S, et al. Utility of gallium-67 scintigraphy for evaluation of cardiac sarcoidosis with ventricular tachycardia. Int J Cardiovasc Imaging 2006;22(3–4):443–8.

66. Winters SL, Cohen M, Greenberg S, et al. Sustained ventricular tachycardia associated with sarcoidosis: assessment of the underlying cardiac anatomy and the prospective utility of programmed ventricular stimulation, drug therapy and an implantable antitachycardia device. J Am Coll Cardiol 1991;18(4): 937–43.

67. Furushima H, Chinushi M, Sugiura H, et al. Ventricular tachyarrhythmia associated with cardiac sarcoidosis: its mechanisms and outcome. Clin Cardiol 2004;27(4):217–22.

68. Hiramitsu S, Morimoto S, Uemura A, et al. National survey on status of steroid therapy for cardiac sarcoidosis in Japan. Sarcoidosis Vasc Diffuse Lung Dis 2005;22(3):210–3.

69. Betensky BP, Tschabrunn CM, Zado ES, et al. Long-term follow-up of patients with cardiac sarcoidosis and implantable cardioverter-defibrillators. Heart Rhythm 2012;9(6):884–91.

70. Schuller JL, Zipse M, Crawford T, et al. Implantable cardioverter defibrillator therapy in patients with cardiac sarcoidosis. J Cardiovasc Electrophysiol 2012; 23(9):925–9.

71. Kron J, Sauer W, Schuller J, et al. Efficacy and safety of implantable cardiac defibrillators for treatment of ventricular arrhythmias in patients with cardiac sarcoidosis. Europace 2013;15(3):347–54.

72. Patel AR, Klein MR, Chandra S, et al. Myocardial damage in patients with sarcoidosis and preserved left ventricular systolic function: an observational study. Eur J Heart Fail 2011;13(11):1231–7.

73. Viles-Gonzalez JF, Pastori L, Fischer A, et al. Supraventricular arrhythmias in patients with cardiac sarcoidosis prevalence, predictors, and clinical implications. Chest 2013;143(4):1085–90.

74. Namboodiri N, Stiles MK, Young GD, et al. Electrophysiological features of atrial flutter in cardiac sarcoidosis: a report of two cases. Indian Pacing Electrophysiol J 2012;12(6):284–9.

75. Srivatsa UN, Rogers J. Sarcoidosis and atrial fibrillation: a rare association and interlink with inflammation. Indian Pacing Electrophysiol J 2012;12(6): 290–1.

Ocular Sarcoidosis

Sirichai Pasadhika, MD[a],*, James T. Rosenbaum, MD[b]

KEYWORDS

- Sarcoidosis • Eye • Uveitis • Dry eye • Optic neuropathy • Orbital inflammation

KEY POINTS

- Ocular sarcoidosis can involve any part of the eye and its adnexal tissues.
- The most common ocular manifestations are uveitis, dry eye, and conjunctival nodules.
- Ocular involvement is the presenting symptom in approximately 20% to 30% of patients with sarcoidosis.
- Multidisciplinary approaches are required to achieve the best treatment outcomes for both ocular and systemic manifestations.
- With appropriate treatment, visual prognosis is generally good.

Sarcoidosis can involve almost any structure within or around the eye. In addition, the first recognized clinical manifestation of sarcoidosis often is eye disease. Both ophthalmologists and nonophthalmologists need to be aware of the protean ocular manifestations of sarcoidosis.

EPIDEMIOLOGY

Ocular involvement of sarcoidosis has been known since the early 1900s and has become more recognized since the mid-1900s.[1] Variability in the diagnostic criteria has made epidemiologic studies of ocular sarcoidosis challenging.

The prevalence of ocular involvement in different series ranges widely from 13% (Turkish study) to 79% (Japanese study) in patients with systemic sarcoidosis.[2–4] Ocular involvement is the presenting symptom in approximately 20% to 30%.[5,6] Uveitis was reported in 30% to 70%, and conjunctival nodules were found in 40%.[2] In patients with systemic sarcoidosis, females (56%) were more likely to develop ocular involvement compared with males (23%) in a study of 121 patients with biopsy-proven sarcoidosis.[6]

Sarcoidosis reportedly may affect children, and most of these cases begin between the ages of 8 and 15 years.[7] Many patients, however, previously diagnosed as having early-onset sarcoidosis are now recognized as having Blau syndrome with de novo mutations.[8] Age distributions of ocular sarcoidosis in adults are bimodal. Two peaks of incidence are 20 to 30 years and 50 to 60 years.[2] The mean age at presentation of uveitis is 42 years (range, 4–82 years).[9] African Americans with biopsy-proven sarcoidosis have a higher likelihood of developing ocular involvement compared with Caucasians.[10] Race may also influence the age of onset of uveitis. Blacks tend to develop uveitis at a mean age of 35 to 44 years, whereas whites are more likely to have uveitis at a mean age of 43 to 52 years.[9,11]

Sarcoidosis accounted for approximately 1% to 3% of pediatric uveitis in referral centers,[12,13] whereas approximately 10% of adult uveitis was found to be associated with sarcoidosis.[14,15] An epidemiologic study in the southeastern United States showed that sarcoidosis was the cause of uveitis in 11% of the studied population (385 patients: 67% Caucasian and 31% African

Dr S. Pasadhika has no conflict of interests to disclose.
Dr J.T. Rosenbaum is a consultant for Abbvie, UCB, Genentech, Medimmune, Xoma, Portage, Auventx, Santen, Sanofi, and Regeneron.
[a] Vitreoretinal and Uveitis Service, Legacy Devers Eye Institute, 1040 Northwest 22nd Avenue Suite 168, Portland, OR 97210, USA; [b] Legacy Devers Eye Institute, 1040 Northwest 22nd Avenue Suite 168, Portland, OR 97210, USA
* Corresponding author.
E-mail address: spasadhi@LHS.ORG

American). Subgroup analysis demonstrated that sarcoidosis accounted for 25% of uveitis among the African American patients.[15]

Most sarcoid uveitis is bilateral, and approximately 90% are chronic.[9] The prevalence of uveitis subtype based on anatomic location varies among different studies, partly because of the different terminologies used. Dana and colleagues[9] reported that of 112 eyes with sarcoid uveitis, 28% were anterior, 38% were intermediate, 12% were posterior, and 22% were panuveitis. A Turkish study reported 46% as intermediate, 15% as anterior, and 38% as panuveitis.[16] Another study from Japan described 75% eyes with iritis and 67% eyes with retinal vasculitis.[4]

The rate of sarcoidosis in patients with multifocal chorioretinitis is variable because of the different diagnostic criteria and the extent of investigations among different studies. A study by Abad and colleagues[17] of 37 patients with multifocal chorioretinitis demonstrated a prevalence (68%) of biopsy-proven and presumed sarcoidosis, while Ossewaarde-Van Norel and colleagues[18] reported a 39% rate. Of note, 62% of patients in the former study received a chest computed tomographic (CT) scan,[17] but only 26% did in the latter.[18]

A Case-Control Etiologic Study of Sarcoidosis (ACCESS) presented evidence for the allelic variation at the HLA-DRB1 locus as a significant contributing factor for sarcoidosis. HLA-DRB1*0401 allele was associated with ocular involvement in both blacks and whites (odds ratio 3.49).[19]

CLINICAL MANIFESTATIONS OF OCULAR SARCOIDOSIS

Ocular disease may be the initial manifestation in patients with sarcoidosis and may cause severe visual impairment. The involvement may be characterized by granulomatous inflammation, which can affect any part of the eye and its adnexa. Examples of the clinical presentations of ocular sarcoidosis are listed in **Table 1**. The most common ocular manifestations are uveitis, dry eye, and conjunctival nodules.

Uveitis and Fundoscopic Abnormalities

Uveitis is the term used to describe an inflammation of the uveal tissues, which are composed of the iris, ciliary body, and choroid. Uveitis commonly affects tissue or space adjacent to the

Table 1
Examples of clinical manifestations of ocular sarcoidosis

Ocular Structures	Ophthalmic Manifestations
Eyelids	Eyelid granuloma, madarosis (loss of eyelashes), poliosis (whitening of lashes), entropion, trichiasis, lagoghthalmos (if associated with facial palsy)
Conjunctiva	Conjunctival nodules or granuloma, conjunctivitis, symblepharon, conjunctival cicatrization
Episclera/sclera	Episcleritis, scleritis
Cornea	Peripheral ulcerative keratitis, interstitial keratitis, exposure keratopathy, band keratopathy
Trabecular meshwork and anterior chamber angle	Trabecular granuloma, peripheral anterior synechiae, ocular hypertension, glaucoma
Iris	Anterior uveitis (iritis), iris nodules/granuloma, posterior synechiae, pupillary abnormalities
Lens	Cataract
Pars plana/vitreous	Intermediate uveitis
Retina	Retinitis, retinal vasculitis, macular edema
Choroid	Choroiditis, granuloma
Optic nerve	Papillitis, papilledema (increased intracranial pressure due to neurosarcoid), granuloma, optic neuropathy (compressive or infiltrative), optic atrophy
Lacrimal gland	Granuloma, dacryoadenitis, keratoconjunctivitis sicca (dry eye)
Nasolacrimal drainage system	Nasolacrimal duct obstruction
Extraocular muscles and other orbital tissues	Granuloma, strabismus, proptosis, optic nerve compression
Intracranial lesions involving visual pathway	Decreased vision, visual field defects, abnormal pupillary response, abnormal eye movement

uvea such as the anterior chamber, vitreous humor, or retina. Uveitis is most commonly classified by the anatomic location of the observed inflammation using slit lamp biomicroscopy and fundus examination. Uveitis associated with sarcoidosis can present as anterior, intermediate, posterior, or panuveitis. The most universally accepted uveitis classification, grading, and terminologies are published by the Standardization of Uveitis Nomenclature (SUN) Working Group.[20]

In fact, sarcoidosis is well known as a cause of granulomatous inflammation. One can be easily confused by multiple investigators who state that sarcoid uveitis can present as either nongranulomatous or granulomatous uveitis. These clinical pathologic terms are essentially misnomers, because they do not represent actual histopathologic studies. Granulomatous uveitis is used when at least one of the following clinical signs are observed: (1) large mutton-fat keratic precipitates (accumulation of inflammatory leukocytes that deposit on the corneal endothelium), (2) iris or trabecular meshwork nodules, or (3) choroidal granuloma. It is not uncommon that typical cases of sarcoid uveitis present with at least one of these findings. However, these signs may not be observed in all cases, especially in those with early onset, those with less-severe inflammation, or those who have been successfully treated. On the other hand, these signs are not specific for sarcoid uveitis because they may be noticed in uveitis related to other causes, such as infections. The study of 112 eyes with sarcoid uveitis depicted 81% with granulomatous pattern.[9]

Anterior chamber inflammation is perhaps the most common sign of sarcoid uveitis, and it was detected in 42 (91%) of 46 patients with biopsy-proven sarcoid uveitis in one study.[1] Of those 42 patients, 16 (38%) had inflammation only in the anterior chamber, without posterior segment involvement.[1] Typical clinical presentations in patients with acute anterior chamber inflammation may include redness, decreased vision, eye pain, and photophobia. The degrees of inflammation may be variable from mild to very severe. However, the development of hypopyon (pus in the anterior chamber) is unlikely.[21] Pain can be caused by ciliary spasm or elevated intraocular pressure (IOP). IOP elevation can be secondary to an obstruction of trabecular meshwork by many inflammatory leukocytes, trabecular meshwork nodules and inflammation, or peripheral anterior synechiae (adhesion of the peripheral iris to the peripheral cornea preventing aqueous outflow through the trabecular meshwork in the affected area). In cases with moderate and severe inflammation, posterior synechiae (adhesion of the iris

to the anterior lens capsule) may form and cause an irregular and poorly dilated pupil, which may prevent detailed examination of the posterior segment. Iris nodules are generally associated with moderate or severe inflammation. Without appropriate treatment, severe anterior uveitis can lead to anterior segment deformity and predispose to cataract formation. However, mild sarcoid uveitis may also be insidious in onset, and the patients can be asymptomatic. The diagnosis may only be made on screening or routine ocular examination. Early detection is crucial to potentially prevent sequelae from chronic inflammation.

Intermediate uveitis is also a common presentation of ocular sarcoidosis. Patients may complain of floaters and/or blurry vision. Vitreous opacity and cystoid macular edema (CME) are the leading causes of decreased vision in patients with intermediate uveitis. Pars plana exudates and accumulation of white blood cells and vitreous debris on the retinal surface may be characterized as snow banks and snow balls (also called, string of pearls) on examination. Neovascularization of the optic disc and peripheral retina can also complicate peripheral retinal involvement[22] and can lead to vitreous hemorrhage in a minority of cases.

In sarcoid posterior uveitis, the retinal lesions usually accompany choroidal inflammation; however, either retinal or choroidal involvement can be isolated (**Fig. 1**). Posterior involvement is generally bilateral, but can be largely asymmetric. Choroidal granulomas may be unifocal or multifocal and may vary in size from small (Dalen-Fuchs-like nodules or sarcoid spots) to large (may simulate choroidal tumors).[23,24] Peripheral granulomas are unlikely to cause visual disturbance, but central lesions may lead to severe visual impairment. Choroidal neovascularization can develop in such lesions.[25] Multifocal choroiditis related to sarcoidosis can present with fundoscopic findings very similar to those seen in birdshot chorioretinopathy.[26] Exudative retinal detachment can rarely be seen in patients with ocular sarcoidosis, particularly in those with large chorioretinal granulomas. Treated or inactive lesions may be noticeable as multifocal peripheral small punched-out chorioretinal scars similar to those observed in idiopathic multifocal choroiditis. Retinal pigment epithelial changes are observed in many cases but do not usually cause visual loss.[22] However, extensive involvement in the posterior pole may cause severe permanent visual disability (**Fig. 2**).

Perivascular sheathing is a common finding representing retinal vasculitis associated with ocular sarcoidosis. Midperipheral periphlebitis is characteristic. In severe forms with scattered

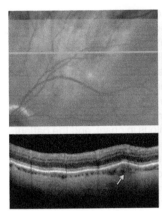
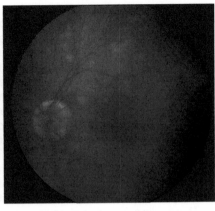

Fig. 1. (*Right*) Color fundus photograph of a 59-year-old male patient with multifocal choroiditis secondary to sarcoidosis demonstrates multiple round, creamy, subretinal lesions in the superotemporal quadrant of the left eye. (*Left*) Optical coherence tomography study through the lesion showed that the lesion primarily involves the choroid (*arrow*).

whitish-yellow perivascular retinal exudates along the retinal veins, the perivascular exudates have been described as candle-wax drippings.[24] Generally, periphlebitis in ocular sarcoidosis is not associated with significant vascular occlusion. However, occlusive retinal vascular diseases, such as branch and central retinal vein occlusion, have been reported. Intraretinal hemorrhages and retinal or optic disc neovascularization with subsequent vitreous hemorrhage may complicate retinal vasculitis secondary to sarcoidosis.

CME is a common cause of vision loss in patients with sarcoid uveitis, and it may accompany severe active inflammation or retinal vasculitis in the posterior pole. CME generally responds to corticosteroid therapy. Epiretinal membrane formation can also occur.

The incidence of central nervous system involvement increased from 2% to 37% when fundoscopic abnormalities of ocular sarcoidosis were observed in a study.[24] However, another study did not find such an association.[22]

Optic Nerve Involvement and Neuroophthalmic Manifestations

Neurosarcoidosis is sometimes called the great imitator because it can cause nonspecific and variable symptoms simulating many other conditions. The symptoms are associated with the location of granuloma formation and related inflammatory sequelae. These symptoms may include decreased vision or visual field defects secondary to involvement of the optic nerve and its visual pathway, papilledema (see below) secondary to increased intracranial pressure, abnormal eye movement, pupillary abnormalities, visual hallucinations, encephalopathy, vasculopathy, peripheral neuropathy, myopathy, seizure, aseptic meningitis, hydrocephalus, spinal cord involvement, and psychiatric symptoms.[27]

Cranial neuropathy is the most frequent manifestation of neurosarcoidosis. The most commonly affected nerves are the optic and facial nerves.[28] Involvement of the optic nerve may be visible as optic nerve granulomas or nodules, optic disc edema, or optic atrophy. Besides resulting from increased intracranial pressure secondary to space-occupying lesions or hydrocephalus, optic disc edema can be associated with either severe posterior uveitis or periphlebitis, or direct involvement of the optic disc, nerve, or nerve sheath by granulomatous tissue.[29] Irreversibly impaired visual acuity occurs in more than half of those with direct optic nerve involvement.[30] Facial paresis is a classic manifestation; it was believed to be related to either inflammation in the parotid gland, a result of a meningitic reaction, or direct compression.[30] Lower motor neuron facial nerve paresis can cause ipsilateral poor eyelid tone and closure, which may lead to exposure keratopathy, epiphora, and ectropion. Severe surface abnormalities can progress to corneal ulcers with permanent blindness.

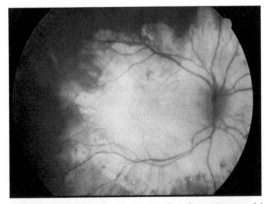

Fig. 2. Color fundus photograph of a 56-year-old male patient with extensive chorioretinal atrophy and scar secondary to long-standing involvement from ocular sarcoidosis.

Acquired abnormal ocular movements such as nystagmus may be observed in neurosarcoidosis.[31] Pupillary abnormalities, such as a relative pupillary defect and light-near dissociation, as well as visual hallucinations have been reported in sarcoidosis with central nervous system involvement.[32]

Eyelid and Ocular Surface Disease

Dermatologic manifestations of sarcoidosis are well known. Partial- or full-thickness involvement of the eyelid may be seen. Periorbital erythematous eyelid swelling can be present as the only sign of ocular sarcoidosis.[33,34] Erythematous eyelid mass lesions may vary in size from small papules[35] to a large mass, which may mimic eyelid tumors or cutaneous scars.[36] Collins and colleagues[37] reported a case of a 50-year-old woman with systemic sarcoidosis, including pulmonary, dermatologic, and articular symptoms. The patient had chronic eyelid nodules, which subsequently caused eye irritation and eyelid deformities with mucocutaneous notching. She had extensive scarring of the posterior lamella causing entropion and trichiasis. The patient underwent full-thickness wedge resection to treat eyelash malposition. Histopathologic study showed full-thickness noncaseating granuloma of the eyelid. A similar case was reported by Moin and coworkers[38] in a 43-year-old African American man. The patient had distorted eyelid architecture with madarosis, marked forniceal foreshortening, and symblepharon. Eyelid, conjunctiva, and facial skin biopsies demonstrated noncaseating granulomatous inflammation. Extensive destruction of the eyelid was partially treated with corticosteroids and methotrexate, before performing reconstruction surgery.[38] Rarely, granulomatous inflammation may selectively involve small eyelid structure such as the Müller muscle, and such lesion may cause eyelid retraction, which is far more commonly seen in patients with thyroid orbitopathy.[39]

Conjunctival involvement is common but may be overlooked because most conjunctival lesions are asymptomatic. Most typical conjunctival nodules are observed at the palpebral conjunctivae; however, they may also be located at the bulbar or perilimbal areas.[40] Early lesions may present as multiple, white, discrete bulbar conjunctival deposits.[41] Some patients may have significant redness and irritation and present as acute follicular conjunctivitis.[42,43] Cases with chronic cicatricial conjunctivitis with progressive scarring and symblepharon have also been reported.[44,45] Large conjunctival granuloma may simulate conjunctival tumors.[46]

Scleritis is uncommonly associated with sarcoidosis, but sarcoidosis should be considered in the differential diagnosis of scleritis. Sarcoidosis-associated scleritis may present as anterior diffuse,[47] anterior nodular,[47–49] or posterior scleritis.[50] All the reported cases were women with age ranging from 53 to 64 years[47–49] who were on average older than most patients with sarcoid uveitis, except 1 patient (42-year-old man) with posterior scleritis who also had annular ciliochoroidal effusion.[50] Sarcoidosis-associated scleritis is more likely nonnecrotizing and tends to respond well to oral corticosteroids. A clinicopathologic study of 55 patients who were diagnosed with necrotizing scleritis showed that only 1 patient (1.8%) had sarcoidosis. Although the patient presented clinically with necrotizing scleritis, the biopsy demonstrated discrete nonnecrotizing granulomatous inflammation.[51]

The cornea can also be affected by ocular sarcoidosis. The most common corneal involvement is superficial punctate keratitis secondary to keratoconjunctivitis sicca (KCS; dry eye). Patients with chronic inflammation may have peripheral band opacities resulting from calcium deposits on the Bowman subepithelial layer, or the so-called band keratopathy.[1] Interstitial keratitis was also reported as a presenting sign of ocular sarcoidosis along with an evidence of posterior uveitis and optic disc edema. The patient was diagnosed with sarcoidosis by transbronchial biopsy 2 years thereafter.[52] Peripheral ulcerative keratitis leading to corneal perforation was also described in a 42-year-old woman in one report.[53]

Lacrimal System and Keratoconjunctivitis Sicca

The lacrimal gland is the most common organ in the orbit affected by sarcoidosis. Histopathologic studies of biopsy-proven orbital sarcoidosis revealed the main lacrimal gland involvement in 42% to 63% cases.[54–56] Patients with lacrimal gland involvement may or may not be symptomatic. If there is significant enlargement of the lacrimal gland, they may present with palpable mass or other symptoms due to mass effects. Typical characteristic features on CT are diffuse enlargement of the gland with homogenous enhancement.[54]

KCS has long been recognized as a common consequence of sarcoidosis.[57] Dry eye syndrome in sarcoidosis is believed to be related primarily to lacrimal gland inflammation/infiltration that results in decreased aqueous tear production. Most studies reported abnormal imaging and biopsy results of the main lacrimal gland, but to the authors' knowledge none has specifically mentioned an involvement of the accessory lacrimal glands. However, full-thickness eyelid skin involvement has been reported.[37] Physiologically, the main lacrimal glands located at the anterolateral part of the orbit are responsible mainly for reflex tear secretion, whereas the small accessory lacrimal glands in the eyelid and conjunctivae produce the majority of basal tear. This knowledge may imply that both the main and accessory lacrimal glands may be affected in those with severe dry eye associated with sarcoidosis. KCS may cause irritation, tearing, corneal epitheliopathy, corneal abrasion, infection, and permanent corneal scars.

The tear is drained via the puncta through the canaliculi, nasolacrimal sac, and duct into the nasal meatus. Granulomatous inflammation due to sarcoidosis may directly affect the lacrimal drainage system causing lacrimal obstruction and lead to symptomatic epiphora (excessive tearing).[58,59]

Orbital Involvement

Besides the lacrimal gland, sarcoidosis can also involve other orbital structures, including orbital fat, extraocular muscles, and the optic nerve sheath.[54] Histopathologic studies showed that the main complaints of patients with orbital sarcoidosis requiring orbital biopsy are palpable mass and eyelid swelling.[54–56] Other symptoms included ptosis, globe displacement, proptosis, redness, pain, vision loss, tearing, and diplopia. The age range of patients with this condition was between 18 and 83 years, with mean age of approximately 45 to 55 years. Most patients were women. Concurrent systemic sarcoidosis was reported in 34% to 50% of biopsy-proven orbital sarcoidosis.[54,56] The lesions were well circumscribed in 85% to 90%, with 10% to 15% of diffuse or infiltrative patterns. The lesions were solid, but rarely cystic.[56] Most of the lesions are located in the anterior orbit, especially anteroinferior.[55] Orbital mass secondary to sarcoidosis can cause central retinal artery occlusion leading to permanent blindness.[60]

Glaucoma and Cataract

Elevated IOP is common in patients with sarcoid uveitis. A retrospective study in 1986 reported a high rate of severe visual loss (vision of 20/200 or worse) in 8 of 11 patients with concurrent sarcoid uveitis and glaucoma.[61] Ocular hypertension and glaucoma may result from trabecular meshwork dysfunction because of edema or obstruction from inflammatory cells. Severe or chronic anterior

chamber inflammation may cause angle closure glaucoma secondary to peripheral anterior synechiae formation. A Japanese study revealed a high incidence of abnormal gonioscopic findings (61% trabecular nodules and 55% tentlike peripheral anterior synechiae) among 159 patients with systemic sarcoidosis.[4] Patients with uveitic glaucoma have a significant risk of surgical failure when requiring a filtering procedure.[62] Elevated IOP can also be related to orbital mass effects or side effects from corticosteroid therapy.

Cataract formation is also common in patients with sarcoid uveitis and leads to visual loss. Any form of corticosteroid therapy, including topical, regional, or systemic corticosteroids, can cause cataract and ocular hypertension.

DIAGNOSIS OF OCULAR SARCOIDOSIS

Sarcoidosis is one of several conditions that may simultaneously involve multiple ocular tissues with various presentations. For example, patients may present with acute anterior uveitis with lacrimal gland enlargement, bilateral multifocal choroiditis with conjunctival nodules, or peripheral ulcerative keratitis with orbital inflammation. Sarcoidosis should be particularly high on differential diagnoses in those with involvement of multiple ocular tissues.

The gold standard for the diagnosis of sarcoidosis is a tissue biopsy. The most common biopsy samples are retrieved from the lungs, lymph nodes, skin, conjunctivae, lacrimal glands, or orbital tissues. However, suspected lesions may not be easily accessible, and biopsy may not be a desirable diagnostic choice from the patient standpoint. The lungs and hilar lymph nodes are the most commonly affected organs. Therefore, imaging studies, including a chest radiograph, a chest CT scan, and occasionally gallium scintigraphy, may help aid the diagnosis. Some patients with sarcoidosis may have elevated serum levels of calcium, angiotensin-converting enzyme (ACE), and/or lysozyme.

The diagnostic criteria for ocular sarcoidosis vary among different experts. In 2009, the first International Workshop on Ocular Sarcoidosis (IWOS) published the international criteria for the diagnosis of ocular sarcoidosis with the aim of universal usage.[63] The members of the IWOS identified 7 clinical signs suggesting ocular sarcoidosis, 5 laboratory investigations in suspected ocular sarcoidosis, and 4 diagnostic terms for ocular sarcoidosis (**Table 2**).

The clinical signs listed are useful for the diagnosis of sarcoid uveitis. However, the IWOS did not discuss the criteria for diagnosis of ocular

Table 2
Summary from international criteria for the diagnosis of ocular sarcoidosis

Ocular signs suggesting ocular sarcoidosis

1. Mutton-flat keratic precipitates and/or iris nodules
2. Trabecular meshwork nodules and/or tent-shaped peripheral anterior synechiae
3. Snowballs or string of pearls in the vitreous
4. Active or inactive multiple chorioretinal peripheral lesions
5. Nodular and/or segmental periphlebitis and/or macroaneurysms in an inflamed eye
6. Optic disc nodule or nodules/granuloma or granulomas and/or solitary choroidal nodule
7. Bilateral involvement

Laboratory investigations in patients with suspected ocular sarcoidosis

1. Negative result of tuberculin test in a BCG-vaccinated patient or with previous positive result of PPD (or Mantoux) skin test
2. Elevated serum level of ACE and/or lysozyme
3. Chest radiograph for bilateral symmetric hilar adenopathy
4. Abnormal results of liver enzyme tests (any 2 of alkaline phosphatase, AST, ALT, LDH, or GGT)
5. Chest CT in patients with negative result of chest radiograph

Diagnostic criteria and terminologies for ocular sarcoidosis

Definite ocular sarcoidosis	Biopsy-proven sarcoidosis with a compatible uveitis
Presumed ocular sarcoidosis	Biopsy not performed; BHL with compatible uveitis
Probable ocular sarcoidosis	Biopsy not performed and no BHL detected; presence of 3 suggestive ocular signs and positive results of 2 above-mentioned laboratory tests
Possible ocular sarcoidosis	Biopsy result negative; presence of 4 suggestive ocular signs and positive results of 2 above-mentioned laboratory tests

Abbreviations: ACE, angiotensin-converting enzyme; ALT, alanine aminotransferase; AST, aspartate aminotransferase; BHL, bilateral hilar adenopathy; GGT, γ-glutamyltransferase; LDH, lactate dehydrogenase; PPD, purified protein derivative.

Adapted from Herbort CP, Rao NA, Mochizuki M, Members of Scientific Committee of First International Workshop on Ocular Sarcoidosis. International criteria for the diagnosis of ocular sarcoidosis: results of the first International Workshop On Ocular Sarcoidosis (IWOS). Ocul Immunol Inflamm 2009;17(3):166–7; with permission.

adnexal involvement, which was mainly diagnosed based on histopathologic studies of the accessible lesions. In the authors' practice, they generally start with a chest radiograph and reserve a chest CT scan for highly suspicious patients or for whom the diagnosis may change their therapy. Owing to the amount of radiation, the authors are less likely to order chest CT scans for younger patients. Elevated serum levels of calcium, ACE, or lysozyme alone are usually neither sensitive nor specific for the diagnosis.

Conjunctival biopsy is a simple and useful procedure when patients present with conjunctival nodules or prominent follicles. Careful examination may reveal these findings. There is largely disagreement regarding the yield of random conjunctival biopsy in those without visible conjunctival lesions. In various studies, the rate of positive random biopsy results ranged from 20% to 71% in patients with positive results of biopsies from other sites, and from 1% to 28% in those with clinically suspected sarcoidosis without histologic confirmation.[1,64–66] Nichols and

colleagues[64] reported 55% positive conjunctival biopsy rate in patients with biopsy-proven sarcoidosis from other tissues but only 1% positive rate in those with negative systemic biopsy. Based on this study, a strip of conjunctival tissue of size at least 3 by 10 mm was removed from the inferior cul-de-sac of each eye. The investigators found no association between the incidence of anterior uveitis and a positive result of conjunctival biopsy. The presence of conjunctival follicles may slightly increase the likelihood of a positive result of biopsy. Crick and colleagues[1] demonstrated 20% positive conjunctival biopsy rate in biopsy-proven sarcoidosis, and the rate was increased to 37% in those with conjunctival follicles. In the authors' practice, a conjunctival biopsy is reserved only for those with visible conjunctival nodules on examination.

Several noninvasive diagnostic imaging techniques have been studied in patients with ocular sarcoidosis. In vivo confocal microscopy of the conjunctiva was successfully used to identify the presence of multinucleated giant cells in patients with sarcoid conjunctival nodules with 100% specificity and 50% sensitivity.[67] The procedure required technical skills and may need an instrument with high resolution and deep penetration ability to improve the sensitivity of the test. Rose-Nussbaumer and colleagues[68] recently reported that anterior segment spectral domain optical coherence tomography (OCT) could differentiate a predominantly mononuclear pattern of anterior chamber cells in active anterior uveitis associated with sarcoidosis or inflammatory bowel disease from a predominantly polymorphonuclear pattern in HLA-B27-related uveitis.[68] Güngör and colleagues[69] revealed that patients with quiescent sarcoid posterior uveitis may have decreased choroidal thickness measurements than normal controls using an enhanced depth imaging OCT.

The authors' group previously studied microarray analysis of gene expression on peripheral blood, lung, and lymph node and found that patients with sarcoidosis (with or without uveitis) had significant increases in signal transducer and activator of transcription 1 (STAT1)- and STAT1-regulated chemokines compared with normal controls. STAT1 is a transcription factor; it can be activated by interferons, which contribute to granuloma formation and which occasionally cause granulomatous adverse reactions.[70] The STAT1 upregulated pattern was not observed in patients with ankylosing spondylitis (with or without uveitis).[71] Subsequent gene expression study on conjunctival granuloma tissues showed that the activated form of STAT1 was more frequently detected in patients with sarcoidosis; however, the activity of STAT1-regulated genes may not be specific to only sarcoidosis because STAT1 may also express on other conjunctival granulomatous diseases.[72] More recently, the authors have analyzed the gene expression pattern from either the lacrimal gland or orbital adipose tissue affected by sarcoidosis.[73] This study confirmed an increased expression of STAT1 and showed that levels of similar transcripts are elevated in the blood and solid tissue from patients with sarcoidosis.[73]

TREATMENT OF OCULAR SARCOIDOSIS

The primary aims for the management of ocular sarcoidosis are to restore vision and to prevent complications from related inflammation. Corticosteroid therapy, including topical, regional, and systemic routes, is the mainstay of treatment. Other immunomodulators may be required in some patients who are dependent, unresponsive, or intolerant to corticosteroid treatment.

Treatment of Sarcoid Uveitis

Topical corticosteroids

The most commonly used topical corticosteroid for anterior uveitis is prednisolone acetate. The dosage can be titrated based on the degree of anterior chamber inflammation from once daily to hourly. The relatively new medication, difluprednate, generally is more potent. Difluprednate 0.05% given 4 times daily may be at least as effective as prednisolone acetate 1% administered 8 times daily for the treatment of anterior uveitis.[74] Their side effects are dose dependent, with the most concern to cause elevated IOP and cataract progression.

Topical corticosteroid drops are used primarily to treat anterior chamber inflammation but are typically insufficient to control posterior segment inflammation. However, it may be effective to treat CME associated with florid anterior uveitis.

Topical cycloplegics

Cycloplegic eye drops are helpful to relieve pain from ciliary spasm and to break or prevent posterior synechiae, which are common in patients with moderate and severe anterior chamber inflammation. Shorter-acting medications such as cyclopentolate 1% are generally used in the acute case, and longer-acting agents such as atropine 1% may be given in those with chronic or severe anterior chamber inflammation.

Regional corticosteroid injections and implants

Regional corticosteroid injections and implants can be considered in uveitis associated with posterior segment involvement or when a patient is poorly responsive or noncompliant to frequent topical corticosteroids. The depot injections can be given periocularly or intravitreally.

Periocular injections can be performed using either a transcutaneous or transconjunctival route, and either a superior or inferior approach. In the authors' practice, an orbital floor injection is typically given through the inferolateral eyelid skin. The most commonly used medication is triamcinolone acetonide, 20 to 40 mg. Examples of other alternatives are betamethasone and methylprednisolone, which both have a shorter duration of effect compared with triamcinolone acetonide. The injection can be repeated as soon as 4 to 6 weeks after the initial therapy.

Intravitreal triamcinolone acetonide (1–4 mg) injections may be given, especially when periocular injections inadequately control inflammation. The effects may last 3 to 6 months after each injection. The patients need to be monitored carefully for elevated IOP. The procedure can be performed in clinic under topical or subconjunctival anesthesia.

A biodegradable intraocular implant containing 700 μg of dexamethasone given through a 22-gauge applicator has been approved for the treatment of uveitis involving the posterior segment of the eye. A study of its efficacy and safety for persistent uveitic CME showed that a single dexamethasone implant was effective in improving vision and macular edema in most patients. However, recurrence of CME can be observed in approximately 65% of the patients at 6 months.[75] A study comparing intravitreal triamcinolone injections with dexamethasone implants in CME secondary to retinal vein occlusion demonstrated similar outcomes and similar incidence of side effects.[76]

A sustained-release fluocinolone acetonide implant has been approved in the United States for chronic noninfectious posterior uveitis. The implant is inserted surgically into the vitreous cavity through a scleral incision and may release drug for a median period of 30 months. The implant is effective in controlling inflammation in most implanted eyes,[77] but it is associated with high rate of complications, especially elevated IOP and cataractogenesis. Approximately 37% of the implanted eyes needed glaucoma surgery in a 3-year follow-up study.[78] A cost-effective study revealed that a fluocinolone implant was reasonably cost-effective compared with systemic immunosuppressive agents in patients with unilateral disease, but not for those who need bilateral implants.[79]

Systemic corticosteroids

Systemic corticosteroids are used in patients with severe bilateral uveitis, when topical and/or regional therapy is insufficient to control inflammation, or when the systemic disease also requires therapy. Systemic corticosteroid therapy generally is rapidly effective, but a high dose such as 60 mg of prednisone daily should be used for a limited duration to avoid both ocular and systemic adverse effects. Prednisone is the most commonly used oral corticosteroids in the United States. This drug is typically prescribed at 1 to 1.5 mg/kg/d initially, and the dose is then tapered gradually to avoid relapse. Short-term intravenous methylprednisolone is sometimes given in patients with vision-threatening retinal or optic nerve lesions, followed by oral prednisone.

Systemic immunosuppressive agents

Systemic immunosuppressive agents are indicated in patients who are corticosteroid dependent or corticosteroid intolerant. A low dose of prednisone such as 5 mg/d may be preferable to an immunosuppressant. In some circumstances, patients may have already received a systemic immunosuppressant to control their systemic manifestations of sarcoidosis. Antimetabolites[80,81] and calcineurin inhibitors[82,83] have been studied for the treatment of sarcoid-related ocular inflammation. Examples and dosage of systemic immunosuppressive drugs that may be used for the treatment of noninfectious uveitis are listed in **Table 3**.[84] The most commonly used medications for chronic eye inflammation including ocular sarcoidosis are methotrexate,[85] mycophenolate mofetil,[86] azathioprine,[87] and cyclosporine.[88]

Biologic agents

Biologics are relatively novel treatment of refractory noninfectious uveitis. The knowledge on ocular indications is mainly based on case reports and series, with the minority of evidence coming from several nonrandomized trials and 1 randomized double-masked trial.[89] To date, biologic agents studied for the treatment of uveitis related to sarcoidosis are tumor necrosis factor (TNF)-α inhibitors, including infliximab, adalimumab, etanercept, and golimumab.

Infliximab has been reported as an effective immunosuppressive agent in most patients with refractory uveitis related to multiple causes in a

Table 3		
Examples of steroid-sparing systemic immunosuppressive agents that may be used for the treatment of ocular sarcoidosis		
Medication	**Dose**	**Expected Onset of Action**
Antimetabolites		
Methotrexate	7.5–25 mg/wk po, SQ, or IM	2–12 wk
Mycophenolate mofetil	500–1500 mg po twice daily	2–12 wk
Azathioprine	1–4 mg/kg/d po daily	4–12 wk
Calcineurin inhibitors		
Cyclosporine	2.5–10 mg/kg/d po twice daily	2–6 wk
Tacrolimus	0.15–0.30 mg/kg/d po	2–6 wk

Abbreviations: IM, intramuscularly; SQ, subcutaneously.

Adapted from Jabs DA, Rosenbaum JT, Foster CS, et al. Guidelines for the use of immunosuppressive drugs in patients with ocular inflammatory disorders: recommendations of an expert panel. Am J Ophthalmol 2000;130(4):496–7; with permission.

prospective trial.[90] However, limited data revealed mixed results on its efficacy to control ocular inflammation in sarcoid uveitis in particular. Suhler and colleagues[90,91] prospectively enrolled 31 patients with refractory uveitis for infliximab therapy as a concomitant immunosuppressant. Of the 31 patients, 3 were diagnosed with sarcoid panuveitis. All 3 patients had improved visual acuity after infliximab therapy, but none of them showed an ability to completely control inflammation or to reduce doses of concomitant prednisone and immunosuppressive treatment by half. In contrast, all 4 patients with sarcoid uveitis from different series (2 of Pritchard and Nadarajah's,[92] 1 of Doty and colleagues',[93] and 1 of Benitez-del-Castillo and colleagues'[94]) had resolution of ocular inflammation several weeks after infliximab therapy but needed continuation of infliximab infusions every 4 to 8 weeks to prevent relapse.

Erckens and coworkers[95] studied the use of adalimumab as an adjunctive therapy in 41 eyes of 26 patients with refractory posterior sarcoidosis secondary to sarcoidosis; 85% of the cases showed improvement of intraocular inflammatory signs, whereas 15% had stable outcomes. The improvement of intraocular inflammation included resolution of vasculitis, choroidal involvement, papillitis, macular edema, and vitreous haze in most patients who had the respective signs at baseline.[95] A study by the authors' group also showed that all 6 patients with sarcoid uveitis, out of 31 patients with various uveitic diagnoses, were defined as clinical responders at 10 weeks by demonstrating either improvement of visual acuity, ocular inflammation, or angiographic findings or an ability to taper medications. At 50 weeks, 3 patients (50%) retained clinical success, while the others had secondary failure (1 due to loss of efficacy, 1 due to failure to taper corticosteroids, and 1 due to being lost to follow-up).[96]

Etanercept is generally less effective than infliximab and adalimumab for ocular indications. This drug failed to show significant difference in control of uveitis associated with juvenile idiopathic arthritis compared with placebo in a randomized trial.[97] Baughman and colleagues[98] randomized 18 patients with refractory sarcoid uveitis; 9 received etanercept and 9 were given placebo. The investigators found no significant improvement of ocular inflammation with etanercept therapy compared with placebo.

Golimumab has been reported to be effective for the treatment of various uveitides in several series.[99–103] Calvo-Rio and colleagues[102] reported successful control of inflammation in 2 patients with active sarcoid uveitis having previously failed infliximab; however, the follow-up periods were limited to 1 and 9 months for each patient. Similar findings were reported by Cordero-Coma and coworkers[103] who studied the use of golimumab in uveitis; 2 patients with sarcoid uveitis who previously failed other TNF inhibitors (1 with panuveitis and macular edema and 1 with intermediate uveitis) achieved complete control of inflammation after 6 months of golimumab therapy.

Owing to limited long-term safety and efficacy data, biologic therapy is reserved only as secondary or tertiary treatment of uveitis associated with sarcoidosis. However, rarely, there are multiple reports and series suggesting that anti-TNF agents (infliximab,[104–109] adalimumab,[108–110] etanercept,[107,108] and certolizumab[111]) may cause sarcoidosislike conditions, including uveitis.

Treatment of Scleritis and External Eye Diseases

Nonsteroidal antiinflammatory drugs (NSAIDs) are usually prescribed as a first-line therapy for scleritis. In patients who do not respond to NSAIDs, corticosteroids are typically helpful. Concomitant use of oral corticosteroids and NSAIDs may cause significant gastrointestinal adverse effects. In patients refractory or intolerant to corticosteroids, systemic immunomodulators may be used. The authors' group reported successful treatment of recalcitrant scleritis with rituximab in 75% of patients; however, partly due to rarity, none of those patients had scleritis secondary to sarcoidosis.[112] In one case report, thalidomide was successfully used to treat cutaneous sarcoidosis and nodular scleritis in a patient who failed azathioprine and corticosteroid therapy.[113] Thalidomide is not only considered a sedative, hypnotic agent but also has antiinflammatory activity. This agent is under special regulations because it can cause severe congenital defects.

Besides systemic corticosteroid treatment, cutaneous lesions on the eyelids may be treated with intralesional triamcinolone injection[36] or oral chloroquine.[114] Conjunctival lesions and KCS may respond to topical cyclosporine eye drops.[115,116]

Treatment of Orbital Disease

Orbital inflammation is also typically responsive to oral corticosteroids and/or immunosuppressive agents. In patients with accessible orbital lesions or high suspicion for possible malignancy, biopsy or removal of the lesions should be performed. Along with orbital lesions, strabismus and/or abnormal eyelid position can also be observed. The treatment should initially be maximized with antiinflammatory therapy. If surgical interventions are required, orbital surgery should be carried out first, followed by strabismus and eyelid surgery.

Treatment of Ocular Complications

Treatment of ocular complications secondary to ocular inflammation and adverse effects from therapy should not be overlooked. Glaucoma, cataract, epiretinal membrane formation, and CME are common. The use of corticosteroids should be minimized by using alternative antiinflammatory agents in those with significantly elevated IOP. Cataract surgery may be considered when quiescence of intraocular inflammation has been achieved for at least 3 months to avoid postoperative severe inflammatory reaction. Systemic and/or regional corticosteroids may also be given during the perioperative period.

The most important and effective way for the treatment of CME is to control intraocular inflammation with antiinflammatory therapy.[117] In patients in whom CME persists without active inflammation, intravitreal injections of bevacizumab[118] or ranibizumab[119] have been reported as possibly effective therapy to improve vision and macular anatomy. Epiretinal membrane may be surgically removed in those with visually significant puckers. However, treatment of associated inflammation and/or edema should be maximized before considering surgery to avoid postoperative inflammation and unnecessary surgery.

PROGNOSIS OF OCULAR SARCOIDOSIS

Visual prognosis of ocular sarcoidosis may vary depending on the severity and chronicity of eye inflammation, a delay in presentation to a specialist, and ocular complications secondary to uveitis.[9] A long-term prognostic study of sarcoid uveitis showed that most (54%) patients retained vision of better than 20/40 in both eyes and that only 4.6% had lost vision less than 20/120 in both eyes, at 10 years after the onset of uveitis in a setting of an ophthalmic referral center.[120] The main causes of irreversible vision loss were glaucoma and chronic maculopathy related to posterior segment inflammation. Thirty-five (47%) of 75 patients had extraocular involvement at the uveitis onset, with a further 17% having it during the following 10 years. It was observed that 51% of the patients needed oral corticosteroids and an additional 11% required immunosuppressive drugs for uveitis treatment. Approximately one-fifth of the patients underwent ocular surgery, including cataract extraction (17%), trabeculectomy (4%), retinal detachment repair (1%), and epiretinal membrane peel (1%). The ocular prognosis of sarcoid uveitis seemed unrelated to the presence of extraocular disease.[120]

In Finland, Karma and colleagues[121] studied 281 patients with biopsy-proven sarcoidosis. Of those 281 patients, 21 patients with uveitis were followed up regularly. A total of 8 patients (38%) had a monophasic course of uveitis requiring less than 6 months of treatment, while the remainder (13 patients; 62%) had a relapsing course with multiple recurrences. In the latter group, uveitis was subsequently burned out after several years of treatment in 9 of the 13 patients. This study also showed that the chest radiograph finding of hilar adenopathy could resolve while the ocular findings persisted. This observation suggests that a subset of patients with idiopathic uveitis may have sarcoidosis that is not diagnosable by routine chest radiograph.

A 10-year visual prognostic study of 69 patients with peripheral multifocal chorioretinitis revealed that the presence of systemic sarcoidosis had no influence on the risks of developing CME, epiretinal membrane, cataract, glaucoma, or optic atrophy. CME was the main cause of decreased vision. The presence of an epiretinal membrane may not necessarily affect final vision.[18]

Although ocular sarcoidosis can present with a sudden onset and a limited course, it is most important to educate the patients of the potential chronicity of ocular inflammation. Long-term follow-up and medication compliance are required for treatment success to prevent permanent visual damage from both ocular inflammation and drug-related adverse effects.

REFERENCES

1. Crick RP, Hoyle C, Smellie H. The eyes in sarcoidosis. Br J Ophthalmol 1961;45(7):461–81.
2. Rothova A. Ocular involvement in sarcoidosis. Br J Ophthalmol 2000;84(1):110–6.
3. Atmaca LS, Atmaca-Sonmez P, Idil A, et al. Ocular involvement in sarcoidosis. Ocul Immunol Inflamm 2009;17(2):91–4.
4. Ohara K, Okubo A, Sasaki H, et al. Intraocular manifestations of systemic sarcoidosis. Jpn J Ophthalmol 1992;36(4):452–7.
5. Heiligenhaus A, Wefelmeyer D, Wefelmeyer E, et al. The eye as a common site for the early clinical manifestation of sarcoidosis. Ophthalmic Res 2011;46(1):9–12.
6. Rothova A, Alberts C, Glasius E, et al. Risk factors for ocular sarcoidosis. Doc Ophthalmol 1989;72(3–4):287–96.
7. Hoover DL, Khan JA, Giangiacomo J. Pediatric ocular sarcoidosis. Surv Ophthalmol 1986;30(4):215–28.

8. Rose CD, Wouters CH, Meiorin S, et al. Pediatric granulomatous arthritis: an international registry. Arthritis Rheum 2006;54(10):3337–44.

9. Dana MR, Merayo-Lloves J, Schaumberg DA, et al. Prognosticators for visual outcome in sarcoid uveitis. Ophthalmology 1996;103(11):1846–53.

10. Evans M, Sharma O, LaBree L, et al. Differences in clinical findings between Caucasians and African Americans with biopsy-proven sarcoidosis. Ophthalmology 2007;114(2):325–33.

11. Birnbaum AD, Oh FS, Chakrabarti A, et al. Clinical features and diagnostic evaluation of biopsy-proven ocular sarcoidosis. Arch Ophthalmol 2011; 129(4):409–13.

12. Kump LI, Cervantes-Castaneda RA, Androudi SN, et al. Analysis of pediatric uveitis cases at a tertiary referral center. Ophthalmology 2005;112(7):1287–92.

13. Smith JA, Mackensen F, Sen HN, et al. Epidemiology and course of disease in childhood uveitis. Ophthalmology 2009;116(8):1544–51, 1551.e1.

14. Rodriguez A, Calonge M, Pedroza-Seres M, et al. Referral patterns of uveitis in a tertiary eye care center. Arch Ophthalmol 1996;114(5):593–9.

15. Merrill PT, Kim J, Cox TA, et al. Uveitis in the southeastern United States. Curr Eye Res 1997;16(9): 865–74.

16. Sungur G, Hazirolan D, Bilgin G. Pattern of ocular findings in patients with biopsy-proven sarcoidosis in Turkey. Ocul Immunol Inflamm 2013;21(6):455–61.

17. Abad S, Meyssonier V, Allali J, et al. Association of peripheral multifocal choroiditis with sarcoidosis: a study of thirty-seven patients. Arthritis Rheum 2004;51(6):974–82.

18. Ossewaarde-van Norel J, Ten Dam-van Loon N, de Boer JH, et al. Long-term visual prognosis of peripheral multifocal chorioretinitis. Am J Ophthalmol 2015;159(4):690–7.

19. Rossman MD, Thompson B, Frederick M, et al. HLA-DRB1*1101: a significant risk factor for sarcoidosis in blacks and whites. Am J Hum Genet 2003;73(4):720–35.

20. Jabs DA, Nussenblatt RB, Rosenbaum JT, Standardization of Uveitis Nomenclature Working Group. Standardization of uveitis nomenclature for reporting clinical data. Results of the First International Workshop. Am J Ophthalmol 2005;140(3): 509–16.

21. Zaidi AA, Ying GS, Daniel E, et al, Systemic Immunosuppressive Therapy for Eye Diseases Cohort Study. Hypopyon in patients with uveitis. Ophthalmology 2010;117(2):366–72.

22. Spalton DJ, Sanders MD. Fundus changes in histologically confirmed sarcoidosis. Br J Ophthalmol 1981;65(5):348–58.

23. Letocha CE, Shields JA, Goldberg RE. Retinal changes in sarcoidosis. Can J Ophthalmol 1975; 10(2):184–92.

24. Gould H, Kaufman HE. Sarcoid of the fundus. Arch Ophthalmol 1961;65:453–6.

25. Hoogstede HA, Copper AC. A case of macular subretinal neovascularisation in chronic uveitis probably caused by sarcoidosis. Br J Ophthalmol 1982;66(8):530–5.

26. Khurana RN, Parikh JG, Rao NA. Sarcoid choroiditis simulating birdshot chorioretinopathy. Retin Cases Brief Rep 2008;2(4):301–3.

27. Delaney P. Neurologic manifestations in sarcoidosis: review of the literature, with a report of 23 cases. Ann Intern Med 1977;87(3):336–45.

28. Phillips YL, Eggenberger ER. Neuro-ophthalmic sarcoidosis. Curr Opin Ophthalmol 2010;21(6): 423–9.

29. Gass JD, Olson CL. Sarcoidosis with optic nerve and retinal involvement. Arch Ophthalmol 1976; 94(6):945–50.

30. Zajicek JP, Scolding NJ, Foster O, et al. Central nervous system sarcoidosis–diagnosis and management. QJM 1999;92(2):103–17.

31. Oie K, Tanigawa K, Suganuma Y, et al. A case of CNS sarcoidosis -case report of hydrocephalus due to mechanical obstruction secondary to sarcoid granulomata at the outlet of the fourth ventricle (author's transl). No Shinkei Geka 1981; 9(1):75–8 [in Japanese].

32. Zhang J, Waisbren E, Hashemi N, et al. Visual hallucinations (Charles Bonnet syndrome) associated with neurosarcoidosis. Middle East Afr J Ophthalmol 2013;20(4):369–71.

33. Yaosaka M, Abe R, Ujiie H, et al. Unilateral periorbital oedema due to sarcoid infiltration of the eyelid: an unusual presentation of sarcoidosis with facial nerve palsy and parotid gland enlargement. Br J Dermatol 2007;157(1):200–2.

34. Pessoa de Souza Filho J, Martins MC, Sant'Anna AE, et al. Eyelid swelling as the only manifestation of ocular sarcoidosis. Ocul Immunol Inflamm 2005;13(5):399–402.

35. Hall JG, Cohen KL. Sarcoidosis of the eyelid skin. Am J Ophthalmol 1995;119(1):100–1.

36. Kim YJ, Kim YD. A case of scar sarcoidosis of the eyelid. Korean J Ophthalmol 2006;20(4):238–40.

37. Collins ME, Petronic-Rosic V, Sweiss NJ, et al. Full-thickness eyelid lesions in sarcoidosis. Case Rep Ophthalmol Med 2013;2013:579121.

38. Moin M, Kersten RC, Bernardini F, et al. Destructive eyelid lesions in sarcoidosis. Ophthal Plast Reconstr Surg 2001;17(2):123–5.

39. Behbehani R, Nipper KS, Eagle RC Jr, et al. Systemic sarcoidosis manifested as unilateral eyelid retraction. Arch Ophthalmol 2006;124(4):599–600.

40. Hegab SM, al-Mutawa SA, Sheriff SM. Sarcoidosis presenting as multilobular limbal corneal nodules. J Pediatr Ophthalmol Strabismus 1998; 35(6):323–6.

41. Dithmar S, Waring GO 3rd, Goldblum TA, et al. Conjunctival deposits as an initial manifestation of sarcoidosis. Am J Ophthalmol 1999;128(3):361–2.

42. Papadaki TG, Kafkala C, Zacharopoulos IP, et al. Conjunctival non-caseating granulomas in a human immunodeficiency virus (HIV) positive patient attributed to sarcoidosis. Ocul Immunol Inflamm 2006;14(5):309–11.

43. Manrique Lipa RK, de los Bueis AB, De los Rios JJ, et al. Sarcoidosis presenting as acute bulbar follicular conjunctivitis. Clin Exp Optom 2010;93(5):363–5.

44. Geggel HS, Mensher JH. Cicatricial conjunctivitis in sarcoidosis: recognition and treatment. Ann Ophthalmol 1989;21(3):92–4.

45. Flach A. Symblepharon in sarcoidosis. Am J Ophthalmol 1978;85(2):210–4.

46. Schilgen G, Sundmacher R, Pomjanski N, et al. Bilateral large conjunctival tumours as primary manifestation of sarcoidosis–successful treatment with steroid-depot-injections. Klin Monbl Augenheilkd 2006;223(4):326–9 [in German].

47. Dursun D, Akova YA, Bilezikci B. Scleritis associated with sarcoidosis. Ocul Immunol Inflamm 2004;12(2):143–8.

48. Heiligenhaus A, Michel D, Koch JM. Nodular scleritis in a patient with sarcoidosis. Br J Ophthalmol 2003;87(4):507–8.

49. Babu K, Kini R, Mehta R. Scleral nodule and bilateral disc edema as a presenting manifestation of systemic sarcoidosis. Ocul Immunol Inflamm 2010;18(3):158–61.

50. Dodds EM, Lowder CY, Barnhorst DA, et al. Posterior scleritis with annular ciliochoroidal detachment. Am J Ophthalmol 1995;120(5):677–9.

51. Riono WP, Hidayat AA, Rao NA. Scleritis: a clinicopathologic study of 55 cases. Ophthalmology 1999;106(7):1328–33.

52. Lennarson P, Barney NP. Interstitial keratitis as presenting ophthalmic sign of sarcoidosis in a child. J Pediatr Ophthalmol Strabismus 1995;32(3):194–6.

53. Siracuse-Lee D, Saffra N. Peripheral ulcerative keratitis in sarcoidosis: a case report. Cornea 2006;25(5):618–20.

54. Mavrikakis I, Rootman J. Diverse clinical presentations of orbital sarcoid. Am J Ophthalmol 2007;144(5):769–75.

55. Prabhakaran VC, Saeed P, Esmaeli B, et al. Orbital and adnexal sarcoidosis. Arch Ophthalmol 2007;125(12):1657–62.

56. Demirci H, Christianson MD. Orbital and adnexal involvement in sarcoidosis: analysis of clinical features and systemic disease in 30 cases. Am J Ophthalmol 2011;151(6):1074–80.e1.

57. Jones BR, Stevenson CJ. Keratoconjunctivitis sicca due to sarcoidosis. Br J Ophthalmol 1957;41(3):153–60.

58. Chapman KL, Bartley GB, Garrity JA, et al. Lacrimal bypass surgery in patients with sarcoidosis. Am J Ophthalmol 1999;127(4):443–6.

59. Kay DJ, Saffra N, Har-El G. Isolated sarcoidosis of the lacrimal sac without systemic manifestations. Am J Otolaryngol 2002;23(1):53–5.

60. Kim DS, Korgavkar K, Zahid S, et al. Vision loss after central retinal artery occlusion secondary to orbital sarcoid mass. Ophthal Plast Reconstr Surg 2014. [Epub ahead of print].

61. Jabs DA, Johns CJ. Ocular involvement in chronic sarcoidosis. Am J Ophthalmol 1986;102(3):297–301.

62. Shimizu A, Maruyama K, Yokoyama Y, et al. Characteristics of uveitic glaucoma and evaluation of its surgical treatment. Clin Ophthalmol 2014;8:2383–9.

63. Herbort CP, Rao NA, Mochizuki M, Members of Scientific Committee of First International Workshop on Ocular Sarcoidosis. International criteria for the diagnosis of ocular sarcoidosis: results of the first International Workshop on Ocular Sarcoidosis (IWOS). Ocul Immunol Inflamm 2009;17(3):160–9.

64. Nichols CW, Eagle RC Jr, Yanoff M, et al. Conjunctival biopsy as an aid in the evaluation of the patient with suspected sarcoidosis. Ophthalmology 1980;87(4):287–91.

65. Karcioglu ZA, Brear R. Conjunctival biopsy in sarcoidosis. Am J Ophthalmol 1985;99(1):68–73.

66. Bornstein JS, Frank MI, Radner DB. Conjunctival biopsy in the diagnosis of sarcoidosis. N Engl J Med 1962;267:60–4.

67. Wertheim MS, Mathers WD, Lim L, et al. Non-invasive detection of multinucleated giant cells in the conjunctiva of patients with sarcoidosis by in-vivo confocal microscopy. Ocul Immunol Inflamm 2006;14(4):203–6.

68. Rose-Nussbaumer J, Li Y, Lin P, et al. Aqueous cell differentiation in anterior uveitis using Fourier-domain optical coherence tomography. Invest Ophthalmol Vis Sci 2015;56(3):1430–6.

69. Güngör SG, Akkoyun I, Reyhan NH, et al. Choroidal thickness in ocular sarcoidosis during quiescent phase using enhanced depth imaging optical coherence tomography. Ocul Immunol Inflamm 2014;22(4):287–93.

70. Ma J, Chen T, Mandelin J, et al. Regulation of macrophage activation. Cell Mol Life Sci 2003;60(11):2334–46.

71. Rosenbaum JT, Pasadhika S, Crouser ED, et al. Hypothesis: sarcoidosis is a STAT1-mediated disease. Clin Immunol 2009;132(2):174–83.

72. Rosenbaum JT, Hessellund A, Phan I, et al. The expression of STAT-1 and phosphorylated STAT-1 in conjunctival granulomas. Ocul Immunol Inflamm 2010;18(4):261–4.

73. Rosenbaum JT, Choi D, Wilson DJ, et al. Parallel gene expression changes in sarcoidosis involving

the lacrimal gland, orbital tissue, or blood. JAMA Ophthalmol 2015;133(7):770–7.

74. Sheppard JD, Toyos MM, Kempen JH, et al. Difluprednate 0.05% versus prednisolone acetate 1% for endogenous anterior uveitis: a phase III, multicenter, randomized study. Invest Ophthalmol Vis Sci 2014;55(5):2993–3002.

75. Khurana RN, Porco TC. Efficacy and safety of dexamethasone intravitreal implant for persistent uveitic cystoid macular edema. Retina 2015; 35(8):1640–6.

76. Ozkok A, Saleh OA, Sigford DK, et al. THE OMAR STUDY: comparison of ozurdex and triamcinolone acetonide for refractory cystoid macular edema in retinal vein occlusion. Retina 2015; 35(7):1393–400.

77. Jaffe GJ, Martin D, Callanan D, et al, Fluocinolone Acetonide Uveitis Study Group. Fluocinolone acetonide implant (Retisert) for noninfectious posterior uveitis: thirty-four-week results of a multicenter randomized clinical study. Ophthalmology 2006; 113(6):1020–7.

78. Goldstein DA, Godfrey DG, Hall A, et al. Intraocular pressure in patients with uveitis treated with fluocinolone acetonide implants. Arch Ophthalmol 2007; 125(11):1478–85.

79. Multicenter Uveitis Steroid Treatment Trial Research Group, Sugar EA, Holbrook JT, et al. Cost-effectiveness of fluocinolone acetonide implant versus systemic therapy for noninfectious intermediate, posterior, and panuveitis. Ophthalmology 2014;121(10):1855–62.

80. Dev S, McCallum RM, Jaffe GJ. Methotrexate treatment for sarcoid-associated panuveitis. Ophthalmology 1999;106(1):111–8.

81. Bhat P, Cervantes-Castaneda RA, Doctor PP, et al. Mycophenolate mofetil therapy for sarcoidosis-associated uveitis. Ocul Immunol Inflamm 2009; 17(3):185–90.

82. Walton RC, Nussenblatt RB, Whitcup SM. Cyclosporine therapy for severe sight-threatening uveitis in children and adolescents. Ophthalmology 1998; 105(11):2028–34.

83. Murphy CC, Greiner K, Plskova J, et al. Cyclosporine vs tacrolimus therapy for posterior and intermediate uveitis. Arch Ophthalmol 2005;123(5): 634–41.

84. Jabs DA, Rosenbaum JT, Foster CS, et al. Guidelines for the use of immunosuppressive drugs in patients with ocular inflammatory disorders: recommendations of an expert panel. Am J Ophthalmol 2000;130(4):492–513.

85. Gangaputra S, Newcomb CW, Liesegang TL, et al, Systemic Immunosuppressive Therapy for Eye Diseases Cohort Study. Methotrexate for ocular inflammatory diseases. Ophthalmology 2009;116(11): 2188–98.e2.

86. Daniel E, Thorne JE, Newcomb CW, et al. Mycophenolate mofetil for ocular inflammation. Am J Ophthalmol 2010;149(3):423–32.e1–2.

87. Pasadhika S, Kempen JH, Newcomb CW, et al. Azathioprine for ocular inflammatory diseases. Am J Ophthalmol 2009;148(4):500–9.e2.

88. Kacmaz RO, Kempen JH, Newcomb C, et al. Cyclosporine for ocular inflammatory diseases. Ophthalmology 2010;117(3):576–84.

89. Jaffe GJ, Thorne JE, Scales D, et al. Adalimumab in patients with active, non-infectious uveitis requiring high-dose corticosteroids: the VISUAL-1 trial. ARVO 2015 Annual Meeting Abstracts by Scientific Section/Group - Immunology/Microbiology. Denver, May 3–7, 2015.

90. Suhler EB, Smith JR, Wertheim MS, et al. A prospective trial of infliximab therapy for refractory uveitis: preliminary safety and efficacy outcomes. Arch Ophthalmol 2005;123(7):903–12.

91. Suhler EB, Smith JR, Giles TR, et al. Infliximab therapy for refractory uveitis: 2-year results of a prospective trial. Arch Ophthalmol 2009;127(6):819–22.

92. Pritchard C, Nadarajah K. Tumour necrosis factor alpha inhibitor treatment for sarcoidosis refractory to conventional treatments: a report of five patients. Ann Rheum Dis 2004;63(3):318–20.

93. Doty JD, Mazur JE, Judson MA. Treatment of sarcoidosis with infliximab. Chest 2005;127(3): 1064–71.

94. Benitez-del-Castillo JM, Martinez-de-la-Casa JM, Pato-Cour E, et al. Long-term treatment of refractory posterior uveitis with anti-TNFalpha (infliximab). Eye (Lond) 2005;19(8):841–5.

95. Erckens RJ, Mostard RL, Wijnen PA, et al. Adalimumab successful in sarcoidosis patients with refractory chronic non-infectious uveitis. Graefes Arch Clin Exp Ophthalmol 2012;250(5):713–20.

96. Suhler EB, Lowder CY, Goldstein DA, et al. Adalimumab therapy for refractory uveitis: results of a multicentre, open-label, prospective trial. Br J Ophthalmol 2013;97(4):481–6.

97. Smith JA, Thompson DJ, Whitcup SM, et al. A randomized, placebo-controlled, double-masked clinical trial of etanercept for the treatment of uveitis associated with juvenile idiopathic arthritis. Arthritis Rheum 2005;53(1):18–23.

98. Baughman RP, Lower EE, Bradley DA, et al. Etanercept for refractory ocular sarcoidosis: results of a double-blind randomized trial. Chest 2005;128(2): 1062–147.

99. William M, Faez S, Papaliodis GN, et al. Golimumab for the treatment of refractory juvenile idiopathic arthritis-associated uveitis. J Ophthalmic Inflamm Infect 2012;2(4):231–3.

100. Cordero-Coma M, Salom D, Diaz-Llopis M, et al. Golimumab for uveitis. Ophthalmology 2011; 118(9):1892.e3–4.

101. Miserocchi E, Modorati G, Pontikaki I, et al. Golimumab treatment for complicated uveitis. Clin Exp Rheumatol 2013;31(2):320–1.

102. Calvo-Rio V, de la Hera D, Blanco R, et al. Golimumab in uveitis previously treated with other anti-TNF-alpha drugs: a retrospective study of three cases from a single centre and literature review. Clin Exp Rheumatol 2014;32(6):864–8.

103. Cordero-Coma M, Calvo-Rio V, Adan A, et al. Golimumab as rescue therapy for refractory immune-mediated uveitis: a three-center experience. Mediators Inflamm 2014;2014:717598.

104. Izzi S, Francesconi F, Visca P, et al. Pulmonary sarcoidosis in a patient with psoriatic arthritis during infliximab therapy. Dermatol Online J 2010; 16(5):16.

105. Olivier A, Gilson B, Lafontaine S, et al. Pulmonary and renal involvement in a TNFalpha antagonist drug-induced sarcoidosis. Rev Med Interne 2012; 33(5):e25–7 [in French].

106. Takahashi H, Kaneta K, Honma M, et al. Sarcoidosis during infliximab therapy for Crohn's disease. J Dermatol 2010;37(5):471–4.

107. Clementine RR, Lyman J, Zakem J, et al. Tumor necrosis factor-alpha antagonist-induced sarcoidosis. J Clin Rheumatol 2010;16(6):274–9.

108. Daien CI, Monnier A, Claudepierre P, et al, Club Rhumatismes et Inflammation. Sarcoid-like granulomatosis in patients treated with tumor necrosis factor blockers: 10 cases. Rheumatology (Oxford) 2009;48(8):883–6.

109. Dhaille F, Viseux V, Caudron A, et al. Cutaneous sarcoidosis occurring during anti-TNF-alpha treatment: report of two cases. Dermatology 2010; 220(3):234–7.

110. Metyas SK, Tadros RM, Arkfeld DG. Adalimumab-induced noncaseating granuloma in the bone marrow of a patient being treated for rheumatoid arthritis. Rheumatol Int 2009;29(4):437–9.

111. Moisseiev E, Shulman S. Certolizumab-induced uveitis: a case report and review of the literature. Case Rep Ophthalmol 2014;5(1):54–9.

112. Suhler EB, Lim LL, Beardsley RM, et al. Rituximab therapy for refractory scleritis: results of a phase I/II dose-ranging, randomized, clinical trial. Ophthalmology 2014;121(10):1885–91.

113. Huddleston SM, Houser KH, Walton RC. Thalidomide for recalcitrant nodular scleritis in sarcoidosis. JAMA Ophthalmol 2014;132(11):1377–9.

114. Brownstein S, Liszauer AD, Carey WD, et al. Sarcoidosis of the eyelid skin. Can J Ophthalmol 1990;25(5):256–9.

115. Oh JY, Wee WR. Cyclosporine for conjunctival sarcoidosis. Ophthalmology 2008;115(1):222.

116. Akpek EK, Ilhan-Sarac O, Green WR. Topical cyclosporin in the treatment of chronic sarcoidosis of the conjunctiva. Arch Ophthalmol 2003;121(9): 1333–5.

117. Pasadhika S, Smith JR. Treatment of uveitic macular edema: an overview and update. Ophthalmol Int 2008;97–103.

118. Cordero Coma M, Sobrin L, Onal S, et al. Intravitreal bevacizumab for treatment of uveitic macular edema. Ophthalmology 2007;114(8):1574–9.e1.

119. Acharya NR, Hong KC, Lee SM. Ranibizumab for refractory uveitis-related macular edema. Am J Ophthalmol 2009;148(2):303–9.e2.

120. Edelsten C, Pearson A, Joynes E, et al. The ocular and systemic prognosis of patients presenting with sarcoid uveitis. Eye (Lond) 1999;13(Pt 6):748–53.

121. Karma A, Huhti E, Poukkula A. Course and outcome of ocular sarcoidosis. Am J Ophthalmol 1988;106(4):467–72.

Cutaneous Sarcoidosis

Karolyn A. Wanat, MD[a,b], Misha Rosenbach, MD[c],*

KEYWORDS

- Cutaneous sarcoidosis • Granulomas • Noncaseating • Lupus pernio • Erythema nodosum
- Löfgren syndrome

KEY POINTS

- Skin is the second most common organ affected after the pulmonary system.
- Cutaneous sarcoidosis can be the presenting sign of systemic sarcoidosis, and work-up is indicated in all patients with cutaneous manifestations. Certain presentations can provide clues to prognosis and underlying systemic involvement.
- The skin is readily accessible for evaluation and biopsy. Biopsy of cutaneous disease is helpful and may be essential for diagnosis of systemic sarcoidosis; it can sometimes obviate more invasive testing.
- Health-related quality of life measures and objective assessment tools can help standardize evaluation.
- Treatment of cutaneous sarcoidosis should follow a therapeutic ladder with potential treatments based on additional organ involvement and extent of cutaneous disease with weighing of potential risks of therapy.

INTRODUCTION

Sarcoidosis is a multisystem, noncaseating granulomatous disorder of unknown cause with skin as the second most common organ affected, occurring in 25% to 30% of cases reported.[1–8] Cutaneous sarcoidosis may be the presenting sign of systemic disease and a high clinical index of suspicion is critical because there can be protean manifestations.[9,10] Sarcoidosis may affect patients of all races and at any age, although the clinical presentation may vary by ethnic background. African Americans are more often affected by chronic skin sarcoidosis compared with white people. Sarcoidosis is more common in women than in men, with African American women having the highest rates of sarcoidosis in the United States, including the highest rates of chronic cutaneous sarcoidosis. There is also a higher incidence of erythema nodosum in women.[2] Lesions can range from minimal skin involvement to extensive disease that results in significant morbidity and dramatic impact on quality of life. By strict definition, a diagnosis of sarcoidosis can only be rendered when there is more than 1 organ involved, and requires the presence of granulomatous inflammation in multiple systems.[11] If cutaneous involvement only is present, then a diagnosis of sarcoidlike granulomatous disease of unknown significance may be more precise, although some clinicians describe it as isolated cutaneous sarcoidosis; this is an area of active debate.[12]

SKIN PATHOPHYSIOLOGY

The exact inciting cause of sarcoidosis remains unknown. Sarcoidal inflammation is caused by a complex interplay of multiple factors, including genetics; environmental and/or infectious antigens;

Disclosure: The authors have nothing to disclose.
[a] Department of Dermatology, University of Iowa, 200 Hawkins Drive, Iowa City, IA 52242, USA; [b] Department of Pathology, University of Iowa, 200 Hawkins Drive, Iowa City, IA 52242, USA; [c] Department of Dermatology, University of Pennsylvania, 3400 Spruce Street, Philadelphia, PA 19104, USA
* Corresponding author.
E-mail address: misha.rosenbach@uphs.upenn.edu

and the immune system, involving Th1 predominant response with interferon-gamma and tumor necrosis factor (TNF) playing an important role, and with emerging evidence suggesting a role of Th17 inflammation and interplay with the innate immune system.[13,14] Although sarcoidosis can affect any site on the skin, including the mucosa, cutaneous sarcoidosis preferentially occurs in sites of prior injury, such as scars, as well as in tattoos. Patients with sarcoidosis and tattoos may have none, some, or all of their tattoos affected, and cutaneous sarcoidosis can affect multiple tattoo pigments. Notably, polarizable material may be seen in approximately 25% (ranges of 20%–78% have been reported) of skin biopsies of sarcoidosis, suggesting that in some patients foreign material serves as a nidus for granuloma formation.[15–20] Although not the sole cause of disease, foreign bodies, scars, and trauma may affect the distribution of skin lesions in patients with sarcoidosis.

CLINICAL PRESENTATION

Cutaneous sarcoidosis can present in various ways and is often considered an imitator of other skin diseases. Skin disease is often present at disease onset and activity correlates with systemic inflammation in many cases, although cutaneous sarcoidal inflammation may be discordant with internal involvement as well. Skin manifestations can be divided into specific lesions and nonspecific lesions: specific manifestations refer to the presence of noncaseating granulomas observed within skin biopsies, and nonspecific lesions are considered reactive to systemic sarcoidosis but do not have granulomas on biopsy (this refers primarily to erythema nodosum).

Although specific lesions of cutaneous sarcoidosis are widely variable, certain manifestations are observed more frequently than others. In addition, some morphologies may be associated with better or worse prognosis, and in some cases may be a clue as to particular patterns of internal organ involvement.

Common Morphologies

Macules/papules

One of the commonest morphologies affecting the skin includes lesions smaller than a centimeter, either macules (flat lesions) or papules (raised lesions).[21] These lesions can range in color and may be red/violaceous, skin colored to brown, and even hypopigmented (**Fig. 1**A). Often, there are numerous macules or papules that can be disseminated or concentrated in certain areas, such as the central face, extremities, and areas of trauma.[21–23] Papular sarcoidosis shows a predilection for knees or sites of repetitive trauma in some patients (**Fig. 1**B).[22] Macules and papules have been described as more common in acute forms of sarcoidosis and may be seen in association with erythema nodosum; they may also occur in patients with chronic disease.[1,24] Overall, these lesions portend a good prognosis with on average less than 2 years of active systemic sarcoidosis, and often self-resolve without scarring.[24]

Plaque

As skin lesions become larger than 1 cm, they are defined as plaque sarcoidosis. In addition to papular sarcoidosis, this is one of the commonest lesions and can be found on face, back, buttocks, and often on the extensor surfaces of arms (**Fig. 2**).[2,8,24,25] Compared with macules/papules, plaque sarcoidosis is less often associated with acute presentation of disease, does not occur in conjunction with erythema nodosum as frequently, and often predicts a more chronic course with a higher likelihood of recurrence.[2,8,24] In addition, systemic symptoms also seem to be more chronic, lasting longer than 2 years in most cases, and individuals can have persistent symptoms, including bilateral hilar lymphadenopathy, splenomegaly, pulmonary fibrosis, and uveitis, although these associations are based on small studies (**Fig. 3**).[1,7,9,10,24,26,27] Compared with macules/papules, plaque sarcoidosis is more likely to leave dyspigmentation and scarring.

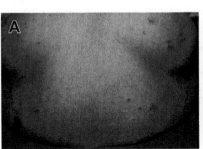
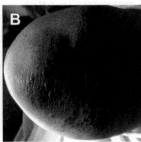

Fig. 1. Papular sarcoidosis. Scattered violaceous papules (<1 cm) on the back (*A*) and erythematous papules on the elbow (*B*), most likely reflecting a site of trauma.

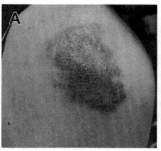 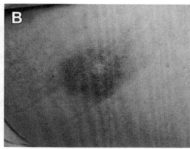

Fig. 2. Plaque sarcoidosis. Erythematous to violaceous, indurated plaque (*A, B*).

Annular sarcoidosis is a type of plaque sarcoidosis in which there is central clearing in the center of the plaques (**Fig. 4**). This morphology has similar prognosis to other forms of plaque sarcoidosis but the clinical differential diagnosis includes other annular lesions (**Table 1**).

Lupus pernio

Lupus pernio is a specific presentation of cutaneous sarcoidosis that is most strictly defined by chronic, red to violaceous, indurated plaques with occasional superficial scaling of the nose, central face, and cheeks (**Figs. 5** and **6**). Involvement of the ears and digits also has been reported. This term is a source of some confusion, because nondermatologists sometimes incorrectly refer to any chronic cutaneous lesion as lupus pernio. The origin of the term lupus pernio is attributed to Ernest Besnier in 1889, using the term to signify lesions on the nose (lupus meaning wolflike) that are different from lupus vulgaris (tuberculosis) or lupus erythematosus (systemic lupus).[28] The definition is important, because lupus pernio carries prognostic significance. This morphology is most common in African Americans, with a female predominance.[29–31] This morphology can be extremely cosmetically disfiguring and consequently emotionally disturbing for patients (see **Fig. 5**B). Strict morphologic characterization can

be helpful with potential prognostic implications. Lupus pernio is highly predictive of involvement of the sinuses and oropharynx, and may be more associated with bone cysts, pulmonary fibrosis, and uveitis.[25,29,31–33] Within the nasal cavity, involvement of the nasal mucosa can occur, resulting in ulceration and potential septal perforation.[29] Severe, recalcitrant arthritis also has been reported in association with lupus pernio.[32] This clinical manifestation also portends a prolonged (>2 years and up to 25 years in some cases[33]), chronic, and often treatment-resistant course, requiring more aggressive systemic therapy (discussed later).[7,24,25,31]

Subcutaneous sarcoidosis

Subcutaneous sarcoidosis (also known as Darier-Roussy) is a form of cutaneous sarcoidosis that affects the deep dermis and subcutaneous tissue. Clinically, lesions present as firm, nontender, mobile subcutaneous nodules, often 0.5 to 2 cm in size, and often do not have associated redness (**Fig. 7**). Unlike erythema nodosum, the most

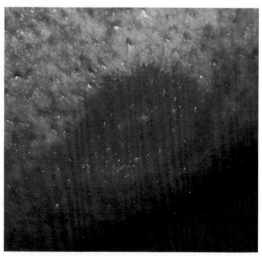

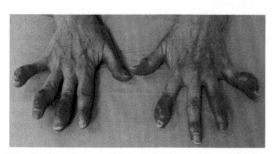

Fig. 3. Chronic, severe sarcoidosis. In this case, nodules and plaques affected the digits and correlated with a chronic course of systemic disease.

Fig. 4. Annular sarcoidosis. Plaque sarcoidosis with more heaped-up borders and central clearing.

Table 1
Clinical differential diagnosis for cutaneous sarcoidosis based on morphology

Frequency	Morphology	Clinical Differential
Common	Macules/papules	Acne, rosacea, syringoma, angiofibroma, xanthelasma, lichen planus, granuloma annulare, adnexal tumors
	Plaque	Lichen planus, granuloma annulare, necrobiosis lipoidica, morphea, psoriasis, syphilis, leprosy, discoid lupus. Annular lesions: granuloma annulare, tinea corporis, subacute cutaneous lupus, leprosy
	Lupus pernio	Cutaneous lupus, rosacea (rhinophyma), cutaneous malignancy (basal cell carcinoma, squamous cell carcinoma), lymphoma, leishmaniasis, systemic/deep fungal infections, granulomatosis with polyangiitis (if nasal destruction)
	Subcutaneous	Erythema nodosum, lupus panniculitis, panniculitis T-cell lymphoma, granuloma annulare, lipomas, deep cysts, rheumatoid nodule
	Scar/tattoo	Hypertrophic scar, keloids, atypical mycobacterial infections
Uncommon	Psoriasiform	Psoriasis, secondary syphilis
	Lichenoid	Lichen planus, lichen nitidus, lichen striatus
	Verrucous	Hypertrophic lichen planus, hypertrophic lupus, squamous cell carcinoma, verruca vulgaris
	Ichthyosiform	Ichthyosis vulgaris, acquired ichthyosis
	Lymphedematous	Other causes of lymphedema: congestive heart failure, Kaposi sarcoma (if lymph nodes involved), lymphoma
	Atrophic	Necrobiosis lipoidica, morphea, scar
	Ulcerative	Necrobiosis lipoidica, atypical mycobacterial infection, malignancy (squamous cell carcinoma), trauma
	Hypopigmented	Postinflammatory hypopigmentation, tinea versicolor, vitiligo, pityriasis alba, leprosy
	Angiolupoid	Basal cell carcinoma, rosacea, cutaneous lymphoma, fungal infections
Rare	Erythroderma	Medication reactions, cutaneous T-cell lymphoma, psoriasis, atopic dermatitis
	Pigmented purpuric	Pigmented purpuric dermatosis, cutaneous T-cell lymphoma
	Photodistributed	Actinic granuloma, granuloma annulare, cutaneous lupus
	Scalp	Central centrifugal cicatricial alopecia, lichen planopilaris, alopecia areata, atypical necrobiosis lipoidica
	Nails	Lichen planus, psoriasis, onychomycosis
	Mucosal	Crohn disease, Melkersson-Rosenthal, mucosal neuromas, foreign body reaction, lichen planus
	Genital	Crohn disease, infection (cellulitis), lymphatic blockage, foreign body reaction
Nonspecific lesions	Erythema nodosum	Subcutaneous sarcoidosis, lupus panniculitis, panniculitis T-cell lymphoma, granuloma annulare, lipomas, deep cysts
	Calcinosis cutis	Gouty tophi, rheumatoid nodule, milia
	Digital clubbing	Other causes of lung disease
	Neutrophilic dermatoses	Deep fungal infection, mycobacterial infection, malignancy, vasculitis

common location for subcutaneous sarcoidosis is the arms, and lesions are not painful.[34–39] Woman are affected more than men.[40] Subcutaneous sarcoidosis may occur either early in the disease course or later in the course of disease, and is often associated with nonsevere forms of systemic disease, such as hilar lymphadenopathy, and uncommonly with pulmonary fibrosis.[34,38,40]

Scar/tattoo
Sarcoidosis has a predilection for sites of prior trauma and scars, and all patients presenting with concerns for sarcoidosis should have their scars examined closely for any infiltration. This condition can be the sole cutaneous manifestation of sarcoidosis but also can be seen in association with other morphologies, including erythema

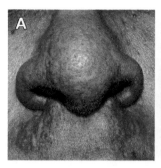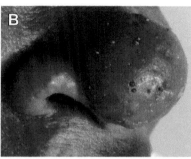

Fig. 5. Lupus pernio. Characteristic violaceous plaques involving the nose and central upper lip in an African American woman (*A*). A more severe presentation with a pedunculated nodule protruding from the dorsum and causing severe nasal destruction and leading to disfigurement (*B*).

nodosum.[1,24,25] This characteristic feature of scar involvement with sarcoidosis can include increased nodularity or red to violaceous discoloration but can be difficult to diagnose because it can clinically mimic hypertrophic scars or keloids and is subtle in some patients.[1,41] Scar sarcoidosis may be the initial presentation of disease and has variable association with systemic disease, with some reports of scar sarcoidosis with quick resolution of disease with a good prognosis and others reporting a more chronic disease course.[24,42]

As a variant of scar sarcoidosis, it is well recognized that cutaneous sarcoidosis can occur within tattoos and can be the presenting sign of disease (**Fig. 8**).[43–49] Patients with sarcoidosis should be advised to avoid tattoos to help prevent development of disease. In addition, sarcoidosis also occurs at sites of other injections, including silicone, insulin injections, desensitizing injections, and cosmetic filler.[43,50–53] Note that patients may develop granulomatous tattoo reactions in the absence of systemic inflammation; in such cases, they are best diagnosed simply with granulomatous tattoo reactions and not sarcoidosis, but a

systemic work-up to exclude sarcoidosis is suggested.

Less Common Morphologies

Cutaneous sarcoidosis can have numerous other morphologies on the skin and can simulate several dermatologic diseases.

Psoriasiform sarcoidosis clinically resembles psoriasis and can be clinically indistinguishable, with erythematous plaques with overlying silvery scale.[54–57] Although this variant may represent a unique presentation of cutaneous sarcoidosis, it may just localize to psoriatic lesions, as occurs with scar sarcoidosis or prior sites of trauma. The coexistence of sarcoidosis and psoriasis also has been reported in both case series and population-based cohorts, which is hypothesized to occur as a result of overlapping pathogenetic mechanisms.[58–60]

Lichenoid sarcoidosis can present as small, flat-topped, skin-colored to erythematous papules; however, it can be differentiated from lichen planus by a lack of overlying white lacy marks (Wickham striae). This cutaneous presentation has been reported most often in children, can be localized or extensive, and can be eruptive in nature.[61–64]

Verrucous sarcoidosis presents most often on the lower legs of African American men and clinically appears as warty papules and plaques with overlying thick scale (hyperkeratotic) (**Fig. 9**).

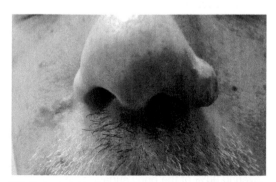

Fig. 6. Lupus pernio. Although less common in white people, the presence of erythematous, indurated plaques along the nasal rim is diagnostic for lupus pernios, which portends a more chronic course and can indicate nasal and pulmonary involvement, uveitis, and bony cysts.

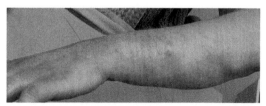

Fig. 7. Subcutaneous sarcoidosis. Firm, mobile, often noninflammatory (no overlying redness) nodules on the extremity, which can sometimes be differentiated from erythema nodosum, which is inflammatory.

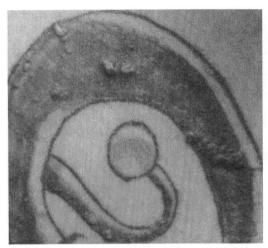

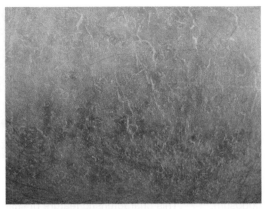

Fig. 10. Ichthyosiform sarcoidosis presents with overlying dry, flaking, fishlike scale with erythema; underlying induration can be a clue.

Fig. 8. Tattoo sarcoidosis. Sarcoidosis has a tendency to occur in scars or affect sites of prior trauma, including tattoos or piercings.

Lesions can be mistaken for malignancies or other skin conditions, such as lichen planus.[65–68]

Ichthyosiform sarcoidosis also is common on the lower legs of African Americans and presents as dry, thick, variably sized polygonal flakes of skin; however, it can be extensive and lead to diffuse red skin (**Fig. 10**).[69–71]

Lymphedema can be the presenting sign of sarcoidosis (lymphedematous sarcoidosis), which occurs secondary to extensive, granulomatous

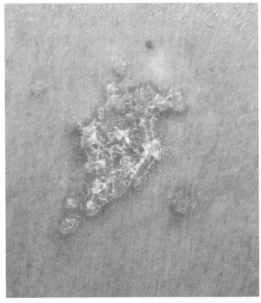

Fig. 9. Hyperkeratotic or verrucous sarcoidosis. This morphology is uncommon but can be seen with plaque sarcoidosis.

involvement of subcutaneous tissue as well as the draining lymph node basin.[72,73] Imaging often reveals extensive lymphadenopathy and biopsy of indurated areas of the skin (or where there are subcutaneous nodules) shows noncaseating granulomas.[72]

Atrophic and ulcerative sarcoidosis may be similar presentations on the same spectrum of disease and can occur as the presenting signs of systemic sarcoidosis, occurring de novo or in conjunction with macular, papular, or atrophic lesions, most often on the lower legs.[74,75] These lesions preferentially occur in African Americans and Japanese people.[74–76] The ulcerations often heal with scarring, and trauma is hypothesized to be the inciting factor (**Fig. 11**).

Hypopigmented macules can be seen occasionally in darker skinned patients with sarcoidosis as well-defined, circular or oval hypopigmented macules, often on the face (**Fig. 12**). Granulomas are often seen on biopsy, but in some cases represent postinflammatory skin changes.[77,78]

Angiolupoid sarcoidosis is an uncommon variant of sarcoidosis characterized by prominent telangiectasias within a plaque or nodule. These lesions are most often located on the face of women and are unlikely to self-resolve.[79–81] Although uncommon in the United States, angiolupoid sarcoidosis was reported in 38% of patients in a recent series from Taiwan; this variant also was associated with eye involvement.[79]

Erythroderma is defined as erythema (redness) covering 90% of the body surface area. This condition can be seen in sarcoidosis when other morphologies become extensive in disease (widespread involvement of papules, lichenoid papules, plaques), or the acquired ichthyosis.[61,70,82] When a significant amount of skin is involved, then

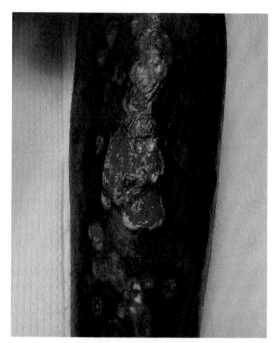

Fig. 11. Ulcerative sarcoidosis. Large areas of ulceration with surrounding dyspigmentation; areas of atrophy often correspond with previously ulcerative lesions.

systemic medications are necessary to control cutaneous disease.

Another unusual presentation of sarcoidosis is pigmented purpuric dermatosis–like sarcoidosis, which presents as brown to slightly purple macules and papules symmetrically on the lower legs.[83,84] A photoinduced variant of sarcoidosis with seasonal variation in clinical disease also has been reported.[85]

Special sites

Scalp Sarcoidosis of the scalp can result in both scarring and nonscarring alopecia. Scarring

alopecia occurs more frequently and involves destruction of the hair follicles with granulomas, resulting in smooth surfaces on the scalp and an inability for hair to regrow.[86–90] Scaling, erythema, indurated plaques, nodules, and diffuse or localized disease can occur, with some presentations mimicking discoid lupus erythematosus.[90] African American women are most commonly affected, and most patients concurrently have other cutaneous sarcoidosis, with the frequent involvement of the face.[86,90] Nonscarring alopecia (retention of the underlying hair follicles) is much less common, with infrequent reports of both localized disease on scalp and nonscalp sites and 1 report of diffuse total body involvement.[90,91] Histopathology of both scarring and nonscarring alopecia shows granulomas on biopsy.[90] Because sarcoidosis has been reported in association with alopecia areata (a Th1-mediated autoimmune nonscarring alopecia), biopsy of the affected area may be helpful in diagnosis.[92]

Nails Nail changes seen in sarcoidosis are highly variable and can include splinter hemorrhages, thinning, pitting, onycholysis, subungual debris, scarring, trachyonychia, color changes, or complete absence of the nail (anonychia) (**Fig. 13**).[93–99] The presence of significant nail changes has a high association with underlying bony cysts, most often in the distal phalynx and may signify a chronic course of systemic disease.[95]

Mucosal disease Oral involvement of sarcoidosis is rare and morphologically can simulate cutaneous diseases with the presence of papules; nodules; erythema, including strawberry gums; and ulcerations.[100–103] Any portion of the oral cavity can be affected, and this can be the presenting sign of systemic disease.[102] Within the oral cavity, the buccal mucosa, gingiva, lips, tongue, and floor of mouth were most commonly affected, followed

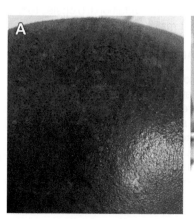
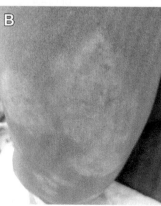

Fig. 12. Hypopigmented sarcoidosis. Macules and papules (*A*) and plaques (*B*) can be seen in African American patients.

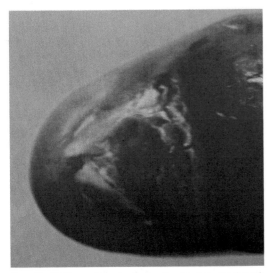

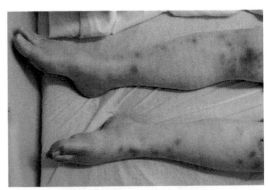

Fig. 14. Erythema nodosum. Nonspecific (ie, reactive, without sarcoidal granulomas on biopsy) manifestation of sarcoidosis that can be associated with fever and lymphadenopathy, known as Löfgren syndrome.

Fig. 13. Nail sarcoidosis. Nails can be involved with sarcoidosis with multiple manifestations; pterygium (scarring) is shown here, which can lead to anonychia.

by the palate and submandibular glands.[103] Genital involvement in sarcoidosis also is rare and can present as infiltrative plaques, nodules, masses, or swelling in these areas.[104–108] Few cases of vulvar sarcoidosis have been reported in the literature to date and 1 case of vaginal sarcoidosis.[104–106] Similarly, scrotal, penile, testicular, or epididymal involvement of sarcoidosis is rarely reported.[107,108] Patients with mucosal or genital sarcoidosis must be evaluated for underlying inflammatory bowel disease, because Crohn disease may present similarly and cases of coexistant sarcoidosis and Crohn disease have been reported.[109]

Nonspecific

The most common nonspecific lesion seen with sarcoidosis is erythema nodosum, which presents as painful, bright red, subcutaneous nodules that are typically symmetric on the anterior shins (**Fig. 14**). These nodules can range in size from 0.5 cm to several centimeters, last for several days up to several weeks, and often evolve by flattening and healing with brown discoloration. Erythema nodosum is often associated with fever, arthralgias, and malaise, and is a reaction pattern observed in association not only with sarcoidosis but also with numerous other causes, including medication-induced causes, infections such as streptococcus and pulmonary endemic fungal infections, and other systemic inflammatory diseases (inflammatory bowel disease, lupus), and it may be idiopathic. Of all erythema nodosum cases, approximately 10% to 22% are associated with

sarcoidosis.[110] When associated with systemic sarcoidosis, this presentation portends an excellent prognosis. This presentation is common in Scandinavians, seen in up to one-third of patients.[111] The association of erythema nodosum with hilar lymphadenopathy and fever is referred to as Löfgren syndrome and represents an acute form of the disease with an overall excellent prognosis.[112,113]

Other nonspecific lesions that have been reported in association with sarcoidosis include digital clubbing, which may be related to underlying pulmonary disease and represents a poor prognostic factor; and calcinosis, which reflects changes in calcium homeostasis with this disease.[114,115] Digital clubbing differs from distal phalynx involvement of sarcoidosis and it is important to differentiate the two. Neutrophilic dermatoses (Sweet syndrome and pyoderma gangrenosum) also have been reported in association with sarcoidosis and may represent either a nonspecific manifestation of sarcoidosis or a concomitant dermatologic disease.[116,117] A sarcoidosis-lymphoma syndrome has been described, highlighting the potential increased rates of malignancy in patients with sarcoidosis; atypical lesions or presentations warrant additional biopsies to rule out concomitant malignancy.

DIAGNOSIS AND WORK-UP

The diagnosis of cutaneous sarcoidosis requires a biopsy and histopathologic examination. Clinical clues were previously discussed and clinicians should include sarcoidosis on the differential diagnosis of numerous skin lesions. Diascopy can be performed on cutaneous lesions by pressing on a papule or plaque with a clear blank slide; the findings of apple-jelly or yellow-brown coloration with diascopy are suggestive but not specific for sarcoidosis.

The characteristic histopathology described for cutaneous sarcoidosis shows noncaseating granulomas composed of epithelioid histiocytes with giant cells surrounded by a mild lymphocytic inflammatory infiltrate (**Fig. 15**). The mild surrounding lymphocytic infiltrate has led to the description of sarcoidal granulomas as naked granulomas. Although naked, noncaseating granulomas are highly specific for sarcoidosis, these histopathologic features are not always present and have been estimated to be seen in 71% to 89% of cases.[118–120] Necrosis within granulomas is very rare in cutaneous sarcoidosis. Different eosinophilic inclusions, including asteroid bodies, Schumann bodies, and crystalline inclusions, can be seen, but are neither specific nor sensitive for sarcoidosis.[121] Biopsies can have variable features, including dense lymphocytes, neutrophils, perineural invasion, caseation, and vasculitis.[8,118,119] Polarization of specimens for foreign material is important, but the presence of foreign material does not exclude the diagnosis of sarcoidosis (**Fig. 16**). Stains to detect microorganisms (Gram stain, periodic acid-Schiff stain for fungal organisms, and acid-fast bacilli stains for mycobacterial organisms) should be performed to exclude an infection.

Systemic evaluation is necessary in any patient when the skin biopsy is concerning for sarcoidosis or a diagnosis of sarcoidosis is expected. Systemic work-up includes in-depth history, physical examination, and laboratory and radiographic evaluation (**Box 1**). Thyroid function also should be considered after a diagnosis has been made, because thyroid dysfunction has been reported in association with cutaneous disease.[122]

Given the potential for disfigurement and the impact on quality of life, health-related quality-of-life indicators and clinical assessment tools can be useful.[123–126] Clinical assessment tools are becoming increasingly important to help quantify active versus nonactive cutaneous disease and standardize baseline characteristics as well as response to treatment.[123–125] Using these in conjunction with quality-of-life metrics can help guide therapeutic decisions and standardize assessment. Several tools have been developed and are available for clinicians to use.[123–126]

DIFFERENTIAL DIAGNOSIS

Given the protean manifestations of cutaneous sarcoidosis, there is a broad clinical differential, and physicians should have a low threshold to involve experienced dermatologists and to biopsy skin lesions. Clinical differential diagnosis of sarcoidosis can be wide and depends on the presenting clinical manifestations (**Table 2**). The histopathologic differential diagnosis includes other granulomatous diseases, including granuloma annulare; necrobiosis lipoidica; foreign body reactions to tattoos; siliconosis; cutaneous Crohn disease; necrobiotic xanthogranuloma; and infections, specifically mycobacterial infections, including tuberculosis, leprosy, and atypical mycobacterial infections (see **Box 1**; **Table 3**).[8]

TREATMENT

Therapeutic decisions for sarcoidosis should be dictated by the organ most severely affected or that has the potential to lead to the most serious disease. Medications for systemic organ involvement often control cutaneous disease; at other times, the skin disease fails to respond and needs targeted therapy. Skin-directed treatment of sarcoidosis is often necessary as an adjuvant to systemic therapy for underlying organ involvement or when cutaneous disease is destructive and disfiguring. A stepwise approach for cutaneous sarcoidosis often is used with the consideration of risks versus benefit of therapy compared with treatment of cutaneous disease: topical treatments, low-risk/nonimmunosuppressive immunomodulators, systemic immunosuppressants, and biologics (TNF inhibitors) (**Table 3**). However, there

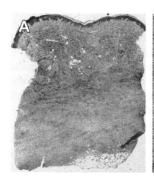
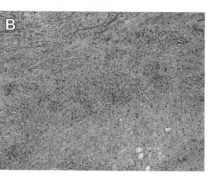

Fig. 15. Histopathology of sarcoidosis. On lower power (2× original magnification), there is a proliferation of granulomas within the dermis (*A*). On higher power (Hematoxylin-eosin stain, magnification × 20), there are collections of histiocytes and multinucleated giant cells with an associated mild lymphocytic infiltrate (*B*, Hematoxylin-eosin stain, magnification × 100).

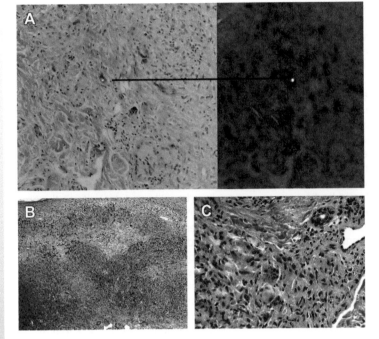

Fig. 16. Foreign material within sarcoidal granulomas. Foreign material seen engulfed in histiocytes and multinucleated giant cells does not rule out sarcoidosis; this foreign material can be polarized (*A*, Hematoxylin-eosin stain, magnification × 200; arrow demonstrates the polarizable particle both under normal light (*left*) and polarized light (*right*). Tattoo pigment can also be seen within the histiocytes and multinucleated giant cells in tattoo-associated sarcoidosis (*B*, Hematoxylin-eosin, magnification × 100) (*C*, Hematoxylin-eosin, magnification × 400).

Box 1
Suggested systemic work-up in patient with cutaneous sarcoidosis
History (occupational/environmental exposure, complete review of systems)
Physical examination
Chest radiograph (posterior-anterior and lateral)
Pulmonary function tests (including diffusion capacity for carbon monoxide)
Ophthalmologic examination
Complete blood count
Comprehensive serum chemistries (including calcium, liver function tests, creatinine)
Electrocardiogram, transthoracic echocardiogram, Holter monitor (consider additional testing if symptomatic)
Urinalysis (if history of stone, then 24-hour urine calcium)
Tuberculin skin test or interferon-gamma release assay
Thyroid testing
Vitamin D_{25} & Vitamin $D_{1,25}$

is a shortage of evidence for treatment and no US Food and Drug Administration–approved treatments. Most treatments take 2 to 3 months to begin to show efficacy, and counseling patients about appropriate expectations is essential.

Topical treatment options for sarcoidosis include steroids (topical and intralesional), topical immunomodulators such as tacrolimus, and topical retinoids. These therapies should be considered for limited skin disease or as adjuvants to other systemic therapy. High-potency topical steroids (clobetasol, halobetasol, betamethasone) applied once to twice daily can lead to clinical resolution of disease.[127,128] Intralesional injections (triamcinolone, 5–40 mg) also can be used for thicker plaques to provide additional penetration.[129] The major risks of these medications, especially when used on thin skin (such as the face) include atrophy, dyspigmentation, and development of telangiectasias. Similarly, topical tacrolimus (used alone or alternating with topical corticosteroids) applied once to twice daily also has been reported to be beneficial and is advantageous, because it does not lead to skin atrophy as can occur with topical steroids.[130,131] Topical retinoids also can be used as an adjuvant therapy to help with dyspigmentation or scaling.

Table 2
Histopathologic differential diagnosis of cutaneous sarcoidosis

Entity	Histopathologic Features
Sarcoidosis	Noncaseating granulomas composed of epithelioid histiocytes surrounded by a mild lymphocytic infiltrate (naked)
Granuloma annulare	Palisading granulomatous inflammatory infiltrate surrounding collagen with mucin
Necrobiosis lipoidica	Horizontally layered, palisading granulomas with necrobiotic collagen interspersed between histiocytes; associated plasma cells are seen
Necrobiotic xanthogranuloma	Palisading xanthogranulomas with associated caseation, neutrophilic debris, and cholesterol clefting; associated lymphocytes and plasma cells are seen
Foreign body reaction	Granulomas composed of multinucleated giant cells and histiocytes with haphazardly arranged nuclei; material is birefringent and can be highlighted with polarization
Infections	Necrotic granulomas composed of histiocytes, lymphocytes, and neutrophilic inflammation; stains for microorganisms can be positive

Table 3
Therapeutic options for cutaneous sarcoidosis

	Medication	Dosing
Topical therapy	Clobetasol	Twice daily (can alternately use with tacrolimus)
	Betamethasone dipropionate	Twice daily
	Halobetasol	Twice daily
	Tacrolimus	Twice daily (can alternately use with topical steroids)
	Tretinoin, Tazarotene	Once daily
Intralesional	Triamcinolone (10–40 mg/kg)	Every 4–8 weeks as needed
Physical	Phototherapy (UVA)	Three times weekly
	Photodynamic therapy	—
	Laser	Pulsed dye, CO_2, ruby, KTP
	Surgery	—
Immunomodulatory	Hydroxychloroquine	200–400 mg daily
	Chloroquine	250–500 mg daily
	Minocycline (or doxycycline or tetracycline)	100 mg twice daily
	Pentoxifylline	400 mg 3 times daily
	Apremilast	20 mg twice daily
	Isotretinoin	20–60 mg daily
	Acitretin	25 mg daily
	Thalidomide	50–200 mg nightly
Immunosuppressants	Prednisone	10–60 mg daily
	Methotrexate	7.5–25 mg weekly
	Azathioprine	50–200 mg daily
	Mycophenolate mofetil	500–1500 mg twice daily
TNF inhibitors	Adalimumab	40 mg weekly (or every other week)
	Infliximab	3–5 mg IV week 0, 2, 6, then every 4–8 wk

Abbreviations: IV, intravenous; KTP, potassium titanyl phosphate; UVA, ultraviolet A.

Other skin-directed therapies reported to be beneficial include photodynamic therapy, phototherapy, laser therapy, and surgical excision. Photodynamic therapy involves the use of a photosensitizing chemical applied to involved areas of the skin, followed by the use of a specific wavelength of light to help induce reactive oxygen species. The use of aminolevulinic and methyl aminolevulinate acid in combination with both blue and red light has yielded beneficial results, but often with recurrence after discontinuation.[132–134] Ultraviolet A phototherapy also has been used with demonstrated improvement with 30 to 50 treatments.[135] With both photodynamic therapy and ultraviolet A phototherapy, risks include burning, erythema, and skin discomfort. Certain lasers have also been reported to be helpful for cutaneous sarcoidosis, with pulsed dye, CO_2 for laryngeal lesions, ruby, and potassium titanyl phosphate lasers being reported.[136–141] In addition, surgical excision can be used on inactive skin lesions in certain circumstances. Because cutaneous sarcoidosis can have a predilection for areas of trauma or scars, lasers and surgical removal should be used with caution.[142]

After localized skin therapy, the next tier of medications often used for cutaneous sarcoidosis includes immunomodulatory therapies, with overall lower potential risks. This category includes antimalarials, tetracycline-class antibiotics (specifically minocycline), pentoxifylline, apremilast, and systemic retinoids. If a patient fails topical therapy or has more than limited skin disease, then the antimalarials (hydroxychloroquine or chloroquine) often are the next line of treatment. Response to these medications often takes at least 3 months, but they can be beneficial for cutaneous sarcoidosis in approximately two-thirds to three-quarters of cases.[143–146] The main side effects and risks include gastrointestinal distress, potential for skin dyspigmentation, and risks of ocular toxicity. Tetracycline antibiotics (minocycline, doxycycline, tetracycline) are used for their antiinflammatory properties with cutaneous sarcoidosis.[147,148] Similar to antimalarials, the effect of these medications can take up to 3 months. Other immunomodulators reported to be effective in cutaneous sarcoidosis include pentoxifylline, apremilast, and retinoids.[149–151] This group of medications may be used alone or in combination, and for more extensive skin disease in cases in which patients are on systemic suppression for extracutaneous disease, or wish to avoid immunosuppression, the use of hydroxychloroquine, minocycline and pentoxifylline may be appropriate.

Traditional, systemic immunosuppressive therapies for both cutaneous and systemic sarcoidosis include systemic corticosteroids (prednisone), methotrexate, and thalidomide. These medications all have potential systemic side effects and require frequent patient follow-up and monitoring. Systemic corticosteroids have been studied in pulmonary sarcoidosis and can be used to obtain rapid control of disease in disfiguring or rapidly progressing cutaneous disease given their immunosuppressant and antiinflammatory properties; dosages can vary and may start at 20 to 40 mg/kg/d with subsequent tapering.[152–155] Systemic corticosteroids can have numerous, well-documented side effects (discussed earlier).

Methotrexate is considered the first-line systemic medication for extensive or recalcitrant cutaneous sarcoidosis.[156–159] Typically dosed at 7.5 to 25 mg/kg/wk depending on response, methotrexate may be used concomitantly with systemic corticosteroids, because the steroids confer rapid resolution of disease and methotrexate can take up to 3 months to show improvement; laboratory monitoring is essential with systemic methotrexate (discussed earlier).

Thalidomide, hypothesized to be effective secondary to its TNF inhibitory properties, has been studied and is beneficial for treatment of cutaneous sarcoidosis.[160–164] Because of its side effect profile, including teratogenicity, neuropathy, and venous thrombosis, it often is reserved for recalcitrant or severe skin disease. A recent double-blind placebo-controlled trial failed to show efficacy in patients with severe cutaneous disease.[165]

Less frequently used but reportedly steroid-sparing agents for cutaneous sarcoidosis include mycophenolate mofetil and azathioprine.[157,166] A small case series of mycophenolate mofetil showed its use as a steroid-sparing agent in cutaneous sarcoidosis, and azathioprine has been used in other forms of sarcoidosis. There may be a publication bias toward positive results, because patients treated with mycophenolate mofetil or azathioprine for extracutaneous disease often fail to show improvement in their skin lesions. Given the limited data, these should be considered options when methotrexate and other agents are not feasible.[157,166]

TNF inhibitors, specifically adalimumab and infliximab, have shown clearance of chronic, recalcitrant, and severe disease, including lupus pernio, ulcerative sarcoidosis, and lesions not responsive to systemic steroids.[167–176] Infliximab (dosed at 3–7 mg/kg at 0, 2, and 6 weeks, with maintenance every 4–8 weeks) has been documented to provide rapid control of cutaneous sarcoidosis when systemic steroids were not helpful and for refractory lupus pernio.[171,173–175,177] Similarly, adalimumab (40 mg weekly) has been studied in a prospective, randomized control trial and in case series with documented improvement in refractory skin disease.[167–170] Etanercept has not been as well studied, although reports of improvement in skin disease exist.[178,179] There is a suggestion of etanercept being less effective for sarcoidosis because a trial for pulmonary disease was discontinued early secondary to lack of efficacy and worse side effects associated with treatment.[180] In addition, it has been ineffective in cases of cutaneous sarcoidosis, when subsequent treatment with other TNF inhibitors has worked.[167,181] Treatment of cutaneous sarcoidosis with TNF inhibitors is complicated and not well understood, because worsening skin disease and development of sarcoidosis when using a TNF inhibitor for other diseases have been reported.[182–185] Clinicians should be aware and consider discontinuation of TNF inhibitors if worsening disease is noted. Evaluation for latent tuberculosis and hepatitis, laboratory monitoring, and consideration of other comorbidities need to be considered in all patients before the initiation of TNF inhibitors.

SUMMARY

Cutaneous sarcoidosis is a common manifestation of systemic sarcoidosis with protean manifestations. Certain skin manifestations can provide clues to underlying organ involvement and potential prognostic information, which can help clinicians guide therapeutic decisions. Systemic evaluation for underlying organ involvement is of paramount importance, and skin-directed therapies can be used as sole therapy or adjuvant therapy.

REFERENCES

1. Mana J, Marcoval J. Skin manifestations of sarcoidosis. Presse Med 2012;41:e355–74.
2. Baughman RP, Teirstein AS, Judson MA, et al. Clinical characteristics of patients in a case control study of sarcoidosis. Am J Respir Crit Care Med 2001;164:1885–9.
3. Lofgren S. Diagnosis and incidence of sarcoidosis. Br J Tuberc Dis Chest 1957;51:8–13.
4. Longcope WT, Freiman DG. A study of sarcoidosis; based on a combined investigation of 160 cases including 30 autopsies from The Johns Hopkins Hospital and Massachusetts General Hospital. Medicine (Baltimore) 1952;31:1–132.
5. Mayock RL, Bertrand P, Morrison CE, et al. Manifestations of sarcoidosis. Analysis of 145 patients, with a review of nine series selected from the literature. Am J Med 1963;35:67–89.
6. Siltzbach LE, James DG, Neville E, et al. Course and prognosis of sarcoidosis around the world. Am J Med 1974;57:847–52.
7. Yanardag H, Pamuk ON, Karayel T. Cutaneous involvement in sarcoidosis: analysis of the features in 170 patients. Respir Med 2003;97:978–82.
8. Ishak R, Kurban M, Kibbi AG, et al. Cutaneous sarcoidosis: clinicopathologic study of 76 patients from Lebanon. Int J Dermatol 2015;54:33–41.
9. Hanno R, Callen JP. Sarcoidosis: a disorder with prominent cutaneous features and their interrelationship with systemic disease. Med Clin North Am 1980;64:847–66.
10. Hanno R, Needelman A, Eiferman RA, et al. Cutaneous sarcoidal granulomas and the development of systemic sarcoidosis. Arch Dermatol 1981;117:203–7.
11. Statement on sarcoidosis. Joint statement of the American Thoracic Society (ATS), the European Respiratory Society (ERS) and the World Association of Sarcoidosis and Other Granulomatous Disorders (WASOG) adopted by the ATS Board of Directors and by the ERS Executive Committee, February 1999. Am J Respir Crit Care Med 1999;160:736–55.
12. Judson MA, Baughman RP. How many organs need to be involved to diagnose sarcoidosis? An unanswered question that, hopefully, will become irrelevant. Sarcoidosis Vasc Diffuse Lung Dis 2014;31:6–7.
13. Celada LJ, Hawkins C, Drake WP. The etiologic role of infectious antigens in sarcoidosis pathogenesis. Clin Chest Med 2015, in press.
14. Fingerlin TE, Hamzeh N, Maier LA. Genetics of sarcoidosis. Clin Chest Med 2015, in press.
15. Callen JP. The presence of foreign bodies does not exclude the diagnosis of sarcoidosis. Arch Dermatol 2001;137:485–6.
16. Lofgren S, Snellman B, Nordenstam H. Foreign-body granulomas and sarcoidosis; a clinical and histo-pathological study. Acta Chir Scand 1955;108:405–18.
17. Marcoval J, Mana J, Moreno A, et al. Foreign bodies in granulomatous cutaneous lesions of patients with systemic sarcoidosis. Arch Dermatol 2001;137:427–30.
18. Marcoval J, Moreno A, Mana J. Foreign bodies in cutaneous sarcoidosis. J Cutan Pathol 2004;31:516.
19. Val-Bernal JF, Sanchez-Quevedo MC, Corral J, et al. Cutaneous sarcoidosis and foreign bodies. An electron probe roentgenographic microanalytic study. Arch Pathol Lab Med 1995;119:471–4.
20. Walsh NM, Hanly JG, Tremaine R, et al. Cutaneous sarcoidosis and foreign bodies. Am J Dermatopathol 1993;15:203–7.

21. Elgart ML. Cutaneous sarcoidosis: definitions and types of lesions. Clin Dermatol 1986;4:35–45.

22. Marcoval J, Moreno A, Mana J. Papular sarcoidosis of the knees: a clue for the diagnosis of erythema nodosum-associated sarcoidosis. J Am Acad Dermatol 2003;49:75–8.

23. Elgart ML. Cutaneous lesions of sarcoidosis. Prim Care 1978;5:249–62.

24. Marcoval J, Mana J, Rubio M. Specific cutaneous lesions in patients with systemic sarcoidosis: relationship to severity and chronicity of disease. Clin Exp Dermatol 2011;36:739–44.

25. Mana J, Marcoval J, Rubio M, et al. Granulomatous cutaneous sarcoidosis: diagnosis, relationship to systemic disease, prognosis and treatment. Sarcoidosis Vasc Diffuse Lung Dis 2013;30:268–81.

26. Callen JP. Relationship of cutaneous sarcoidosis to systemic disease. Clin Dermatol 1986;4:46–53.

27. Olive KE, Kataria YP. Cutaneous manifestations of sarcoidosis. Relationships to other organ system involvement, abnormal laboratory measurements, and disease course. Arch Intern Med 1985;145:1811–4.

28. Sharma OP, Papanikolaou IC. Lupus pernio: a tale of four characters in search of a malady. Sarcoidosis Vasc Diffuse Lung Dis 2009;26:167–71.

29. Spiteri MA, Matthey F, Gordon T, et al. Lupus pernio: a clinico-radiological study of thirty-five cases. Br J Dermatol 1985;112:315–22.

30. Stagaki E, Mountford WK, Lackland DT, et al. The treatment of lupus pernio: results of 116 treatment courses in 54 patients. Chest 2009;135:468–76.

31. Yanardag H, Pamuk ON, Pamuk GE. Lupus pernio in sarcoidosis: clinical features and treatment outcomes of 14 patients. J Clin Rheumatol 2003;9:72–6.

32. Efthimiou P, Kukar M. Lupus pernio: sarcoid-specific cutaneous manifestation associated with chronic sarcoid arthropathy. J Clin Rheumatol 2011;17:343.

33. Neville E, Mills RG, Jash DK, et al. Sarcoidosis of the upper respiratory tract and its association with lupus pernio. Thorax 1976;31:660–4.

34. Ahmed I, Harshad SR. Subcutaneous sarcoidosis: is it a specific subset of cutaneous sarcoidosis frequently associated with systemic disease? J Am Acad Dermatol 2006;54:55–60.

35. Dalle Vedove C, Colato C, Girolomoni G. Subcutaneous sarcoidosis: report of two cases and review of the literature. Clin Rheumatol 2011;30:1123–8.

36. El Sayed F, Dhaybi R, Ammoury A. Subcutaneous nodular sarcoidosis and systemic involvement successfully treated with doxycycline. J Med Liban 2006;54:42–4.

37. Higgins EM, Salisbury JR, Du Vivier AW. Subcutaneous sarcoidosis. Clin Exp Dermatol 1993;18:65–6.

38. Marcoval J, Mana J, Moreno A, et al. Subcutaneous sarcoidosis–clinicopathological study of 10 cases. Br J Dermatol 2005;153:790–4.

39. Marcoval J, Moreno A, Mana J, et al. Subcutaneous sarcoidosis. Dermatol Clin 2008;26:553–6, ix.

40. Meyer-Gonzalez T, Suarez-Perez JA, Lopez-Navarro N, et al. Subcutaneous sarcoidosis: a predictor of systemic disease? Eur J Intern Med 2011;22:e162–3.

41. Marchell RM, Judson MA. Cutaneous sarcoidosis. Semin Respir Crit Care Med 2010;31:442–51.

42. Veien NK, Stahl D, Brodthagen H. Cutaneous sarcoidosis in Caucasians. J Am Acad Dermatol 1987;16:534–40.

43. Antonovich DD, Callen JP. Development of sarcoidosis in cosmetic tattoos. Arch Dermatol 2005;141:869–72.

44. Corbaux C, Fauconneau A, Doutre MS, et al. Systemic sarcoidosis revealed by sarcoidal granulomas on tattoo. J Eur Acad Dermatol Venereol 2015. [Epub ahead of print].

45. Kluger N. Sarcoidosis on tattoos: a review of the literature from 1939 to 2011. Sarcoidosis Vasc Diffuse Lung Dis 2013;30:86–102.

46. Morales-Callaghan AM Jr, Aguilar-Bernier M Jr, Martinez-Garcia G, et al. Sarcoid granuloma on black tattoo. J Am Acad Dermatol 2006;55:S71–3.

47. Post J, Hull P. Tattoo reactions as a sign of sarcoidosis. CMAJ 2012;184:432.

48. Psaltis NM, Gardner RG, Denton WJ. Systemic sarcoidosis and red dye granulomatous tattoo inflammation after influenza vaccination: a case report and review of literature. Ocul Immunol Inflamm 2014;22:314–21.

49. Sowden JM, Cartwright PH, Smith AG, et al. Sarcoidosis presenting with a granulomatous reaction confined to red tattoos. Clin Exp Dermatol 1992;17:446–8.

50. Marcoval J, Mana J. Silicone granulomas and sarcoidosis. Arch Dermatol 2005;141:904.

51. Marcoval J, Moreno A, Mana J. Subcutaneous sarcoidosis localised to sites of previous desensitizing injections. Clin Exp Dermatol 2008;33:132–4.

52. Marcoval J, Fanlo M, Penin RM, et al. Systemic sarcoidosis with specific cutaneous lesions located at insulin injection sites for diabetes mellitus. J Eur Acad Dermatol Venereol 2014;28:1259–60.

53. Marcoval J, Mana J, Penin RM, et al. Sarcoidosis associated with cosmetic fillers. Clin Exp Dermatol 2014;39:397–9.

54. Burgoyne JS, Wood MG. Psoriasiform sarcoidosis. Arch Dermatol 1972;106:896–8.

55. Mitsuishi T, Nogita T, Kawashima M. Psoriasiform sarcoidosis with ulceration. Int J Dermatol 1992;31:339–40.

56. Mittal RR, Singh SP, Gill SS. Psoriasiform sarcoidosis associated with depigmentation. Indian J Dermatol Venereol Leprol 1996;62:103–5.

57. Sakemi H, Oiwa H. Psoriasiform plaques of sarcoidosis. Intern Med 2009;48:391.

58. Khalid U, Gislason GH, Hansen PR. Sarcoidosis in patients with psoriasis: a population-based cohort study. PLoS One 2014;9:e109632.

59. Wanat KA, Schaffer A, Richardson V, et al. Sarcoidosis and psoriasis: a case series and review of the literature exploring co-incidence vs coincidence. JAMA Dermatol 2013;149:848–52.

60. Marcella S, Welsh B, Foley P. Development of sarcoidosis during adalimumab therapy for chronic plaque psoriasis. Australas J Dermatol 2011;52:e8–11.

61. Nishizawa A, Igawa K, Teraki H, et al. Diffuse disseminated lichenoid-type cutaneous sarcoidosis mimicking erythroderma. Int J Dermatol 2014;53:e369–70.

62. Nakahigashi K, Miyachi Y, Utani A. Extensive lichenoid sarcoidosis intermingled with white papules. J Dermatol 2011;38:829–32.

63. Vano-Galvan S, Fernandez-Guarino M, Carmona LP, et al. Lichenoid type of cutaneous sarcoidosis: great response to topical tacrolimus. Eur J Dermatol 2008; 18:89–90.

64. Tsuboi H, Yonemoto K, Katsuoka K. A 14-year-old girl with lichenoid sarcoidosis successfully treated with tacrolimus. J Dermatol 2006;33:344–8.

65. Stockman DL, Rosenberg J, Bengana C, et al. Verrucous cutaneous sarcoidosis: case report and review of this unusual variant of cutaneous sarcoidosis. Am J Dermatopathol 2013;35:273–6.

66. Pezzetta S, Zarian H, Agostini C, et al. Verrucous sarcoidosis of the skin simulating squamous cell carcinoma. Sarcoidosis Vasc Diffuse Lung Dis 2013;30:70–2.

67. Koch LH, Mahoney MH, Pariser RJ. Cutaneous sarcoidosis manifesting as extensive verrucous plaques. Int J Dermatol 2010;49:1458–9.

68. Glass LA, Apisarnthanarax P. Verrucous sarcoidosis simulating hypertrophic lichen planus. Int J Dermatol 1989;28:539–41.

69. Kelley BP, George DE, LeLeux TM, et al. Ichthyosiform sarcoidosis: a case report and review of the literature. Dermatol Online J 2010;16:5.

70. Zhang H, Ma HJ, Liu W, et al. Sarcoidosis characterized as acquired ichthyosiform erythroderma. Eur J Dermatol 2009;19:516–7.

71. Gangopadhyay AK. Ichthyosiform sarcoidosis. Indian J Dermatol Venereol Leprol 2001;67:91–2.

72. Tomoda F, Oda Y, Takata M, et al. A rare case of sarcoidosis with bilateral leg lymphedema as an initial symptom. Am J Med Sci 1999;318:413–4.

73. Nathan MP, Pinsker R, Chase PH, et al. Sarcoidosis presenting as lymphedema. Arch Dermatol 1974; 109:543–4.

74. Ichiki Y, Kitajima Y. Ulcerative sarcoidosis: case report and review of the Japanese literature. Acta Derm Venereol 2008;88:526–8.

75. Yoo SS, Mimouni D, Nikolskaia OV, et al. Clinicopathologic features of ulcerative-atrophic sarcoidosis. Int J Dermatol 2004;43:108–12.

76. Albertini JG, Tyler W, Miller OF 3rd. Ulcerative sarcoidosis. Case report and review of the literature. Arch Dermatol 1997;133:215–9.

77. Schmitt CE, Fabi SG, Kukreja T, et al. Hypopigmented cutaneous sarcoidosis responsive to minocycline. J Drugs Dermatol 2012;11:385–9.

78. Hall RS, Floro JF, King LE Jr. Hypopigmented lesions in sarcoidosis. J Am Acad Dermatol 1984; 11:1163–4.

79. Wu MC, Lee JY. Cutaneous sarcoidosis in southern Taiwan: clinicopathologic study of a series with high proportions of lesions confined to the face and angiolupoid variant. J Eur Acad Dermatol Venereol 2013;27:499–505.

80. Arias-Santiago S, Fernandez-Pugnaire MA, Aneiros-Fernandez J, et al. Recurrent telangiectasias on the cheek: angiolupoid sarcoidosis. Am J Med 2010;123:e7–8.

81. Rongioletti F, Bellisomi A, Rebora A. Disseminated angiolupoid sarcoidosis. Cutis 1987;40:341–3.

82. Yoon CH, Lee CW. Case 6. Erythrodermic form of cutaneous sarcoidosis. Clin Exp Dermatol 2003; 28:575–6.

83. Sezer E, Yalcin O, Erkek E, et al. Pigmented purpuric dermatosis-like sarcoidosis. J Dermatol 2015; 42:629–31.

84. Bachmeyer C, Eguia B, Callard P, et al. Purpuric papulonodular sarcoidosis mimicking granulomatous pigmented purpura. Eur J Dermatol 2011;21: 110–1.

85. Wong S, Pearce C, Markiewicz D, et al. Seasonal cutaneous sarcoidosis: a photo-induced variant. Photodermatol Photoimmunol Photomed 2011;27: 156–8.

86. House NS, Welsh JP, English JC 3rd. Sarcoidosis-induced alopecia. Dermatol Online J 2012;18:4.

87. Cho HR, Shah A, Hadi S. Systemic sarcoidosis presenting with alopecia of the scalp. Int J Dermatol 2004;43:520–2.

88. Douri T, Chawaf AZ, Alrefaee BA. Cicatricial alopecia due to sarcoidosis. Dermatol Online J 2003;9:16.

89. Takahashi H, Mori M, Muraoka S, et al. Sarcoidosis presenting as a scarring alopecia: report of a rare cutaneous manifestation of systemic sarcoidosis. Dermatology 1996;193:144–6.

90. Katta R, Nelson B, Chen D, et al. Sarcoidosis of the scalp: a case series and review of the literature. J Am Acad Dermatol 2000;42:690–2.

91. Dan L, Relic J. Sarcoidosis presenting as non-scarring non-scalp alopecia. Australas J Dermatol 2015. [Epub ahead of print].

92. Melnick L, Wanat KA, Novoa R, et al. Coexistent sarcoidosis and alopecia areata or vitiligo: a case

series and review of the literature. J Clin Exp Dermatol Res 2014;5.

93. Kawaguchi M, Suzuki T. Nail dystrophy without bony involvement in a patient with chronic sarcoidosis. J Dermatol 2014;41:194–5.

94. Bekkali N, Boui M. Nail dystrophy: a rare sign of sarcoidosis. Pan Afr Med J 2014;19:67.

95. Santoro F, Sloan SB. Nail dystrophy and bony involvement in chronic sarcoidosis. J Am Acad Dermatol 2009;60:1050–2.

96. Cohen PD, Lester RS. Sarcoidosis presenting as nail dystrophy. J Cutan Med Surg 1999;3:302–5.

97. Wakelin SH, James MP. Sarcoidosis: nail dystrophy without underlying bone changes. Cutis 1995;55: 344–6.

98. Cox NH, Gawkrodger DJ. Nail dystrophy in chronic sarcoidosis. Br J Dermatol 1988;118:697–701.

99. Mann RJ, Allen BR. Nail dystrophy due to sarcoidosis. Br J Dermatol 1981;105:599–601.

100. Motswaledi MH, Khammissa RA, Jadwat Y, et al. Oral sarcoidosis: a case report and review of the literature. Aust Dent J 2014;59:389–94.

101. Bouaziz A, Le Scanff J, Chapelon-Abric C, et al. Oral involvement in sarcoidosis: report of 12 cases. QJM 2012;105:755–67.

102. Al-Azri AR, Logan RM, Goss AN. Oral lesion as the first clinical presentation in sarcoidosis: a case report. Oman Med J 2012;27:243–5.

103. Kasamatsu A, Kanazawa H, Watanabe T, et al. Oral sarcoidosis: report of a case and review of literature. J Oral Maxillofac Surg 2007;65:1256–9.

104. Watkins S, Ismail A, McKay K, et al. Systemic sarcoidosis with unique vulvar involvement. JAMA Dermatol 2014;150:666–7.

105. Vera C, Funaro D, Bouffard D. Vulvar sarcoidosis: case report and review of the literature. J Cutan Med Surg 2013;17:287–90.

106. Xu F, Cheng Y, Diao R, et al. Sarcoidosis: vaginal wall and vulvar involvement. Sarcoidosis Vasc Diffuse Lung Dis 2012;29:151–4.

107. Mahmood N, Afzal N, Joyce A. Sarcoidosis of the penis. Br J Urol 1997;80:155.

108. Chaowattanapanit S, Aiempanakit K, Silpa-Archa N. Etanercept-induced sarcoidosis presented with scrotal lesion: a rare manifestation in genital area. J Dermatol 2014;41:267–8.

109. Chung J, Rosenbach M. Extensive cutaneous sarcoidosis and coexistant Crohn disease with dual response to infliximab: case report and review of the literature. Dermatol Online J 2014;21(3).

110. Garcia-Porrua C, Gonzalez-Gay MA, Vazquez-Caruncho M, et al. Erythema nodosum: etiologic and predictive factors in a defined population. Arthritis Rheum 2000;43:584–92.

111. Hillerdal G, Nou E, Osterman K, et al. Sarcoidosis: epidemiology and prognosis. A 15-year European study. Am Rev Respir Dis 1984;130:29–32.

112. Ponhold W. The Lofgren syndrome: acute sarcoidosis (author's transl). Rontgenblatter 1977;30:325–7 [in German].

113. James DG, Thomson AD, Willcox A. Erythema nodosum as a manifestation of sarcoidosis. Lancet 1956;271:218–21.

114. Shah A, Bhagat R. Digital clubbing in sarcoidosis. Indian J Chest Dis Allied Sci 1992;34:217–8.

115. Carter JD, Warner E. Clinical images: tumoral calcinosis associated with sarcoidosis. Arthritis Rheum 2003;48:1770.

116. Dadban A, Hirschi S, Sanchez M, et al. Association of Sweet's syndrome and acute sarcoidosis: report of a case and review of the literature. Clin Exp Dermatol 2009;34:189–91.

117. Herrero JE, Mascaro JM Jr, Llambrich A, et al. Sarcoidosis and pyoderma gangrenosum: an exceptional association. The role of trauma and immunosuppressive agents. J Eur Acad Dermatol Venereol 2005;19:97–9.

118. Ball NJ, Kho GT, Martinka M. The histologic spectrum of cutaneous sarcoidosis: a study of twenty-eight cases. J Cutan Pathol 2004;31:160–8.

119. Cardoso JC, Cravo M, Reis JP, et al. Cutaneous sarcoidosis: a histopathological study. J Eur Acad Dermatol Venereol 2009;23:678–82.

120. Jung YJ, Roh MR. Clinical and histopathological analysis of specific lesions of cutaneous sarcoidosis in Korean patients. J Dermatolog Treat 2011;22:11–7.

121. Mangas C, Fernandez-Figueras MT, Fite E, et al. Clinical spectrum and histological analysis of 32 cases of specific cutaneous sarcoidosis. J Cutan Pathol 2006;33:772–7.

122. Anolik RB, Schaffer A, Kim EJ, et al. Thyroid dysfunction and cutaneous sarcoidosis. J Am Acad Dermatol 2012;66:167–8.

123. Baughman RP, Judson MA, Teirstein A, et al. Chronic facial sarcoidosis including lupus pernio: clinical description and proposed scoring systems. Am J Clin Dermatol 2008;9:155–61.

124. Cox CE, Donohue JF, Brown CD, et al. The Sarcoidosis Health Questionnaire: a new measure of health-related quality of life. Am J Respir Crit Care Med 2003;168:323–9.

125. Rosenbach M, Yeung H, Chu EY, et al. Reliability and convergent validity of the cutaneous sarcoidosis activity and morphology instrument for assessing cutaneous sarcoidosis. JAMA Dermatol 2013; 149:550–6.

126. Victorson DE, Choi S, Judson MA, et al. Development and testing of item response theory-based item banks and short forms for eye, skin and lung problems in sarcoidosis. Qual Life Res 2013;23: 1301–13.

127. Khatri KA, Chotzen VA, Burrall BA. Lupus pernio: successful treatment with a potent topical corticosteroid. Arch Dermatol 1995;131:617–8.

128. Wise RD. Clinical resolution of facial cutaneous sarcoidosis with systemic colchicine and a topical corticosteroid ointment. Compr Ther 2008;34: 105–10.

129. Singh SK, Singh S, Pandey SS. Cutaneous sarcoidosis without systemic involvement: response to intralesional corticosteroid. Indian J Dermatol Venereol Leprol 1996;62:273–4.

130. Green CM. Topical tacrolimus for the treatment of cutaneous sarcoidosis. Clin Exp Dermatol 2007; 32:457–8.

131. Katoh N, Mihara H, Yasuno H. Cutaneous sarcoidosis successfully treated with topical tacrolimus. Br J Dermatol 2002;147:154–6.

132. Karrer S, Abels C, Wimmershoff MB, et al. Successful treatment of cutaneous sarcoidosis using topical photodynamic therapy. Arch Dermatol 2002;138:581–4.

133. Penrose C, Mercer SE, Shim-Chang H. Photodynamic therapy for the treatment of cutaneous sarcoidosis. J Am Acad Dermatol 2011;65:e12–4.

134. Wilsmann-Theis D, Bieber T, Novak N. Photodynamic therapy as an alternative treatment for cutaneous sarcoidosis. Dermatology 2008;217:343–6.

135. Mahnke N, Medve-Koenigs K, Berneburg M, et al. Cutaneous sarcoidosis treated with medium-dose UVA1. J Am Acad Dermatol 2004;50:978–9.

136. Frederiksen LG, Jorgensen K. Sarcoidosis of the nose treated with laser surgery. Rhinology 1996; 34:245–6.

137. Grema H, Greve B, Raulin C. Scar sarcoidosis–treatment with the Q-switched ruby laser. Lasers Surg Med 2002;30:398–400.

138. Holzmann RD, Astner S, Forschner T, et al. Scar sarcoidosis in a child: case report of successful treatment with the pulsed dye laser. Dermatol Surg 2008;34:393–6.

139. James JC, Simpson CB. Treatment of laryngeal sarcoidosis with CO_2 laser and mitomycin-C. Otolaryngol Head Neck Surg 2004;130:262–4.

140. Roos S, Raulin C, Ockenfels HM, et al. Successful treatment of cutaneous sarcoidosis lesions with the flashlamp pumped pulsed dye laser: a case report. Dermatol Surg 2009;35:1139–40.

141. Ruff T, Bellens EE. Sarcoidosis of the larynx treated with CO_2 laser. J Otolaryngol 1985;14:245–7.

142. Green JJ, Lawrence N, Heymann WR. Generalized ulcerative sarcoidosis induced by therapy with the flashlamp-pumped pulsed dye laser. Arch Dermatol 2001;137:507–8.

143. Jones E, Callen JP. Hydroxychloroquine is effective therapy for control of cutaneous sarcoidal granulomas. J Am Acad Dermatol 1990;23:487–9.

144. Marchetti M, Baker MG, Noland MM. Treatment of subcutaneous sarcoidosis with hydroxychloroquine: report of 2 cases. Dermatol Online J 2014; 20:21250.

145. Modi S, Rosen T. Micropapular cutaneous sarcoidosis: case series successfully managed with hydroxychloroquine sulfate. Cutis 2008;81:351–4.

146. Zic JA, Horowitz DH, Arzubiaga C, et al. Treatment of cutaneous sarcoidosis with chloroquine. Review of the literature. Arch Dermatol 1991;127:1034–40.

147. Miyazaki E, Ando M, Fukami T, et al. Minocycline for the treatment of sarcoidosis: is the mechanism of action immunomodulating or antimicrobial effect? Clin Rheumatol 2008;27:1195–7.

148. Steen T, English JC. Oral minocycline in treatment of cutaneous sarcoidosis. JAMA Dermatol 2013; 149:758–60.

149. Zabel P, Entzian P, Dalhoff K, et al. Pentoxifylline in treatment of sarcoidosis. Am J Respir Crit Care Med 1997;155:1665–9.

150. Baughman RP, Judson MA, Ingledue R, et al. Efficacy and safety of apremilast in chronic cutaneous sarcoidosis. Arch Dermatol 2012;148:262–4.

151. Georgiou S, Monastirli A, Pasmatzi E, et al. Cutaneous sarcoidosis: complete remission after oral isotretinoin therapy. Acta Derm Venereol 1998;78: 457–9.

152. Baughman RP, Lower EE. Evidence-based therapy for cutaneous sarcoidosis. Clin Dermatol 2007;25: 334–40.

153. Baughman RP, Nunes H. Therapy for sarcoidosis: evidence-based recommendations. Expert Rev Clin Immunol 2012;8:95–103.

154. Doherty CB, Rosen T. Evidence-based therapy for cutaneous sarcoidosis. Drugs 2008;68:1361–83.

155. Mosam A, Morar N. Recalcitrant cutaneous sarcoidosis: an evidence-based sequential approach. J Dermatolog Treat 2004;15:353–9.

156. Veien NK, Brodthagen H. Cutaneous sarcoidosis treated with methotrexate. Br J Dermatol 1977;97: 213–6.

157. Vorselaars AD, Wuyts WA, Vorselaars VM, et al. Methotrexate vs azathioprine in second-line therapy of sarcoidosis. Chest 2013;144:805–12.

158. Webster GF, Razsi LK, Sanchez M, et al. Weekly low-dose methotrexate therapy for cutaneous sarcoidosis. J Am Acad Dermatol 1991;24:451–4.

159. Webster GF, Razsi LK, Sanchez M, et al. Methotrexate therapy in cutaneous sarcoidosis. Ann Intern Med 1989;111:538–9.

160. Baughman RP, Lower EE. Newer therapies for cutaneous sarcoidosis: the role of thalidomide and other agents. Am J Clin Dermatol 2004;5: 385–94.

161. Carlesimo M, Giustini S, Rossi A, et al. Treatment of cutaneous and pulmonary sarcoidosis with thalidomide. J Am Acad Dermatol 1995;32:866–9.

162. Fazzi P, Manni E, Cristofani R, et al. Thalidomide for improving cutaneous and pulmonary sarcoidosis in patients resistant or with contraindications to corticosteroids. Biomed Pharmacother 2012;66:300–7.

163. Lee JB, Koblenzer PS. Disfiguring cutaneous manifestation of sarcoidosis treated with thalidomide: a case report. J Am Acad Dermatol 1998;39:835–8.

164. Nguyen YT, Dupuy A, Cordoliani F, et al. Treatment of cutaneous sarcoidosis with thalidomide. J Am Acad Dermatol 2004;50:235–41.

165. Droitcourt C, Rybojad M, Porcher R, et al. A randomized, investigator-masked, double-blind, placebo-controlled trial on thalidomide in severe cutaneous sarcoidosis. Chest 2014;146:1046–54.

166. Kouba DJ, Mimouni D, Rencic A, et al. Mycophenolate mofetil may serve as a steroid-sparing agent for sarcoidosis. Br J Dermatol 2003;148:147–8.

167. Field S, Regan AO, Sheahan K, et al. Recalcitrant cutaneous sarcoidosis responding to adalimumab but not to etanercept. Clin Exp Dermatol 2010;35:795–6.

168. Heffernan MP, Smith DI. Adalimumab for treatment of cutaneous sarcoidosis. Arch Dermatol 2006;142:17–9.

169. Pariser RJ, Paul J, Hirano S, et al. A double-blind, randomized, placebo-controlled trial of adalimumab in the treatment of cutaneous sarcoidosis. J Am Acad Dermatol 2013;68:765–73.

170. Philips MA, Lynch J, Azmi FH. Ulcerative cutaneous sarcoidosis responding to adalimumab. J Am Acad Dermatol 2005;53:917.

171. Heffernan MP, Anadkat MJ. Recalcitrant cutaneous sarcoidosis responding to infliximab. Arch Dermatol 2005;141:910–1.

172. Meyerle JH, Shorr A. The use of infliximab in cutaneous sarcoidosis. J Drugs Dermatol 2003;2:413–4.

173. Sene T, Juillard C, Rybojad M, et al. Infliximab as a steroid-sparing agent in refractory cutaneous sarcoidosis: single-center retrospective study of 9 patients. J Am Acad Dermatol 2012;66:328–32.

174. Tu J, Chan J. Cutaneous sarcoidosis and infliximab: evidence for efficacy in refractory disease. Australas J Dermatol 2013;55:279–81.

175. Tuchinda P, Bremmer M, Gaspari AA. A case series of refractory cutaneous sarcoidosis successfully treated with infliximab. Dermatol Ther (Heidelb) 2012;2:11.

176. Wanat KA, Rosenbach M. Case series demonstrating improvement in chronic cutaneous sarcoidosis following treatment with TNF inhibitors. Arch Dermatol 2012;148:1097–100.

177. Rosen T, Doherty C. Successful long-term management of refractory cutaneous and upper airway sarcoidosis with periodic infliximab infusion. Dermatol Online J 2007;13:14.

178. Khanna D, Liebling MR, Louie JS. Etanercept ameliorates sarcoidosis arthritis and skin disease. J Rheumatol 2003;30:1864–7.

179. Tuchinda C, Wong HK. Etanercept for chronic progressive cutaneous sarcoidosis. J Drugs Dermatol 2006;5:538–40.

180. Utz JP, Limper AH, Kalra S, et al. Etanercept for the treatment of stage II and III progressive pulmonary sarcoidosis. Chest 2003;124:177–85.

181. Thielen AM, Barde C, Saurat JH, et al. Refractory chronic cutaneous sarcoidosis responsive to dose escalation of TNF-alpha antagonists. Dermatology 2009;219:59–62.

182. Dhaille F, Viseux V, Caudron A, et al. Cutaneous sarcoidosis occurring during anti-TNF-alpha treatment: report of two cases. Dermatology 2010;220:234–7.

183. Tong D, Manolios N, Howe G, et al. New onset sarcoid-like granulomatosis developing during anti-TNF therapy: an under-recognised complication. Intern Med J 2012;42:89–94.

184. Santos G, Sousa LE, Joao AM. Exacerbation of recalcitrant cutaneous sarcoidosis with adalimumab - a paradoxical effect? A case report. An Bras Dermatol 2013;88:26–8.

185. Fok KC, Ng WW, Henderson CJ, et al. Cutaneous sarcoidosis in a patient with ulcerative colitis on infliximab. J Crohns Colitis 2012;6:708–12.

Pulmonary Hypertension in Sarcoidosis

Robert P. Baughman, MD[a],*, Peter J. Engel, MD[b], Steven Nathan, MD[c]

KEYWORDS

- Bosentan • Sarcoidosis • Pulmonary hypertension • Dyspnea

KEY POINTS

- Pulmonary hypertension is recognized as a complication of advanced pulmonary sarcoidosis and is associated with increasing morbidity and mortality.
- Pulmonary hypertension should be suspected in patients with persistent dyspnea, reduced 6-minute walk (6MW), or desaturation with exercise. Echocardiography and pulmonary artery (PA) size as assessed by computed tomographic (CT) scan may suggest pulmonary hypertension. However, right heart catheterization remains the definitive test for confirming pulmonary hypertension.
- There is increasing evidence that sarcoidosis-associated pulmonary hypertension (SAPH) may respond to treatment, including agents that lead to PA vasodilation.

INTRODUCTION

Sarcoidosis is a worldwide disease. Although the prognosis of sarcoidosis is usually quite good,[1] some patients will still succumb to the disease. In referral sarcoidosis clinics, the mortality is around 5%, with most patients dying of respiratory failure.[2] Despite the introduction of newer antiinflammatory treatments for sarcoidosis, the mortality from sarcoidosis appears to be rising over the past 20 years.[3,4] Patients with advanced, chronic sarcoidosis have an increased risk for death.[5] SAPH is a major cause of death in patients with advanced pulmonary disease.

Sarcoidosis leading to pulmonary hypertension has been recognized as a complication of advanced disease for many years.[6,7] Over the past 10 years, the condition has been more widely studied, which is partly because of the recognition that it has a major impact on the outcome of disease.[8] Also, as treatments for pulmonary arterial hypertension became available, these have been used to treat SAPH. In this review, the authors discuss the cause, risk factors, diagnosis, and treatment of SAPH.

CAUSE OF SARCOIDOSIS-ASSOCIATED PULMONARY HYPERTENSION

Sarcoidosis is an interstitial lung disease that can lead to pulmonary fibrosis. Other interstitial lung diseases such as idiopathic pulmonary fibrosis and hypersensitivity pneumonitis can lead to pulmonary hypertension.[9–11] In studies of SAPH, patients often have fibrosis on chest roentgenogram and low forced vital capacity (FVC).[6,12] In some cases, not only fibrosis but also emphysematous type changes are present (Fig. 1).[7] This combination of fibrosis and emphysema is similar to what has been observed in combined

Disclosures: Dr. R.P. Baughman is a consultant and receives grant support from Actelion, Gilead, United Therapeutics, and Bayer. Dr. P.J. Engel is a consultant and speaker for Actelion, Gilead, United Therapeutics, Lung Biotechnology, Inc., and Bayer. He receives grant support from Actelion. Dr. S. Nathan is a consultant, speaker and receives grant support from Gilead, United Therapeutics, and Bayer.
a Department of Medicine, University of Cincinnati, 1001 Holmes Eden Avenue, Cincinnati, OH 45220, USA;
b Ohio Heart and Cardiovascular Center, Christ Hospital, Auburn Avenue, Cincinnati, OH 45219, USA;
c Advanced Lung Disease, INOVA Medical Care, 3300 Gallows Road, Falls Church, VA 22042, USA
* Corresponding author.
E-mail address: bob.baughman@uc.edu

Clin Chest Med 36 (2015) 703–714
http://dx.doi.org/10.1016/j.ccm.2015.08.011
0272-5231/15/$ – see front matter © 2015 Elsevier Inc. All rights reserved.

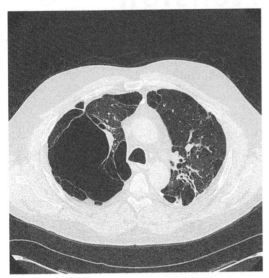

Fig. 1. High-resolution CT scan demonstrating emphysematous as well as fibrotic changes in a patient with chronic sarcoidosis and pulmonary hypertension.

pulmonary fibrosis and emphysema syndrome.[13] This combination may lead to quite severe pulmonary hypertension as a result of the 2 pathologic processes causing severe destruction of lung vasculature.

As opposed to most interstitial lung disease, sarcoidosis can lead to pulmonary hypertension by several other mechanisms beyond just fibrotic lung disease (**Box 1**).[14,15] One mechanism is compression of pulmonary vasculature by enlarged lymph nodes and associated mediastinal fibrosis.[16,17] **Fig. 2** shows the example of a patient with cutaneous and pulmonary sarcoidosis who was found to have severe pulmonary hypertension. Her chest radiograph and CT scan

---

Box 1
Causes of pulmonary hypertension in sarcoidosis

- Fibrotic: obliteration of the pulmonary vascular bed
- Pulmonary vascular compression due to adenopathy
- Granulomatous arteritis
- Pulmonary venoocclusive disease
- Sarcoidosis-associated cirrhosis and portopulmonary hypertension
- Left ventricular systolic and/or diastolic dysfunction
- Hypoxia/pulmonary vasoconstriction

---

demonstrated adenopathy and fibrosis in the hilum and mediastinum, especially in the area of the right upper lobe. On pulmonary angiogram, there was reduced flow to the right upper lobe as a result of extrinsic compression of the PA.

In some cases such as this, PA stenting can be used to improve pulmonary blood flow,[17] However, this could not be performed in this case because of technical reasons.

Pulmonary arteritis can occur as a result of sarcoidosis[14,18]; this may be responsive to corticosteroids or other antiinflammatory drugs.[14,19,20] The incidence of pulmonary hypertension responding to antiinflammatory drugs alone is unknown, but it seems to be fairly rare. However, it may be underrecognized because most patients with chronic pulmonary sarcoidosis will have received corticosteroids for treatment of their pulmonary disease. Workup for pulmonary hypertension is usually reserved for when a patient has failed antiinflammatory therapy and has ongoing symptoms. In studying pulmonary sarcoidosis with early disease using exercise testing, evidence for mild pulmonary hypertension may be seen in patients with no clinical evidence for pulmonary hypertension.[21,22] Pulmonary arterial hypertension due to portopulmonary hypertension has also been reported,[23] but it seems to be rare.

Pulmonary venoocclusive disease has also been reported in SAPH and may be more common than appreciated clinically.[14,18,24] This condition does not seem to respond to antiinflammatory drugs. In general, patients with pulmonary venoocclusive disease may develop pulmonary edema when treated with pulmonary vasodilators such as epoprostenol and bosentan.[25] However, some patients with pulmonary venoocclusive disease have been treated successfully with PA vasodilators.[26] One should consider clinically significant pulmonary venoocclusive disease in a patient with SAPH who is failing to respond or who develops worsening oxygenation of new infiltrates during treatment of their pulmonary hypertension.

Left ventricular (LV) dysfunction can lead to pulmonary hypertension[27]; this can be due to LV dysfunction from myocardial sarcoidosis, resulting in heart failure with reduced ejection fraction. Notably, heart failure with preserved ejection fraction can also occur in patients with sarcoidosis. In both of these cases, the cause may well be LV infiltration from sarcoidosis itself.[15,28] In some cases, MRI scanning of heart may be useful in predicting who has LV dysfunction related to sarcoidosis.[29]

In summary, pulmonary hypertension in sarcoidosis can be caused by pathologic changes similar to those that cause pulmonary arterial hypertension alone (World Health Organization [WHO]

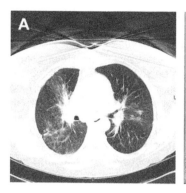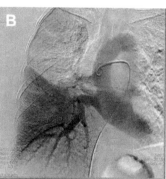

Fig. 2. CT of patient with chronic cutaneous and pulmonary sarcoidosis. (*A*) Upper hilum including the take-off of the right upper lobe (*circled*). This area is compressed by hilar adenopathy and fibrosis. (*B*) Pulmonary angiogram of the right PA. There is normal filling of the right lower lobe; there is marked diminution of flow into the area of the right upper lobe.

Group 1), pulmonary hypertension due to left heart disease (WHO Group 2), and/or pulmonary hypertension associated with lung disease (WHO Group 3). There is also an increased incidence of pulmonary embolism in patients with sarcoidosis[30,31] (WHO Group 4). As a result, the WHO has placed SAPH into WHO Group 5. Although this may be a useful system for epidemiologic purposes, it does not account for the possible implications that the cause of the pulmonary hypertension has on the disease. For example, it is known that patients with SAPH who are in Group 2, that is, LV dysfunction, have a better prognosis than other patients with SAPH.[27] In addition, more precise classification will have implications regarding treatment.

EPIDEMIOLOGY

The reported incidence of SAPH has varied between centers. **Fig. 3** summarizes some of the reported rates of pulmonary hypertension. The prevalence depends on the population studied and the method of confirming the diagnosis of pulmonary hypertension. However, there are some conclusions one can make based on these studies from across the world.

For the studies of unselected patients seen at one clinic, the overall rate of SAPH was 5% to 20%.[32–34] Two of these studies relied on echocardiography alone to make the diagnosis, whereas one study required right heart catheterization to confirm the diagnosis.[33] The study from Kyoto may have included a higher proportion of patients with cardiac sarcoidosis because Japanese patients have an increased incidence of cardiac disease.[32] All 3 studies were performed by tertiary sarcoidosis centers, so the incidence of pulmonary hypertension may be overestimated in a general sarcoidosis clinic. These studies are more likely to reflect the incidence of pulmonary hypertension in patients with pulmonary disease. However, pulmonary disease is the most common manifestation of sarcoidosis.[35,36]

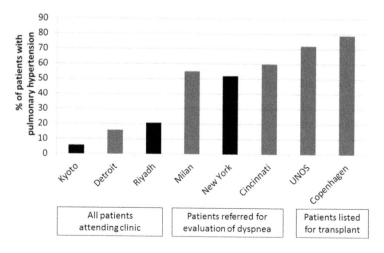

Fig. 3. The incidence of pulmonary hypertension for patients with sarcoidosis. The reports were grouped based on the study population. Black bars indicate those studies that used echocardiography to diagnose pulmonary hypertension. All other series used right heart catheterization to confirm the diagnosis. Three investigators studied all patients seen at a clinic in Kyoto,[32] Detroit,[33] or Riyadh.[34] The next group was composed of patients who were evaluated for persistent or unexplained dyspnea at a clinic in Milan,[6] New York,[12] or Cincinnati.[27] The final group involved patients who had been listed for lung transplant in the United States (United Network for Organ Sharing [UNOS])[38] or Copenhagen.[39]

Patients with persistent or unexplained dyspnea who underwent evaluation for pulmonary hypertension had a greater than 50% chance of having pulmonary hypertension. This fact was true whether the study reported on patients in Italy[6] or the United States.[12,27] Two studies performed right heart catheterization to confirm pulmonary hypertension, which also allowed for a clarification of whether the pulmonary hypertension was pre-capillary or due to LV disease. It was reported that 20% of the patients with pulmonary hypertension had LV disease as the cause of their pulmonary hypertension,[27] and this has also been noted by others.[37]

Patients listed for lung transplant in the United States become part of the United Network for Organ Sharing database. Shorr and colleagues[38] reviewed this database and were able to determine that over 70% of patients awaiting lung transplant had pulmonary hypertension. A similar high percentage was reported from the Copenhagen lung transplant center.[39] Indeed, patients who are listed for lung transplant have the highest reported incidence of pulmonary hypertension.

These studies also give some insight into the risk factors for pulmonary hypertension (**Box 2**). As shown in **Fig. 3**, patients with significant dyspnea were more likely to have pulmonary hypertension. Fibrotic lung disease is one of the causes of SAPH. Therefore the presence of pulmonary fibrosis is a risk factor for pulmonary hypertension. Many reports of patients with SAPH found that most patients had pulmonary fibrosis demonstrated on chest radiograph (Scadding stage 4).[6,12,32,40] For patients being evaluated for pulmonary hypertension, stage 4 chest radiograph was indicative twice as often in those with pulmonary hypertension than in the normal pressure group.[12,40]

Studies reporting pulmonary function testing in SAPH have consistently demonstrated a reduction in the FVC.[12,33,40–43] **Fig. 4**A demonstrates the mean FVC% predicted for patients with SAPH

Box 2
Factors associated with pulmonary hypertension in sarcoidosis

- Dyspnea
- Advanced lung disease by chest radiograph
- Reduced D$_{LCO}$
- Hypoxemia at rest
- Desaturation with 6MW
- Shorter 6MW distance

Abbreviation: D$_{LCO}$, diffusing capacity of lung for carbon monoxide.

---

versus those without SAPH in 3 such studies. The study from Detroit reported on all patients seen at their clinic,[33] whereas the other 2 studies only compared those patients who were undergoing evaluation for persistent dyspnea.[12,40] Similarly, a reduction in the diffusing capacity of lung for carbon monoxide (D$_{LCO}$) has also been reported in patients with SAPH.[12,32,33,40,41] **Fig. 4**B shows the mean percent predicted for patients with and without SAPH at these same 3 centers. A reverse correlation between the PA pressure and the D$_{LCO}$ has been noted in SAPH.[32,40] In one study, patients who died in follow-up of SAPH had significantly lower D$_{LCO}$ than those who survived.[41] A reduction in the DLCO can be the result of either pulmonary fibrosis or pulmonary vascular disease. In patients with sarcoidosis, the synergistic effect of fibrosis and pulmonary vascular disease, as manifest physiologically by a disproportionately reduced D$_{LCO}$, can lead to increased symptoms. In one model for predicting mortality from advanced pulmonary sarcoidosis, the D$_{LCO}$ was an independent factor.[44]

Hypoxia at rest has been found to be more common in those with sarcoidosis with pulmonary hypertension who are being evaluated for dyspnea.[12,38] However, in patients with more advanced disease and listed for lung transplant, the need for supplemental oxygen at rest was no longer predictive of SAPH.[38] Most patients with SAPH require supplemental oxygen at rest or with exercise.[38,41,42,45] The 6MW test is commonly performed to assess cardiopulmonary performance during exercise. In assessing patients with possible SAPH, it has been found to be quite useful. Patients with SAPH tend to have a shorter 6MW distance and often desaturate during the test.[34,46,47] Therefore this test has utility as both a screening tool for SAPH and a prognostic indicator.[48]

DIAGNOSIS OF SARCOIDOSIS-ASSOCIATED PULMONARY HYPERTENSION

As in most types of pulmonary hypertension, the most important factor in diagnosing SAPH is considering the diagnosis in the first place. For the clinician, the first clue is usually unexplained dyspnea. This dyspnea may not correlate with either pulmonary function testing or chest radiograph stage.[49] **Fig. 5** depicts a proposed evaluation algorithm of dyspnea in sarcoidosis. As alluded to previously, the 6MW test has been suggested as a useful way to screen for pulmonary hypertension. Most patients with SAPH will have a 6MW distance of less than 450 m.[33,34,41,42,45,46] However, it is important to bear in mind that the

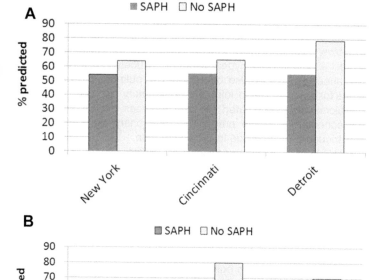

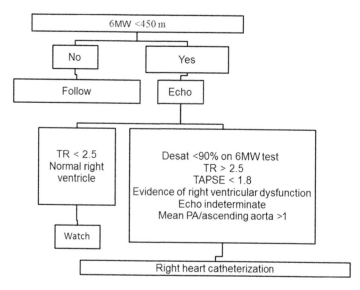

Fig. 4. Comparison of pulmonary function testing for those with and without SAPH at 3 centers in New York,[12] Cincinnati,[40] and Detroit.[33] (*A*) The mean FVC% predicted for the patients with SAPH versus for those without SAPH in these 3 studies. (*B*) Mean percent predicted for patients with and without SAPH at these same 3 centers.

6MW test result may be reduced in sarcoidosis because of various factors, including airway disease, cardiac disease, fatigue, and muscle involvement.[50] In a prospective study of nonselected patients with sarcoidosis, fatigue and general quality-of-life instruments were as predictive of 6MW distance as the FVC% predicted.[46] Although some patients with SAPH may have a 6MW distance of greater than 450 m, these patients are unlikely to require treatment of their

Fig. 5. Proposed evaluation for pulmonary hypertension in the dyspneic sarcoidosis test. The 6MW test determines the distance walked and whether oxygen desaturation (Desat) has occurred. Echocardiogram evaluates for tricuspid regurgitation (TR), tricuspid annular plane systolic excursion (TAPSE) score, and presence of right ventricular dysfunction.

pulmonary hypertension and would just be followed up clinically. Therefore, it seems that a 6MW test would be a reasonable screening test for SAPH. In addition, the 6MW test allows one to determine if desaturation has occurred.

For patients with a reduced 6MW distance, an echocardiogram is the next test to evaluate for pulmonary hypertension. There are several pieces of information that can be determined by echocardiogram. For those patients in whom a tricuspid regurgitant flow can be visualized, an estimate of the PA pressure can be made. In addition, evidence for right ventricular dysfunction can be made by assessing right ventricular size and contractility. However, this is a subjective assessment, while other more sophisticated measures such as the tricuspid annular plane systolic excursion (TAPSE) score allow for a quantifiable number to assess right ventricular dysfunction more objectively.[51]

The most commonly reported echocardiographic parameter for assessing the presence of pulmonary hypertension is based on the finding of tricuspid regurgitation. Although this has proved a useful noninvasive method, it has been found to be less accurate in patients with interstitial lung disease such as idiopathic pulmonary fibrosis.[52,53] In sarcoidosis, there is a correlation between the measured PA systolic pressure and that estimated by echocardiography.[40] **Fig. 6** demonstrates the relationship between estimated PA systolic pressure by echocardiography and direct measurement by right heart catheterization.[27] In this study, 80 patients underwent echocardiography but only 56 (70%) had an identifiable tricuspid regurgitant jet to enable a PA systolic pressure estimate. There was a significant correlation between the 2 measurements (r = 0.62, P<.0001); however,

with a 30 mm Hg echocardiographic cutoff, several patients would have been misclassified. Although increasing the cutoff value for the echocardiography increases its specificity for pulmonary hypertension, it reduces the sensitivity; this has also been noted in pulmonary hypertension due to idiopathic pulmonary fibrosis.[53] Also, the estimated PA systolic does not distinguish between precapillary pulmonary hypertension and that due to LV dysfunction.

Echocardiographic evidence for right ventricular dysfunction may help the clinician detect pulmonary hypertension and the impact thereof.[54] However, most of these measurements are quite subjective and difficult to reproduce in the oddly shaped right ventricle. The TAPSE score has proved to be a reliable indicator of right ventricular dysfunction.[51] This score has been useful in detecting pulmonary hypertension in interstitial lung disease.[55] In one study of patients with SAPH, low TAPSE scores were routinely found.[41]

CT scan of the chest allows one to also visualize the PA. Although PA enlargement has been noted in pulmonary hypertension, measurement of the ratio of the main PA to the ascending aorta might be more accurate in this regard. Specifically, a ratio greater than 1 has been reported as a CT sign of pulmonary hypertension and has been found to be present in many patients with SAPH.[41,56] This ratio was also found to be an independent predictor of mortality from advanced pulmonary sarcoidosis.[44] However, one study did find no correlation between the ratio and the measured PA pressure.[40]

The definitive test for pulmonary hypertension remains right heart catheterization. The results of catheterization are important not only in determining the presence of pulmonary hypertension but also in distinguishing between precapillary

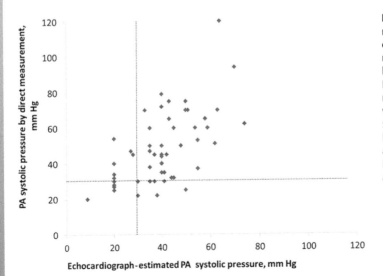

Fig. 6. Correlation between estimated PA systolic pressure by echocardiogram based on the tricuspid regurgitant jet versus the right-heart-catheterization-determined PA systolic pressure. There was a significant correlation between the 2 values (r = 0.62, P<.0001). (*Adapted from* Baughman RP, Engel PJ, Taylor L, et al. Survival in sarcoidosis associated pulmonary hypertension: the importance of hemodynamic evaluation. Chest 2010;138:1078–85.)

and pulmonary hypertension due to LV disease. **Fig. 7** demonstrates the Kaplan-Meier survival curve of 3 groups of patients who underwent right heart catheterization and in whom prolonged follow-up was available. The survival was significantly worse for those with pulmonary hypertension without LV dysfunction compared with the other 2 groups.[27] Other factors that can be determined by right heart catheterization include the right atrial pressure and cardiac output. These factors have been proved to have significant clinical importance in other conditions.

TREATMENT

Many of the available therapies for WHO Group 1 pulmonary arterial hypertension have been used in the treatment of SAPH, although none have been subjected to the necessary large randomized controlled clinical trials to garner the necessary regulatory approval. Therefore the use of these medications, which are summarized in **Table 1**, remains off-label. The first agents used to treat SAPH were the prostanoids.[57] There was some initial concern regarding worsening ventilation perfusion mismatch in patients with lung fibrosis. Also, there was concern that the fibrosis had led to irreversible vessel damage and that there were no further vessels to dilate. However, careful studies identified that many patients with SAPH could still respond to pulmonary vasodilators.[58] In addition, the level of hypoxia was not severe enough to be a contraindication for use of these drugs. An early case series of epoprostenol for moderate to severe SAPH demonstrated response in most patients.[59] This report included 1 patient

who developed congestive heart failure during therapy raising the notion that this patient had pulmonary venoocclusive disease as the cause of pulmonary hypertension, which resulted in pulmonary edema when treated with epoprostenol.[25] Inhaled iloprost is another way to administer a prostanoid for SAPH. In one prospective case series of 15 patients who completed 16 weeks' therapy, 6 had improved hemodynamics and there was a significant improvement in health-related quality of life (HRQoL).[60] However, only 3 patients had a greater than 30 m improvement in their 6MW distance at the end of 16 weeks' therapy.

The endothelin receptor antagonists have also been evaluated as monotherapy for SAPH. The most widely used agent has been bosentan with both case reports and retrospective case series reporting.[41,42,61,62] A double-blind, placebo-controlled trial of bosentan in SAPH has also been reported.[45] In that study, there was significant improvement in the mean PA pressure and the pulmonary vascular resistance (PVR) in the bosentan but not in the placebo-treated group. However, the 16 weeks of therapy was not associated with a significant improvement in the 6MW distance or HRQoL. An increase in the rate of desaturation with exercise was seen for patients treated with bosentan; however, the same rate was seen for those treated with placebo (**Fig. 8**). Of the 23 patients treated with bosentan, 2 required an increase in oxygen supplementation of more than 2 L after 16 weeks of treatment.[45]

Ambrisentan has also been used for SAPH. In a prospective trial, Judson and colleagues[63] reported that less than half of the patients were able to complete the 24 weeks' treatment. The

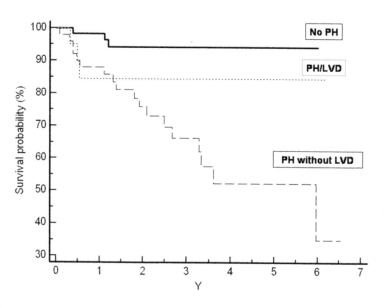

Fig. 7. Comparison of survival of patients with sarcoidosis undergoing right heart catheterization for persistent dyspnea. The patients were divided into 3 groups: normal pulmonary pressure (no PH), pulmonary hypertension with left ventricular dysfunction (PH/LVD), and pulmonary hypertension with no left ventricular dysfunction (PH without LVD). There was a significant difference in survival between groups. (*Adapted from* Baughman RP, Engel PJ, Taylor L, et al. Survival in sarcoidosis associated pulmonary hypertension: the importance of hemodynamic evaluation. Chest 2010;138:1078–85.)

Table 1
Treatment of SAPH

Class/Drug	Evidence	Results
Prostacyclins		
Epoprostenol	CS,[59] CR[57]	CS[59] Clinical improvement
Inhaled iloprost	PCS[60]	PCS[60] Improved hemodynamics in 6/15 Improved HRQoL
Endothelin receptor antagonist		
Bosentan	DBPC[45] CS[40–42]	DBPC[45] Significantly improved hemodynamics after 16 wk vs placebo
Ambrisentan	PCS[63]	PCS[63] Trend for improvement in HRQoL
Phosphodiesterase inhibitor		
Sildenafil	CS[39,41,42]	CS[39] Improvement in hemodynamics but not 6MW distance
Multiple drug therapy	CS[40–42]	—

Abbreviations: CR, case report; CS, case series; DBPC, double-blind placebo controlled; HRQoL, health-related quality of life; PCS, prospective case series.

most common reasons for drop out were edema and/or dyspnea. For the 10 patients who completed the study, there was a trend to improved HRQoL. Unfortunately, the study was underpowered to demonstrate significant changes in HRQoL. In addition, the patients developed edema from ambrisentan and were dropped from the study per protocol. Discontinuation of drug may not have been necessary because analysis of use of ambrisentan in idiopathic pulmonary arterial hypertension has found the drug to be effective in the presence of edema.[64]

The phosphodiesterase 5 inhibitors also have been used as single agents in the treatment of SAPH. Milman and colleagues[39] reported on their use in 12 patients with SAPH awaiting lung transplant. He found an improvement in hemodynamics but no change in 6MW distance in this group of patients with advanced disease. However, there are reports suggesting that this class of drugs may prove more useful in treating patients with less-severe SAPH.[42,62]

In the routine management of pulmonary hypertension, combination therapy is often used for patients failing single-drug treatment. This approach has also been used in managing patients with SAPH, but is difficult to study in the context of randomized clinical trials.[40–42] Nonetheless, it does

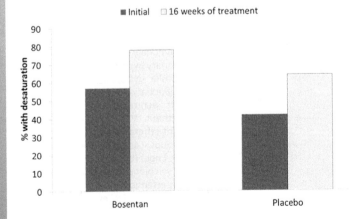

Fig. 8. Percentage of patients with desaturation with exercise during 6MW test before and after 16 weeks of bosentan treatment. Desaturation was defined as a greater than 5% decrease in oxygen saturation compared with rest, increase in supplemental oxygen of greater than 2 L/min, or both. Over time, there was an increase in the rate of desaturation. There was no difference in the rate of desaturation initially or after 16 weeks between the 2 groups. (*Adapted from* Baughman RP, Culver DA, Cordova FC, et al. Bosentan for sarcoidosis associated pulmonary hypertension: a double-blind placebo controlled randomized trial. Chest 2014;145: 810–17.)

make intuitive sense and allows for more prolonged treatment of patients who fail single-drug therapy.

The current status of therapy demonstrates that treatment of SAPH may improve hemodynamics in some patients.[42,45,60] However, the effect on 6MW distance may be less dramatic, and it may require longer treatment before improvement in 6MW distance will occur. The 2 studies reporting improvement in 6MW distance[42,62] had much longer follow-up than the 16 to 24 weeks of the clinical trials.[45,60,63] It is also not clear whether the results of the 6MW test are the best predictors of clinical outcome in pulmonary hypertension. In fact, it has been shown that the change in 6MW distance with treatment does not help predict prognosis in PAH. Recent trials have focused on time until clinical worsening as a more meaningful outcome[65,66]; this may be an important end point in future trials of treatment of SAPH.[67]

Another issue is the role of pulmonary fibrosis in determining the response to treatment of SAPH. Barnett and colleagues[42] had noted that overall there was a significant improvement in 6MW distance with treatment of SAPH. The investigators also found that there was a positive correlation between the initial FVC% predicted and the improvement in 6MW distance. When they analyzed the change in 6MW distance versus the FVC% predicted, they found that those patients with an FVC% predicted above their median value of 51% had a higher likelihood of responding. The investigators did note some patients with a lower FVC% predicted who still responded. However, this factor should be considered when deciding about initial or subsequent therapy.

Box 3
Features associated with reduced survival in SAPH

- Proven risk factors from SAPH trial
  - Reduced FVC% predicted
  - Reduced D$_{LCO}$
  - Higher PVR
  - Lower cardiac index
  - PA systolic pressure of greater than 50 mm Hg
- Potential features based on studies in other conditions
  - Advanced fibrosis on CT scan
  - Lower TAPSE score

SURVIVAL

Several factors have been noted to be associated with reduced survival in patients with SAPH. **Box 3** summarizes those features associated with a worse outcome. Patients who died or underwent transplant for their SAPH had lower FVC% and D$_{LCO}$% predicted.[41] Patients with an elevated PVR also were more likely to die from the disease.[27,41] A lower cardiac index was also seen in those who died or underwent transplant.[41] An elevated PA systolic pressure of greater than 50 mm Hg by echo was also found to be associated with increased mortality.[27]

SUMMARY

Pulmonary hypertension in sarcoidosis is a significant clinical problem because it is associated with increased mortality.[27,68] Over the past few years, techniques have been developed to better diagnose the condition. In addition, there is increasing evidence to support treatment of SAPH with pulmonary vasodilators. These treatments have been associated with improved hemodynamics, quality of life, and exercise tolerance in some patients. However, further studies are needed to determine whether these interventions will change the natural course of the disease.

REFERENCES

1. Reich JM. Mortality of intrathoracic sarcoidosis in referral vs population-based settings: influence of stage, ethnicity, and corticosteroid therapy. Chest 2002;121:32–9.
2. Baughman RP, Winget DB, Bowen EH, et al. Predicting respiratory failure in sarcoidosis patients. Sarcoidosis 1997;14:154–8.
3. Mirsaeidi M, Machado RF, Schraufnagel D, et al. Racial difference in sarcoidosis mortality in the United States. Chest 2015;147:438–9.
4. Swigris JJ, Olson AL, Huie TJ, et al. Sarcoidosis-related mortality in the United States from 1988 to 2007. Am J Respir Crit Care Med 2011;183(11): 1524–30.
5. Nardi A, Brillet PY, Letoumelin P, et al. Stage IV sarcoidosis: comparison of survival with the general population and causes of death. Eur Respir J 2011; 38(6):1368–73.
6. Rizzato G, Pezzano A, Sala G, et al. Right heart impairment in sarcoidosis: haemodynamic and echocardiographic study. Eur J Respir Dis 1983; 64(2):121–8.
7. Battesti JP, Georges R, Basset F, et al. Chronic cor pulmonale in pulmonary sarcoidosis. Thorax 1978; 33(1):76–84.

8. Palmero V, Sulica R. Sarcoidosis-associated pulmonary hypertension: assessment and management. Semin Respir Crit Care Med 2010;31(4):494–500.

9. Nathan SD, Shlobin OA, Ahmad S, et al. Serial development of pulmonary hypertension in patients with idiopathic pulmonary fibrosis. Respiration 2008;76(3):288–94.

10. Oliveira RK, Pereira CA, Ramos RP, et al. A haemodynamic study of pulmonary hypertension in chronic hypersensitivity pneumonitis. Eur Respir J 2014;44(2):415–24.

11. Corte TJ, Wort SJ, Wells AU. Pulmonary hypertension in idiopathic pulmonary fibrosis: a review. Sarcoidosis Vasc Diffuse Lung Dis 2009;26(1):7–19.

12. Sulica R, Teirstein AS, Kakarla S, et al. Distinctive clinical, radiographic, and functional characteristics of patients with sarcoidosis-related pulmonary hypertension. Chest 2005;128(3):1483–9.

13. Cottin V, Le PJ, Prevot G, et al. Pulmonary hypertension in patients with combined pulmonary fibrosis and emphysema syndrome. Eur Respir J 2010;35(1):105–11.

14. Nunes H, Humbert M, Capron F, et al. Pulmonary hypertension associated with sarcoidosis: mechanisms, haemodynamics and prognosis. Thorax 2006;61(1):68–74.

15. Cordova FC, D'Alonzo G. Sarcoidosis-associated pulmonary hypertension. Curr Opin Pulm Med 2013;19(5):531–7.

16. Toonkel RL, Borczuk AC, Pearson GD, et al. Sarcoidosis-associated fibrosing mediastinitis with resultant pulmonary hypertension: a case report and review of the literature. Respiration 2010;79(4):341–5.

17. Hamilton-Craig CR, Slaughter R, McNeil K, et al. Improvement after angioplasty and stenting of pulmonary arteries due to sarcoid mediastinal fibrosis. Heart Lung Circ 2009;18(3):222–5.

18. Takemura T, Matsui Y, Saiki S, et al. Pulmonary vascular involvement in sarcoidosis: a report of 40 autopsy cases. Hum Pathol 1992;23(11):1216–23.

19. Rodman DM, Lindenfeld J. Successful treatment of sarcoidosis-associated pulmonary hypertension with corticosteroids. Chest 1990;97(2):500–2.

20. Gluskowski J, Hawrylkiewicz I, Zych D, et al. Effects of corticosteroid treatment on pulmonary haemodynamics in patients with sarcoidosis. Eur Respir J 1990;3(4):403–7.

21. Baughman RP, Gerson M, Bosken CH. Right and left ventricular function at rest and with exercise in patients with sarcoidosis. Chest 1984;85(3):301–6.

22. Gluskowski J, Hawrylkiewicz I, Zych D, et al. Pulmonary haemodynamics at rest and during exercise in patients with sarcoidosis. Respiration 1984;46(1):26–32.

23. Salazar A, Mana J, Sala J, et al. Combined portal and pulmonary hypertension in sarcoidosis. Respiration 1994;61(2):117–9.

24. Hoffstein V, Ranganathan N, Mullen JB. Sarcoidosis simulating pulmonary veno-occlusive disease. Am Rev Respir Dis 1986;134(4):809–11.

25. Montani D, Achouh L, Dorfmuller P, et al. Pulmonary veno-occlusive disease: clinical, functional, radiologic, and hemodynamic characteristics and outcome of 24 cases confirmed by histology. Medicine (Baltimore) 2008;87(4):220–33.

26. Montani D, Jais X, Price LC, et al. Cautious epoprostenol therapy is a safe bridge to lung transplantation in pulmonary veno-occlusive disease. Eur Respir J 2009;34(6):1348–56.

27. Baughman RP, Engel PJ, Taylor L, et al. Survival in sarcoidosis associated pulmonary hypertension: the importance of hemodynamic evaluation. Chest 2010;138:1078–85.

28. Angomachalelis N, Hourzamanis A, Vamvalis C, et al. Doppler echocardiographic evaluation of left ventricular diastolic function in patients with systemic sarcoidosis. Postgrad Med J 1992;68(Suppl 1):S52–6.

29. Ichinose A, Otani H, Oikawa M, et al. MRI of cardiac sarcoidosis: basal and subepicardial localization of myocardial lesions and their effect on left ventricular function. AJR Am J Roentgenol 2008;191(3):862–9.

30. Crawshaw AP, Wotton CJ, Yeates DG, et al. Evidence for association between sarcoidosis and pulmonary embolism from 35-year record linkage study. Thorax 2011;66(5):447–8.

31. Swigris JJ, Olson AL, Huie TJ, et al. Increased risk of pulmonary embolism among US decedents with sarcoidosis from 1988 to 2007. Chest 2011;140(5):1261–6.

32. Handa T, Nagai S, Miki S, et al. Incidence of pulmonary hypertension and its clinical relevance in patients with sarcoidosis. Chest 2006;129(5):1246–52.

33. Bourbonnais JM, Samavati L. Clinical predictors of pulmonary hypertension in sarcoidosis. Eur Respir J 2008;32(2):296–302.

34. Alhamad EH, Idrees MM, Alanezi MO, et al. Sarcoidosis-associated pulmonary hypertension: clinical features and outcomes in Arab patients. Ann Thorac Med 2010;5(2):86–91.

35. Loddenkemper R, Kloppenborg A, Schoenfeld N, et al. Clinical findings in 715 patients with newly detected pulmonary sarcoidosis–results of a cooperative study in former West Germany and Switzerland. WATL study group. Wissenschaftliche Arbeitsgemeinschaft fur die Therapie von Lungenkrankheiten. Sarcoidosis Vasc Diffuse Lung Dis 1998;15(2):178–82.

36. Baughman RP, Teirstein AS, Judson MA, et al. Clinical characteristics of patients in a case control

study of sarcoidosis. Am J Respir Crit Care Med 2001;164:1885–9.

37. Alhamad EH, Cal JG, Alfaleh HF, et al. Pulmonary hypertension in Saudi Arabia: a single center experience. Ann Thorac Med 2013;8(2):78–85.

38. Shorr AF, Helman DL, Davies DB, et al. Pulmonary hypertension in advanced sarcoidosis: epidemiology and clinical characteristics. Eur Respir J 2005;25(5):783–8.

39. Milman N, Burton CM, Iversen M, et al. Pulmonary hypertension in end-stage pulmonary sarcoidosis: therapeutic effect of sildenafil? J Heart Lung Transplant 2008;27(3):329–34.

40. Baughman RP, Engel PJ, Meyer CA, et al. Pulmonary hypertension in sarcoidosis. Sarcoidosis Vasc Diffuse Lung Dis 2006;23:108–16.

41. Keir GJ, Walsh SL, Gatzoulis MA, et al. Treatment of sarcoidosis-associated pulmonary hypertension: a single centre retrospective experience using targeted therapies. Sarcoidosis Vasc Diffuse Lung Dis 2014;31(2):82–90.

42. Barnett CF, Bonura EJ, Nathan SD, et al. Treatment of sarcoidosis-associated pulmonary hypertension: a two-center experience. Chest 2009; 135:1455–61.

43. Steen V, Medsger TA Jr. Predictors of isolated pulmonary hypertension in patients with systemic sclerosis and limited cutaneous involvement. Arthritis Rheum 2003;48(2):516–22.

44. Walsh SL, Wells AU, Sverzellati N, et al. An integrated clinicoradiological staging system for pulmonary sarcoidosis: a case-cohort study. Lancet Respir Med 2014;2(2):123–30.

45. Baughman RP, Culver DA, Cordova FC, et al. Bosentan for sarcoidosis associated pulmonary hypertension: a double-blind placebo controlled randomized trial. Chest 2014;145:810–7.

46. Baughman RP, Sparkman BK, Lower EE. Six-minute walk test and health status assessment in sarcoidosis. Chest 2007;132(1):207–13.

47. Alhamad EH, Shaik SA, Idrees MM, et al. Outcome measures of the 6 minute walk test: relationships with physiologic and computed tomography findings in patients with sarcoidosis. BMC Pulm Med 2010;10:42.

48. Lederer DJ, Arcasoy SM, Wilt JS, et al. Six-minute-walk distance predicts waiting list survival in idiopathic pulmonary fibrosis. Am J Respir Crit Care Med 2006;174(6):659–64.

49. Yeager H, Rossman MD, Baughman RP, et al. Pulmonary and psychosocial findings at enrollment in the ACCESS study. Sarcoidosis Vasc Diffuse Lung Dis 2005;22(2):147–53.

50. Baughman RP, Lower EE. Six-minute walk test in managing and monitoring sarcoidosis patients. Curr Opin Pulm Med 2007;13(5):439–44.

51. Forfia PR, Fisher MR, Mathai SC, et al. Tricuspid annular displacement predicts survival in pulmonary hypertension. Am J Respir Crit Care Med 2006; 174(9):1034–41.

52. Arcasoy SM, Christie JD, Ferrari VA, et al. Echocardiographic assessment of pulmonary hypertension in patients with advanced lung disease. Am J Respir Crit Care Med 2003;167(5):735–40.

53. Nathan SD, Shlobin OA, Barnett SD, et al. Right ventricular systolic pressure by echocardiography as a predictor of pulmonary hypertension in idiopathic pulmonary fibrosis. Respir Med 2008; 102(9):1305–10.

54. Bertoli L, Rizzato G, Merlini R, et al. Can pulmonary hypertension be predicted by non-invasive approach? Echocardiographic and haemodynamic study. Acta Cardiol 1984;39(2):97–106.

55. Ruocco G, Cekorja B, Rottoli P, et al. Role of BNP and echo measurement for pulmonary hypertension recognition in patients with interstitial lung disease: an algorithm application model. Respir Med 2015; 109(3):406–15.

56. Ng CS, Wells AU, Padley SP. A CT sign of chronic pulmonary arterial hypertension: the ratio of main pulmonary artery to aortic diameter. J Thorac Imaging 1999;14(4):270–8.

57. Barst RJ, Ratner SJ. Sarcoidosis and reactive pulmonary hypertension. Arch Intern Med 1985; 145(11):2112–4.

58. Preston IR, Klinger JR, Landzberg MJ, et al. Vasoresponsiveness of sarcoidosis-associated pulmonary hypertension. Chest 2001;120(3):866–72.

59. Fisher KA, Serlin DM, Wilson KC, et al. Sarcoidosis-associated pulmonary hypertension: outcome with long-term epoprostenol treatment. Chest 2006; 130(5):1481–8.

60. Baughman RP, Judson MA, Lower EE, et al. Inhaled iloprost for sarcoidosis associated pulmonary hypertension. Sarcoidosis Vasc Diffuse Lung Dis 2009;26: 110–20.

61. Foley RJ, Metersky ML. Successful treatment of sarcoidosis-associated pulmonary hypertension with bosentan. Respiration 2005;75(2):211–4.

62. Dobarro D, Schreiber BE, Handler C, et al. Clinical characteristics, haemodynamics and treatment of pulmonary hypertension in sarcoidosis in a single centre, and meta-analysis of the published data. Am J Cardiol 2013;111(2):278–85.

63. Judson MA, Highland KB, Kwon S, et al. Ambrisentan for sarcoidosis associated pulmonary hypertension. Sarcoidosis Vasc Diffuse Lung Dis 2011; 28(2):139–45.

64. Shapiro S, Pollock DM, Gillies H, et al. Frequency of edema in patients with pulmonary arterial hypertension receiving ambrisentan. Am J Cardiol 2012; 110(9):1373–7.

65. Ghofrani HA, Galie N, Grimminger F, et al. Riociguat for the treatment of pulmonary arterial hypertension. N Engl J Med 2013;369(4):330–40.

66. Pulido T, Adzerikho I, Channick RN, et al. Macitentan and morbidity and mortality in pulmonary arterial hypertension. N Engl J Med 2013;369(9):809–18.

67. Baughman RP, Drent M, Culver DA, et al. Endpoints for clinical trials of sarcoidosis. Sarcoidosis Vasc Diffuse Lung Dis 2012;29:90–8.

68. Shorr AF, Davies DB, Nathan SD. Predicting mortality in patients with sarcoidosis awaiting lung transplantation. Chest 2003;124(3):922–8.

Severe Sarcoidosis

Vasileios Kouranos, MD, MSc[a], Joe Jacob, MD[b], Athol U. Wells, MD, PhD[a],*

KEYWORDS

- Sarcoidosis • Pulmonary fibrosis • Cardiac sarcoidosis

KEY POINTS

- The indications for initiating therapy in sarcoidosis can be broadly dichotomized as danger from disease and unacceptable loss of quality of life.
- Disease should be viewed as dangerous if it is already severe or if there is a high risk of major progression.
- A multidisciplinary approach is required to identify severe pulmonary disease, with the integration of symptoms, pulmonary function tests, and imaging findings.
- In stratifying risk for future progression to severe disease, duration of disease and short-term disease behavior should also be taken into account.
- Advanced imaging techniques may be helpful in risk stratification in both pulmonary and cardiac sarcoidosis.

INTRODUCTION

In sarcoidosis, the considerable variability in initial presentation, disease evolution, and outcome poses major problems in the formulation of a logical management strategy. The spectrum of disease ranges from asymptomatic imaging abnormalities, encountered as an incidental finding, to prominent symptoms due to systemic disease activity or major organ involvement. Pulmonary involvement (lung or mediastinal involvement) is evident in 90% to 95% of cases, and this is variably associated with respiratory and systemic symptoms, including fatigue, musculoskeletal symptoms, fevers, and weight loss. The natural history and treated course of disease are also highly heterogeneous, ranging from spontaneous remission to progressive pulmonary and extrapulmonary disease, associated with increased morbidity and mortality.[1,2] Respiratory failure is the most frequent cause of death in sarcoidosis, except in Japanese patients, who most commonly die from cardiac involvement.[3,4] Pulmonary hypertension (PH) is an independent predictor of mortality in sarcoidosis, irrespective of specific organ involvement.[5]

Optimal management in sarcoidosis is critically dependent on the clarity of definition of treatment goals. The historical view that all patients with sarcoidosis require therapy was never uniformly accepted and is now widely regarded as wholly inappropriate. However, the indications for initiating therapy are not exact: clinicians less accustomed to managing sarcoidosis are confronted, in many texts, by a long list of indications for treatment but no logical overview of broad treatment objectives readily understood by patients. It has recently been suggested that clinical reasoning in this context should be based on a simple dichotomy of danger from disease and unacceptable loss of quality of life,[6] with the latter not considered further in this review. It can be argued that when disease is not overtly dangerous, decisions on treatment of morbidity should be patient-driven because the impact of symptoms on

Funding Sources: Nil.
Conflict of Interest: Nil.
a Interstitial Lung Disease Unit, Royal Brompton Hospital, Sydney Street, London SW3 6NP, UK; b Department of Radiology, Royal Brompton Hospital, Sydney Street, London SW3 6NP, UK
* Corresponding author.
E-mail address: RBHILD@rbht.nhs.uk

chestmed.theclinics.com

overall quality of life is something that can never be fully grasped by anyone other than the patient and immediate family. However, when there is danger from disease (consisting of a higher risk either of mortality or disability due to major organ involvement) present in a minority of cases, the management strategy should ideally be based on medical expertise and the identification of severe disease or of risk factors predictive of progression to severe disease. Although factors associated with a high likelihood of spontaneous remission have been clearly identified, including erythema nodosum, stage I chest X-radiographic abnormalities, and ocular involvement, stratification for a high risk of future severe disease is relatively imprecise.

Although the age-adjusted mortality is relatively low in sarcoidosis (2.8 per 1 million population from 1999 to 2010),[7] with less than 10% of patients having a reduction in life expectancy due to sarcoidosis, it is critically important to identify such patients as early as possible, but this is often far from straightforward. There is no classification of disease severity in sarcoidosis and no formal definition of severe sarcoidosis. In principle, severe disease might reasonably be classified according to the level of major organ involvement, but this approach has drawbacks. Intensive treatment algorithms centered on the presence of severe disease amount to an admission of defeat, with an implicit inability to anticipate progression to severe disease and initiate a vigorous approach earlier in the disease course. Ideally, patients at high risk of a malignant outcome should be identified at presentation or early during follow-up, based on (a) symptoms that might presage life-threatening manifestations such as sudden cardiac death or significant functional impairment interfering with essential aspects of daily life; (b) the staging of disease severity based on functional tests and imaging modalities, which have established prognostic significance[8,9]; and (c) the careful observation of longitudinal disease behavior with or without initial therapy.

The purposes of this review are first to detail the evaluation of disease severity in patients with pulmonary and cardiac sarcoidosis (because other less prevalent organ involvement, covered in-depth elsewhere in this issue, are less frequent indications for prolonged therapy). Prognostic evaluation to stratify risk, even when disease is not yet overtly severe, is also discussed. Treatment considerations in high-risk patients are detailed. The effect of age, race, and gender on risk and disease severity is not covered in-depth in this review, although also relevant to disease severity and mortality in sarcoidosis.[3,10]

SEVERE PULMONARY INVOLVEMENT

In most patients with sarcoidosis, disease is either self-limited with spontaneous remission, as typically seen in Löfgren syndrome, or treatment is rapidly effective and the long-term outcome is good. However, interstitial lung involvement progresses to significant pulmonary fibrosis in up to a third of cases.[11] Extensive interstitial lung disease with pulmonary fibrosis and PH has been strongly associated with increased morbidity and mortality. PH may develop as a complication of the severe pulmonary fibrosis but also may be evident without significant parenchymal involvement due to pulmonary vascular infiltration and other pathophysiological mechanisms.

The Definition of Severe Pulmonary Fibrosis

The presence of pulmonary fibrosis does not, in itself, result in differences in the range of clinical manifestations of lung involvement, which include cough, shortness of breath, wheeze, and episodes of hemoptysis (especially when Aspergillus and other fungal species have infiltrated segments with bronchiectatic or bronchial distorted areas). Interestingly, inspiratory crackles and clubbing are not present, in contrast to idiopathic pulmonary fibrosis (IPF).[12] A mixed ventilatory defect pattern with moderate to severe impairment in gas transfer is most common in patients with pulmonary fibrosis in sarcoidosis.[13] Airflow limitation is caused by both airway involvement with predominant inflammation of the small airways and, in an important subgroup, extensive fibrotic abnormalities. Staging the severity of pulmonary fibrosis requires confirmation that irreversible interstitial lung disease is present (based on imaging findings or lack of responsiveness to therapy) and the integration of symptoms, pulmonary function tests (PFT), and imaging findings.

It should be stressed that pulmonary disease severity cannot be staged with confidence without the integration of the above mentioned 3 domains, each of which is seriously flawed when considered in isolation. With regard to severe disease in particular, it might be supposed that exercise intolerance should drive treatment decisions, but although this may be broadly correct on quality-of-life grounds, exertional dyspnea does not always correlate with the severity of lung disease. A discussion of the multiplicity of thoracic and extrathoracic causes of exercise limitation in sarcoidosis lies beyond the scope of this review: suffice it to say that disability due to dyspnea may equally result from interstitial lung disease, PH, and cardiac sarcoidosis, in isolation or in combination. Pulmonary function severity thresholds are attractive for their precision but are limited by variation in the normal predicted range: for example, a forced vital capacity (FVC) level of 70% may equally represent minor decline and severe disease progression from premorbid values of 70% and 120%, respectively.[14] Severe pulmonary function impairment, including resting or exertional hypoxia, can be viewed as synonymous with severe disease, whether due to PH or interstitial lung disease, but more often the degree of impairment is indeterminate—neither definitively severe nor definitively mild.

Given these constraints and the frequent difficulty in reconciling symptoms and PFTs in defining disease severity, the assessment of imaging features has an important role. The traditional diagnostic chest radiographic features, consisting of reticular parenchymal changes with or without bilateral mediastinal lymphadenopathy,[15] are not, in themselves, a guide to the global severity of interstitial lung disease. The Scadding staging system draws distinctions between average outcomes in patient cohorts but does not provide prognostic information in individual patients that is sufficiently reliable to inform management decisions; this is well illustrated by the category of stage IV disease, in which chest radiographic appearances are considered to be fibrotic. Major variation between radiologists exists in the designation of stage IV disease depending on whether stringent evidence of irreversible disease is required (ie, major volume loss or lung destruction) or whether more subtle fibrotic abnormalities are also taken into account.[16] The low interobserver agreement and sensitivity in the detection of fibrotic disease on chest radiography have hampered its use in staging severity and focused attention on high-resolution chest computed tomography (HRCT) in the evaluation of the severity of pulmonary disease.[17]

A spectrum of HRCT findings is shown in **Figs. 1–4**. Pulmonary fibrotic phenotypes on HRCT are broadly characterized by linear opacities, traction bronchiectasis, and architectural distortion.[18] However, it should be stressed that HRCT appearances are highly variable in sarcoidosis with fibrotic features varying from ground-glass attenuation, representing fine fibrosis, to coarse reticular change with or without overt honeycombing. Fibrosis is most often evident in the peribronchovascular regions of the upper lobes. Progressive fibrosis may result in abnormal central conglomeration of perihilar bronchi and vessels associated with masses of fibrous tissue typically marked in the upper lobes. Fibrotic changes streaming outwards from the hilar regions are a distinctive feature. Subpleural honeycombing

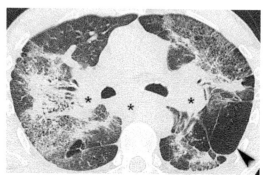

Fig. 1. Widespread pulmonary sarcoidosis in a 38-year-old ex-smoker with a 20-pack-year smoking history. Symmetric lymph node enlargement (*asterisks*) indicates nodal disease coexisting with fibrobullous changes within the lung parenchyma. Fibrosis is characterized by reticulation, traction bronchiectasis, and volume loss and occurs in a typical distribution for sarcoidosis, within the posterior segments of the upper lobes. Conglomerate masses with associated architectural distortion are evident bilaterally as is coexisting bullous disease (*arrowhead*).

occurs in a small percentage of patients involving mainly the upper and middle lobes, especially those with severe fibrosis with the distribution differing from that seen in IPF.[13] Fibrobullous destruction may result in large cystic spaces owing to traction bronchiectasis or bullae, which are the main site of mycetoma formation.[19,20] Patterns of airway involvement include traction bronchiectasis, mosaic attenuation, and isolated tracheobronchial abnormalities.[21] Fibrotic abnormalities are variably admixed with reversible features, including micronodular lesions and ground-glass abnormalities, which in some cases

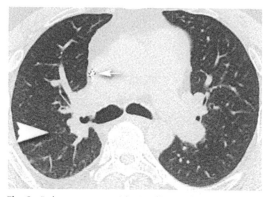

Fig. 2. Pulmonary sarcoidosis of limited extent in a 43-year-old man. Small nodules (*arrowhead*) are the only evidence of lung parenchymal involvement. Coexisting cardiac sarcoidosis required the insertion of a defibrillator, and a defibrillator lead is visible within the superior vena cava (*arrow*).

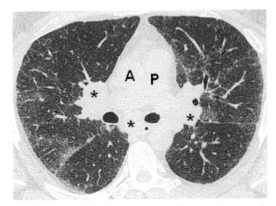

Fig. 3. Sarcoidosis in a 42-year old man. Symmetric lymph node enlargement (*asterisks*) coexists with parenchymal nodules in a perilymphatic distribution with upper lobe predominance. The main pulmonary artery (P) is smaller than the ascending aorta (A), suggesting that the presence of PH is unlikely.

represent inflammatory disease and regress with therapy.

HRCT evaluation of pulmonary involvement is thus a very semiquantitative exercise with conclusions based on both the pattern of abnormalities and the extent of disease. Although no formal HRCT scoring system has been validated in routine practice, accumulated clinical experience indicates that HRCT provides added value when reconciled with PFTs. In this way, it is often possible to conclude that symptoms or functional

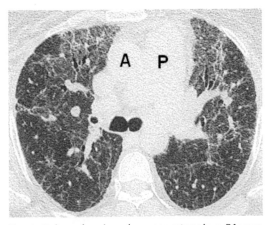

Fig. 4. Enlarged main pulmonary artery in a 54-year-old woman with pulmonary fibrosis secondary to biopsy-proven sarcoidosis. Marked reticulation and traction bronchiectasis in the upper lobes indicate fibrosis. The increased size of the main pulmonary artery (P) relative to the ascending aorta (A) is suggestive of PH.

impairment at an indeterminate level of severity are likely to represent severe disease if associated with overtly extensive fibrotic disease on HRCT. The likelihood of reversibility of severe disease is another important consideration at presentation. However, symptom severity and the level or nature of pulmonary function impairment cast no light on this question. HRCT provides ancillary information that is sometimes helpful but is only an approximate guide. Nodules indicate active granulomatous inflammation and are generally reversible; ground-glass opacities may be reversible or irreversible, and the fibrotic abnormalities discussed earlier do not regress with treatment.[22–24] In a minority of patients, it is possible to conclude that disease is highly likely to be either reversible or irreversible based on HRCT evaluation, but more often HRCT evaluation is inconclusive in this regard with an element of reversibility possible but not definite. This use of HRCT is highlighted only because no other pulmonary or systemic biomarker reliably indicative of the likelihood of reversible pulmonary disease in individual patients (as opposed to patient subgroups) has been identified, despite many studies of disease activity over recent decades.[25]

In the absence of a validated multidisciplinary algorithm for defining severe pulmonary disease, a simple pragmatic approach is to quantify severity using pulmonary function variables as the first step but, importantly, to calibrate these initial impressions against the level of symptoms and imaging findings. In this way, patients with severe or moderately severe pulmonary function impairment (eg, FVC <60%, diffuse lung capacity for carbon dioxide [DLco] <50%) are readily categorized as having severe disease, whereas in those with an indeterminate level of impairment (FVC 60%–80%, DLco 50%–70%), symptoms and imaging abnormalities are more influential in multidisciplinary evaluation. In occasional patients with lesser pulmonary function impairment (FVC >80%, DLco >70%), prominent symptoms in association with extensive disease on HRCT may indicate a high likelihood that premorbid PFTs were supranormal (as often seen in athletes), allowing those individuals to be managed as for severe disease. One important caveat is that in an important patient subgroup, severe pulmonary fibrosis is associated with major airflow obstruction,[21,26] and in this setting, forced expiratory volume in the first second might reasonably replace FVC in the severity thresholds tentatively suggested earlier. In any case, it should be stressed that all thresholds are inherently flawed, providing only very approximate guidance and requiring multidisciplinary calibration.

Pulmonary Risk Factors for Mortality and Future Severe/Dangerous Disease

As implied earlier, the best of all approaches with regard to severe disease is proactive prevention by means of early treatment in patients at higher risk of major future progression. Treatment decisions are often less difficult in advanced pulmonary fibrosis (in which the need for intervention is obvious) than when disease is mild to moderate. Furthermore, the need for long-term treatment is often difficult to judge at presentation when it is not yet clear whether a major proportion of disease is reversible. In this context, it is prudent to defer decisions on the need for ongoing treatment to prevent progression to disability until after an initial trial of corticosteroid therapy and the evaluation (as discussed earlier) of the severity of residual fibrotic disease.

Decisions on the treatment of pulmonary fibrosis are complicated by the failure of various types of biomarker to distinguish reliably between intrinsically stable ("burnt out") and intrinsically progressive irreversible disease (mirroring the lack of guidance provided by current tests in identifying reversible disease). Alone, among a great many markers studied historically,[25] serum IL-2 receptor levels were sufficiently predictive of outcome to suggest added clinical value in one study,[27] but this finding was not reproduced subsequently.[28] Chest radiographic and HRCT evaluation are not equal to demonstrating residual activity within fibrotic disease. However, based on recent data, 2 novel approaches to prognostic evaluation may eventually be fruitful in routine practice.

Fludeoxyglucose-PET /computed tomography (FDG-PET/CT) has been used in sarcoidosis patients with fibrotic lung disease in order to differentiate persistent respiratory symptoms attributed to end-stage irreversible disease from those related to residual disease activity that might benefit from immunomodulation. FDG-PET/CT signal correlates with other markers of disease activity, including bronchoalveolar lavage cell cytology, lung function indices, and serum inflammatory markers.[27–33] A significant reduction of FDG uptake after the initiation or modification of treatment in sarcoidosis patients has been demonstrated, including patients with irreversible disease, suggesting that in fibrotic disease, this modality might be used to identify patients at greater risk of disease progression.[34–36] In a study of 137 sarcoidosis patients, improvements in symptoms, conventional imaging findings, and physiologic data were strongly linked to reduction in maximum standardized uptake values on PET scans after treatment induction.[32]

An alternative approach is to harness HRCT, alone or in combination with PFTs, in an attempt to develop a severity prognostic staging system more accurate in individual patients than the Scadding chest radiographic system. Recently, an easily applicable HRCT/PFT staging protocol has been developed by means of split sample testing in more than 500 patients evaluated at a referral center.[8] In this study, HRCT and PFT markers of interstitial and pulmonary vascular disease were integrated. High- and low-risk subgroups were identified using thresholds for the composite physiologic index (previously developed in IPF,[37] and capturing the combined impact of pulmonary fibrosis and pulmonary vasculopathy), the extent of fibrosis on HRCT, and the main pulmonary artery diameter to ascending aorta diameter ratio as a marker of vasculopathy. In the validation cohort, patients in the high-risk group had a much higher mortality (hazard ratio 5.89, P<.0001). These findings do at least provide proof of concept in the integration of HRCT and PFT, although it is not yet clear whether it is equally accurate in the wider group of sarcoidosis patients not seen at expert centers.

However, both novel approaches discussed require further validation before being used in routine clinical evaluation. Currently, patients with fibrotic disease at higher risk of progressing to disability can only be identified by means of traditional clinical reasoning. Disease severity is the cardinal consideration: the PFT thresholds for severe disease suggested earlier are higher than those widely used to define severe disease in IPF, in the hope of increasing awareness of a higher risk of impending disability in individual patients. The duration of sarcoidosis is also important: a given level of functional impairment has very different implications as to likely future progression in patients with sarcoidosis of recent onset and those with longer-standing disease. Finally, the importance of characterizing longitudinal disease behavior during early follow-up cannot be stressed too strongly. In the recent American Thoracic Society/European Respiratory Society reclassification of the idiopathic interstitial pneumonias,[38] a disease behavior classification was proposed in order to define logical treatment goals in unclassifiable interstitial lung disease, with broad distinctions between major reversible disease (with or without supervening fibrosis) and progressive irreversible disease in which stabilization can be achieved. The underlying principles of this classification are highly applicable to proactive monitoring in the detection of sarcoidosis patients at higher risk of progression to severe disease. In this regard, serial spirometric trends correlate better than DLco or chest radiographic trends with longitudinal morphologic change on HRCT.[39]

Pulmonary Hypertension in Sarcoidosis

PH is increasingly recognized as a significant contributor to morbidity and mortality in patients with sarcoidosis.[5,40] Untreated PH is progressive and can be rapidly fatal, although the rate of progression is highly variable. Although the prevalence of PH is low in unselected patients with sarcoidosis, it increases to approximately 50% in those with chronic exercise intolerance and to even higher levels in patients undergoing evaluation for lung transplantation.[41–45] The underlying pathophysiologic mechanisms are multiple and complex. In a large subgroup, PH occurs in end-stage fibrotic lung disease, due to destruction of the pulmonary vessels, but granulomatous vascular inflammation, extrinsic compression from lymphadenopathy or mediastinal fibrosis, pulmonary veno-occlusive disease, and left heart disease (including cardiac sarcoid involvement) have also been recognized as important contributors to sarcoidosis-associated PH.[46] PH often causes exertional shortness of breath disproportionate to the extent of interstitial lung disease. The detection of PH is a key consideration in severe pulmonary disease.

Echocardiographic variables are widely used as surrogate measures of pulmonary systolic pressure and right ventricular function. Echocardiography is an appropriate initial, noninvasive screening tool for patients with suspected PH. However, the correlation is only moderate between echocardiographic and right heart catheter measurements of pulmonary artery pressure, especially in patients with concomitant parenchymal lung disease: in one meta-analysis, echocardiography had a sensitivity of 83% and a specificity of 72% for the diagnosis of PH.[47] Other noninvasive markers of pulmonary vasculopathy applicable to sarcoidosis patients with interstitial lung disease and severe PFT impairment include reduction in gas transfer disproportionate to lung volumes, and hypoxia at rest or on exercise disproportionate to the severity of interstitial lung disease. HRCT findings can also be helpful in patients with PH due to a pulmonary veno-occlusive process and in indicating that PH might be present when the ratio of the pulmonary artery diameter to the aortic diameter is increased.[46]

SEVERE CARDIAC INVOLVEMENT AND RISK STRATIFICATION

It can be argued that evidence of clinically significant active cardiac involvement should be viewed as indicative of severe disease, simply because of the importance of cardiac morbidity and mortality, including sudden death from cardiac arrhythmias.[48] Therefore, a low threshold for considering cardiac sarcoidosis is warranted in patients with severe exercise intolerance. The lack of a reference for the diagnosis of cardiac sarcoidosis is extremely challenging. Cardiac sarcoidosis is clinically overt in 5% of patients but is present in 20% to 30% at autopsy.[48–51] Myocardial biopsy is seldom performed, based on risk/benefit thinking, mainly because of the patchy distribution of the disease, resulting in both a low sensitivity and difficulties in interpreting the clinical significance of positive findings.[52–54]

With the advent of advanced imaging techniques, including cardiac MRI (CMR) and cardiac FDG-PET, it is now possible to detect subclinical disease underdiagnosed in the past and to explore algorithms to identify patients at future risk of life-threatening cardiac complications. The Japanese Ministry of Health and Welfare (JMHW) diagnostic criteria, which were considered as the established criteria until recently, have been found to be relatively insensitive for detecting cardiac involvement and failed to identify patients at high risk for adverse events when compared with the advanced imaging techniques.[55–58] However, these findings established the pivotal role of CMR and cardiac PET in the diagnosis and the management of cardiac sarcoidosis and led the experts to publish a consensus statement that included both as the noninvasive diagnostic tests of choice in suspected cardiac sarcoidosis.[54] As neither test can yet be viewed as a reference standard in clinical practice, it is appropriate to integrate either or both tests with the clinical presentation of patients, especially when the diagnosis is challenging.

The use of advanced imaging modalities is helpful in the risk stratification of patients with cardiac sarcoidosis. Traditionally, a left ventricular ejection fraction less than 50% has been viewed as a contributor to morbidity and mortality in any heart disease, and this has also been confirmed in sarcoidosis patients.[9] Late gadolinium enhancement (LGE) on CMR, a marker of myocardial fibrosis that is typically focal, involving the subepicardial or midmyocardial walls of the left ventricle, is an independent predictor of mortality and cardiac adverse events.[55,56] Recently, an extent of LGE greater than 20% of the myocardial mass has been linked to a higher incidence of cardiac events, even after adjustment for the degree of left ventricular impairment, which correlates with the extent of myocardial fibrosis.[59] Interestingly, there may be a threshold in the extent of myocardial fibrosis on CMR (greater than 6% of the left ventricular mass) associated with ventricular arrhythmias and cardiac death.[60] In this study, LGE involving the right ventricle was also strongly associated with adverse outcomes.

Cardiac PET has been useful in the diagnosis of cardiac sarcoidosis with a sensitivity and specificity of 89% and 78%, respectively, when compared with the JMHW criteria.[61] In 2 studies assessing the prognostic value of FDG-PET in cardiac sarcoidosis, scan positivity was associated with an increased rate of mortality and adverse outcomes, even after adjusting for the left ventricular ejection fraction.[57,58] As with CMR, increased FDG uptake in the right ventricle is also associated with adverse events.[58,62]

TREATMENT OF SEVERE PULMONARY AND CARDIAC SARCOIDOSIS

It should be acknowledged at the outset that there is a paucity of controlled data relevant to the treatment of severe disease. Thus, the issues discussed later are not addressed by definitive evidence base, but the suggested general approach captures a broad consensus drawn from accumulated clinical experience in expert centers. The principles discussed later with reference to pulmonary sand cardiac sarcoidosis can broadly be applied to other forms of organ involvement, covered elsewhere in this issue.

Use High-Dose Therapy Initially

In severe disease, early treatment should be definitive. In historical statements, it was usual to recommend very high initial doses of corticosteroid therapy, reducing to a maintenance phase of moderately high-dose treatment for 12 months. Without endorsement from formal controlled data, many clinicians now start with much lower steroid doses than used traditionally. However, whilse this approach is amply justified in principle when the main indication for treatment is loss of quality of life, severe/dangerous sarcoidosis should always be treated vigorously at the outset. In favor of this approach is the avoidance of the need to continue to increase corticosteroid doses because lack of efficacy becomes apparent (thereby increasing the total corticosteroid burden) and an early indication that disease is steroid resistant and that immediate recourse to second-line agents is needed. The use of initial parenteral corticosteroid therapy is increasingly widespread in severe sarcoidosis based on rapidity of action and reduction in the side effects expected from long-term high-dose oral therapy. As with other forms of therapy in severe disease, controlled

data are lacking, but this approach has been documented in observational studies.[63–67]

Consider the Early Introduction of Second Line Agents

In severe disease (and in patients at high risk of major progression), it is often appropriate to introduce a second-line/steroid-sparing agent at treatment initiation or shortly afterward. This introduction of a second-line/steroid-sparing agent is especially the case when it is obvious that there is major irreversible disease and that any further progression is likely to be disabling or even life-threatening. In this context, it is imprudent to assume that after initial high-dose treatment, disease progression will be prevented in the longer term by low-dose corticosteroid therapy in isolation. If it is obvious at the outset that a second-line agent is necessary, there is little point in delay because tolerance issues may delay the successful institution of immunosuppressive therapy. Thus, in cardiac sarcoidosis, many clinicians introduce methotrexate or azathioprine, variably in combination with hydroxychloroquine, concurrently with high-dose corticosteroid therapy in the treatment of active disease, especially when associated with major cardiac impairment.

Re-evaluate Treatment Strategies When There Is Major Responsiveness

By contrast, when there is a high likelihood of major reversibility with corticosteroid therapy (ie, prominent signal indicative of cardiac inflammation on CMR or CT-PET or an obvious pulmonary reversible component on HRCT), it may be useful to defer introducing a second-line agent until the degree of reversibility has been quantified. A substantial initial increase in pulmonary or cardiac reserve may allow the adoption of a less aggressive regimen in the longer term, both because disease is no longer severe and because it is clearly very corticosteroid-responsive, suggesting that low-dose maintenance corticosteroid therapy may suffice in a maintenance phase. It should be stressed that this happy outcome applies to only a minority of patients when disease is severe.

Do Not Accept Therapeutic Nihilism in Irreversible Disease

Above all, it is essential that treatments be used in the longer term in severe sarcoidosis to prevent progression of irreversible disease, even when there is no evidence of disease regression with short-term high-dose therapy. Based on partially controlled data in the last century, an unfortunate perception has arisen that sarcoidosis-specific treatments may improve symptoms but do not influence the natural course of disease. This perception has engendered a therapeutic nihilism in some clinicians with the result that progression to severe disease has not been actively combated. To understand why this approach is based on a poverty of evidence, it is necessary to consider the data base from which it was distilled.

In several historical studies, regimens (compared with matched or randomly selected control groups) were studied for 6 months (prednisolone 15 mg daily),[68] 6 months (prednisolone 60 mg daily initially with subsequent reduction),[69] 6 months (prednisolone 30 mg daily initially with subsequent reduction),[70] 3 months (prednisolone 15 mg daily),[71] 7 months (methylprednisolone 24–32 mg daily initially for 2 weeks with subsequent reduction),[72] 6 to 12 months (prednisolone 40 mg daily initially with subsequent reduction),[73] and 18 months (prednisolone 60 mg on alternate days initially, with a gradual reduction over 18 months).[74] In none of these studies was initial efficacy (improvements in chest radiographic or pulmonary function variables) sustained one to 15 years after treatment withdrawal.

Patients included in these trials were not selected because treatment was thought to be warranted clinically: indeed, symptomatic patients tended to be excluded and there were subgroups with bilateral hilar lymphadenopathy without pulmonary infiltration on chest radiography, inactive "burnt out" disease, and mild or transient pulmonary disease with Scadding stage II or stage III chest radiographic appearances. More importantly, the duration of treatment in these studies was simply too brief to apply the findings to patients with severe sarcoidosis. In other disorders driven by immune dysregulation (such as systemic lupus erythematosus), the idea that dangerous disease might become inactive over months rather than years is highly implausible, and there is no reason to imagine that this does not apply to dangerously severe sarcoidosis. A more balanced interpretation is that longer-term treatment for years, rather than months, is required to alter the natural course of disease.

Be Proactive in Identifying and Treating Complications

In severe pulmonary and cardiac disease alike, optimal management depends on the distinction between active sarcoidosis, the complications of fibrotic damage, and comorbidities. In pulmonary disease, a low threshold for suspecting supervening pulmonary embolism, fungal infection, or PH is especially important:

- An increased prevalence of pulmonary embolism, compared with the general population,

has been reported in 2 retrospective studies.[75,76]
- Chronic aspergillus infection, which may cause life-threatening hemoptysis, was present in 2% in a large retrospective study,[77] but is likely to be much higher in severe fibrotic disease: the 2 predisposing factors are immunosuppressive treatment and the presence of upper lobe fibrobullous distortion.[78–81] Antifungal therapy is warranted in symptomatic semi-invasive fungal disease, whereas bronchial artery embolization may be life-saving when there is recurrent major hemoptysis. Surgical mycetoma resection often has a poor outcome[81,82] and is seldom undertaken.
- PH due to occult left heart disease is as frequent as other forms of PH in sarcoidosis and has a much better treated outcome.[83] Because management of these 2 subgroups differs radically, right heart catheterization is strongly indicated in suspected PH and is mandatory before PH treatments are considered. In precapillary PH, there are limited data to suggest beneficial effects from epoprostenol, endothelin receptor antagonists, and phosphodiesterase V inhibitors,[84–87] although access to these agents tends to be restricted to compassionate use and enrollment in treatment trials, due to the lack of definitive proof of efficacy. In occasional patients with an inflammatory pulmonary vascular phenotype, immunomodulation may have an important role.[46]

In cardiac sarcoidosis, optimal management (discussed in greater detail elsewhere in this issue) depends on a clear separation between treatment goals-related active inflammation, cardiac functional impairment, and potentially lethal cardiac arrhythmias. Despite an absence of controlled data, immunomodulation can be viewed as first-line treatment as conduction abnormalities are occasionally reversed and treatment is associated with regression of metabolic activity on CMR and cardiac PET.[88] There are Japanese data suggesting that corticosteroid therapy in patients with cardiac sarcoidosis improves 5-year survival.[9] More extensive LGE is associated with greater improvements in left ventricular ejection fraction with corticosteroid therapy.[59] Anti-inflammatory treatment reduces the burden of myocardial inflammation in PET, with a variable improvement in cardiac function.[89]

Treatment decisions in severe cardiac sarcoidosis should ideally be multidisciplinary with consideration of both immunomodulation and the treatment of the consequences of irreversible disease, including (a) standard treatment of cardiac impairment; (b) antiarrhythmic therapy; (c) catheter ablation for recurrent monomorphic ventricular tachycardia[90]; (d) the insertion of a prophylactic implantable cardioverter defibrillator for ventricular arrhythmias or complete heart block[54]; and (e) referral for cardiac transplantation in patients with severe heart failure not responding to medical therapy.[91]

SUMMARY

Pulmonary and cardiac sarcoidosis are the most frequent causes of death in sarcoidosis, and thus, risk stratification strategies need to be developed with a view to aggressive intervention in both severe and high-risk disease. Pulmonary disease severity is pragmatically defined by the multidisciplinary integration of symptoms, PFTs, and imaging findings. Accurate risk stratification may require the integration of HRCT and PFT in pulmonary disease and advanced imaging techniques in pulmonary disease (PET) and cardiac disease (PET and CMR). Aggressive initial therapy is required for both patients with severe disease and those at high risk of progression to severe disease.

REFERENCES

1. Statement on sarcoidosis. Joint Statement of the American Thoracic Society (ATS), the European Respiratory Society (ERS) and the World Association of Sarcoidosis and Other Granulomatous Disorders (WASOG) adopted by the ATS Board of Directors and by the ERS Executive Committee, February 1999. Am J Respir Crit Care Med 1999; 160(2):736–55.
2. Chappell AG, Cheung WY, Hutchings HA. Sarcoidosis: a long-term follow up study. Sarcoidosis Vasc Diffuse Lung Dis 2000;17:167–73.
3. Swigris JJ, Olson AL, Huie TJ, et al. Sarcoidosis-related mortality in the United States from 1988 to 2007. Am J Respir Crit Care Med 2011;183:1524–30.
4. Morimoto T, Azuma A, Abe S, et al. Epidemiology of sarcoidosis in Japan. Eur Respir J 2008;31:372–9.
5. Shorr AF, Davies DB, Nathan SD. Predicting mortality in patients with sarcoidosis awaiting lung transplantation. Chest 2003;124:922–8.
6. Wells AU, Singh S, Spiro S, et al. Treatment of sarcoidosis. In: Mitchell D, Moller D, Spiro S, et al, editors. Sarcoidosis. 1st edition. London: Hodder & Stoughton; 2012. p. 415–28.
7. Mirsaeidi M, Machado RF, Schraufnagel D, et al. Racial difference in sarcoidosis mortality in the United States. Chest 2015;147(2):438–49.
8. Walsh SL, Wells AU, Sverzellati N, et al. An integrated clinicoradiological staging system for pulmonary sarcoidosis: a case-cohort study. Lancet Respir Med 2014;2(2):123–30.
9. Yazaki Y, Isobe M, Hiroe M, et al. Prognostic determinants of long-term survival in Japanese patients with cardiac sarcoidosis treated with prednisone. Am J Cardiol 2001;88(9):1006–10.
10. Gribbin J, Hubbard RB, Le Jeune I, et al. Incidence and mortality of idiopathic pulmonary fibrosis and sarcoidosis in the UK. Thorax 2006;61:980–5.
11. Iannuzzi MC, Rybicki BA, Teirstein AS. Sarcoidosis. N Engl J Med 2007;357(21):2153–65.
12. Nardi A, Brillet PY, Letoumelin P, et al. Stage IV sarcoidosis: comparison of survival with the general population and causes of death. Eur Respir J 2011; 38:1368–73.
13. Abehsera M, Valeyre D, Grenier P, et al. Sarcoidosis with pulmonary fibrosis: CT patterns and correlation with pulmonary function. AJR Am J Roentgenol 2000;174(6):1751–7.
14. Wells AU, Ward S. Pulmonary function tests in idiopathic pulmonary fibrosis. In: Meyer K, Nathan S, editors. Idiopathic pulmonary fibrosis. A comprehensive clinical guide. 1st edition. New York: Springer Science and Business media; 2014. p. 103–21.
15. Mana J, Gomez-Vaquero C, Montero A, et al. Lofgren's syndrome revisited: a study of 186 patients. Am J Med 1999;107:240–5.
16. Zappala CJ, Desai SR, Copley SJ, et al. Optimal scoring of serial change on chest radiography in sarcoidosis. Sarcoidosis Vasc Diffuse Lung Dis 2011;28(2):130–8.
17. Baughman RP, Shipley R, Desai S, et al. Changes in chest roentgenogram of sarcoidosis patients during a clinical trial of infliximab therapy: comparison of different methods of evaluation. Chest 2009;136: 526–35.
18. Valeyre D, Nunes H, Bernaudin JF. Advanced pulmonary sarcoidosis. Curr Opin Pulm Med 2014; 20(5):488–95.
19. Traill ZC, Maskell GF, Gleeson FV. High-resolution CT findings of pulmonary sarcoidosis. AJR Am J Roentgenol 1997;168(6):1557–60.
20. Hennebicque AS, Nunes H, Brillet PY, et al. CT findings in severe thoracic sarcoidosis. Eur Radiol 2005; 15(1):23–30.
21. Hansell DM, Milne DG, Wilsher ML, et al. Pulmonary sarcoidosis: morphologic associations of airflow obstruction at thin-section CT. Radiology 1998; 209(3):697–704.
22. Müller NL, Miller RR. Ground-glass attenuation, nodules, alveolitis, and sarcoid granulomas. Radiology 1993;189(1):31–2.
23. Baughman RP, Winget DB, Bowen EH, et al. Predicting respiratory failure in sarcoidosis patients. Sarcoidosis Vasc Diffuse Lung Dis 1997;14(2): 154–8.

24. Akira M, Kozuka T, Inoue Y, et al. Long-term follow-up CT scan evaluation in patients with pulmonary sarcoidosis. Chest 2005;127(1):185–91.

25. Keir G, Wells AU. Assessing pulmonary disease and response to therapy: which test? Semin Respir Crit Care Med 2010;31(4):409–18.

26. Handa T, Nagai S, Fushimi Y, et al. Clinical and radiographic indices associated with airflow limitation in patients with sarcoidosis. Chest 2006; 130(6):1851–6.

27. Ziegenhagen MW, Benner UK, Zissel G, et al. Sarcoidosis: TNF-alpha release from alveolar macrophages and serum level of sIL-2R are prognostic markers. Am J Respir Crit Care Med 1997;156(5):1586–92.

28. Grutters JC, Fellrath JM, Mulder L, et al. Serum soluble interleukin-2 receptor measurement in patients with sarcoidosis: a clinical evaluation. Chest 2003; 124(1):186–95.

29. Keijsers RG, Verzijlbergen FJ, Oyen WJ, et al. 18F-FDG-PET, genotype corrected ACE and sIL2R in newly diagnosed sarcoidosis. Eur J Nucl Med Mol Imaging 2009;36:1131–7.

30. Ziegenhagen MW, Rothe ME, Schlaak M, et al. Bronchoalveolar and serological parameters reflecting the severity of sarcoidosis. Eur Respir J 2003;21: 407–13.

31. Mostard RL, Vöö S, van Kroonenburgh MJ, et al. Inflammatory activity assessment by F18 FDG-PET/CT in persistent symptomatic sarcoidosis. Respir Med 2011;105:1917–24.

32. Teirstein AS, Machac J, Almeida O, et al. Results of 188 whole-body fluorodeoxyglucose positron emission tomography scans in 137 patients with sarcoidosis. Chest 2007;132:1949–53.

33. Treglia G, Taralli S, Giordano A. Emerging role of whole-body 18F-fluorodeoxyglucose positron emission tomography as a marker of disease activity in patients with sarcoidosis: a systematic review. Sarcoidosis Vasc Diffuse Lung Dis 2011;28: 87–94.

34. Keijsers RG, van den Heuvel DA, Grutters JC. Imaging the inflammatory activity of sarcoidosis. Eur Respir J 2013;41:743–51.

35. Keijsers RG, Verzijlbergen JF, van Diepen DM, et al. 18F-FDG PET in sarcoidosis: an observational study in 12 patients treated with infliximab. Sarcoidosis Vasc Diffuse Lung Dis 2008;25:143–9.

36. Milman N, Graudal N, Loft A, et al. Effect of the TNF-α inhibitor adalimumab in patients with recalcitrant sarcoidosis: a prospective observational study using FDG-PET. Clin Respir J 2012;6:238–47.

37. Wells AU, Desai SR, Rubens MB, et al. Idiopathic pulmonary fibrosis: a composite physiologic index derived from disease extent observed by computed tomography. Am J Respir Crit Care Med 2003; 167(7):962–9.

38. Travis WD, Costabel U, Hansell DM, et al. An official American Thoracic Society/European Respiratory Society statement: update of the international multidisciplinary classification of the idiopathic interstitial pneumonias. Am J Respir Crit Care Med 2013; 188(6):733–48.

39. Zappala CJ, Desai SR, Copley SJ, et al. Accuracy of individual variables in the monitoring of long-term change in pulmonary sarcoidosis as judged by serial high-resolution CT scan data. Chest 2014; 145(1):101–7.

40. Shorr AF, Helman DL, Davies DB, et al. Pulmonary hypertension in advanced sarcoidosis: epidemiology and clinical characteristics. Eur Respir J 2005;25(5):783–8.

41. Arcasoy SM, Christie JD, Pochettino A, et al. Characteristics and outcomes of patients with sarcoidosis listed for lung transplantation. Chest 2001; 120(3):873–80.

42. Sulica R, Teirstein AS, Kakarla S, et al. Distinctive clinical, radiographic, and functional characteristics of patients with sarcoidosis-related pulmonary hypertension. Chest 2005;128(3):1483–9.

43. Rizzato G, Pezzano A, Sala G, et al. Right heart impairment in sarcoidosis: haemodynamic and echocardiographic study. Eur J Respir Dis 1983; 64(2):121–8.

44. Bourbonnais JM, Samavati L. Clinical predictors of pulmonary hypertension in sarcoidosis. Eur Respir J 2008;32(2):296–302.

45. Baughman RP, Sparkman BK, Lower EE. Six-minute walk test and health status assessment in sarcoidosis. Chest 2007;132(1):207–13.

46. Nunes H, Humbert M, Capron F, et al. Pulmonary hypertension associated with sarcoidosis: mechanisms, haemodynamics and prognosis. Thorax 2006;61(1):68–74.

47. Janda S, Shahidi N, Gin K, et al. Diagnostic accuracy of echocardiography for pulmonary hypertension: a systematic review and meta-analysis. Heart 2011;97(8):612–22.

48. Baughman RP, Teirstein AS, Judson MA, et al. Clinical characteristics of patients in a case control study of sarcoidosis. Am J Respir Crit Care Med 2001;164(10 Pt 1):1885–9.

49. Iwai K, Tachibana T, Takemura T, et al. Pathological studies on sarcoidosis autopsy. I. Epidemiological features of 320 cases in Japan. Acta Pathol Jpn 1993;43(7–8):372–6.

50. Perry A, Vuitch F. Causes of death in patients with sarcoidosis. A morphologic study of 38 autopsies with clinicopathologic correlations. Arch Pathol Lab Med 1995;119(2):167–72.

51. Tavora F, Cresswell N, Li L, et al. Comparison of necropsy findings in patients with sarcoidosis dying suddenly from cardiac sarcoidosis versus dying

suddenly from other causes. Am J Cardiol 2009; 104(4):571–7.

52. Uemura A, Morimoto S, Hiramitsu S, et al. Histologic diagnostic rate of cardiac sarcoidosis: evaluation of endomyocardial biopsies. Am Heart J 1999;138: 299–302.

53. Yoshida A, Ishibashi-Ueda H, Yamada N, et al. Direct comparison of the diagnostic capability of cardiac magnetic resonance and endomyocardial biopsy in patients with heart failure. Eur J Heart Fail 2013;15(2):166–75.

54. Birnie DH, Sauer WH, Bogun F, et al. HRS expert consensus statement on the diagnosis and management of arrhythmias associated with cardiac sarcoidosis. Heart Rhythm 2014;11(7):1305–23.

55. Patel MR, Cawley PJ, Heitner JF, et al. Detection of myocardial damage in patients with sarcoidosis. Circulation 2009;120(20):1969–77.

56. Greulich S, Deluigi CC, Gloekler S, et al. CMR imaging predicts death and other adverse events in suspected cardiac sarcoidosis. JACC Cardiovasc Imaging 2013;6(4):501–11.

57. Ahmadian A, Brogan A, Berman J, et al. Quantitative interpretation of FDG PET/CT with myocardial perfusion imaging increases diagnostic information in the evaluation of cardiac sarcoidosis. J Nucl Cardiol 2014;21(5):925–39.

58. Blankstein R, Osborne M, Naya M, et al. Cardiac positron emission tomography enhances prognostic assessments of patients with suspected cardiac sarcoidosis. J Am Coll Cardiol 2014;63(4): 329–36.

59. Ise T, Hasegawa T, Morita Y, et al. Extensive late gadolinium enhancement on cardiovascular magnetic resonance predicts adverse outcomes and lack of improvement in LV function after steroid therapy in cardiac sarcoidosis. Heart 2014;100(15): 1165–72.

60. Crawford T, Mueller G, Sarsam S, et al. Magnetic resonance imaging for identifying patients with cardiac sarcoidosis and preserved or mildly reduced left ventricular function at risk of ventricular arrhythmias. Circ Arrhythm Electrophysiol 2014;7(6): 1109–15.

61. Youssef G, Leung E, Mylonas I, et al. The use of 18F-FDG PET in the diagnosis of cardiac sarcoidosis: a systematic review and metaanalysis including the Ontario experience. J Nucl Med 2012;53(2):241–8.

62. Manabe O, Yoshinaga K, Ohira H, et al. Right ventricular (18)F-FDG uptake is an important indicator for cardiac involvement in patients with suspected cardiac sarcoidosis. Ann Nucl Med 2014;28(7): 656–63.

63. Wallaert B, Ramon P, Fournier EC, et al. High-dose methylprednisolone pulse therapy in sarcoidosis. Eur J Respir Dis 1986;68(4):256–62.

64. Greos LS, Vichyanond P, Bloedow DC, et al. Methylprednisolone achieves greater concentrations in the lung than prednisolone. A pharmacokinetic analysis. Am Rev Respir Dis 1991;144(3 Pt 1):586–92.

65. Allen RK, Sellars RE, Sandstrom PA. A prospective study of 32 patients with neurosarcoidosis. Sarcoidosis Vasc Diffuse Lung Dis 2003;20(2):118–25.

66. Mahévas M, Lescure FX, Boffa JJ, et al. Renal sarcoidosis: clinical, laboratory, and histologic presentation and outcome in 47 patients. Medicine (Baltimore) 2009;88(2):98–106.

67. Chakrabarti S, Behera D, Varma S, et al. High-dose methyl prednisolone for autoimmune thrombocytopenia in sarcoidosis. Sarcoidosis Vasc Diffuse Lung Dis 1997;14(2):188.

68. Hapke EJ, Meek JC. Steroid treatment in pulmonary sarcoidosis. In: Levinsky L, Macholda F, editors. Proceedings of the 5th International Conference on Sarcoidosis. Prague (Czech Republic): Universita Karlova; 1971. p. 621–5.

69. Young RL, Harkleroad LE, Lordon RE, et al. Pulmonary sarcoidosis: a prospective evaluation of glucocorticoid therapy. Ann Intern Med 1970;73(2): 207–12.

70. Mikami R, Hitagi Y, Iwai K, et al. A double-blind controlled trial on the effect of corticosteroid therapy in sarcoidosis. In: Iwai K, Hosoda Y, editors. Proceedings of the International Conference on Sarcoidosis. Tokyo: University of Tokyo Press; 1974. p. 533–8.

71. Israel HL, Fouts DW, Beggs RA. A controlled trial of prednisone treatment of sarcoidosis. Am Rev Respir Dis 1973;107(4):609–14.

72. Selroos O, Sellergren TL. Corticosteroid therapy of pulmonary sarcoidosis. A prospective evaluation of alternate day and daily dosage in stage II disease. Scand J Respir Dis 1979;60(4):215–21.

73. Eule H, Roth I, Weide W. Clinical and functional results of a controlled clinical trial of the value of prednisolone therapy in sarcoidosis. In: Jones Williams W, Davies BH, editors. Proceedings of the International Conference on Sarcoidosis. Cardiff (United Kingdom): Alpha Omega; 1980. p. 624–31.

74. Yamamoto M, Saito N, Tachibana T, et al. Effects of an 18-month corticosteroid therapy on stage I and stage II sarcoidosis patients (a controlled trial). In: Chretien J, editor. Proceedings of the 9th International Conference on Sarcoidosis. Oxford (United Kingdom): Pergamon Press; 1983. p. 470–4.

75. Swigris JJ, Olson AL, Huie TJ, et al. Increased risk of pulmonary embolism among US decedents with sarcoidosis from 1988 to 2007. Chest 2011;140(5): 1261–6.

76. Vorselaars AD, Snijder RJ, Grutters JC. Increased number of pulmonary embolisms in sarcoidosis patients. Chest 2012;141(3):826–7.

77. Pena TA, Soubani AO, Samavati L. Aspergillus lung disease in patients with sarcoidosis: a case series and review of the literature. Lung 2011;189(2):167–72.

78. Baughman RP, Lower EE. Fungal infections as a complication of therapy for sarcoidosis. QJM 2005; 98(6):451–6.

79. Wollschlager C, Khan F. Aspergillomas complicating sarcoidosis. A prospective study in 100 patients. Chest 1984;86:585–8.

80. Tomlinson JR, Sahn SA. Aspergilloma in sarcoid and tuberculosis. Chest 1987;92(3):505–8.

81. Denning DW, Riniotis K, Dobrashian R, et al. Chronic cavitary and fibrosing pulmonary and pleural aspergillosis: case series, proposed nomenclature change, and review. Clin Infect Dis 2003;37:S265–80.

82. Wex P, Utta E, Drozdz W. Surgical treatment of pulmonary and pleuropulmonary Aspergillus disease. Thorac Cardiovasc Surg 1993;41:64–70.

83. Baughman RP, Engel PJ, Taylor L, et al. Survival in sarcoidosis-associated pulmonary hypertension: the importance of hemodynamic evaluation. Chest 2010;138(5):1078–85.

84. Preston IR, Klinger JR, Landzberg MJ, et al. Vaso-responsiveness of sarcoidosis-associated pulmonary hypertension. Chest 2001;120(3):866–72.

85. Fisher KA, Serlin DM, Wilson KC, et al. Sarcoidosis-associated pulmonary hypertension: outcome with long-term epoprostenol treatment. Chest 2006; 130(5):1481–8.

86. Milman N, Burton CM, Iversen M, et al. Pulmonary hypertension in end-stage pulmonary sarcoidosis: therapeutic effect of sildenafil? J Heart Lung Transplant 2008;27(3):329–34.

87. Keir GJ, Walsh SL, Gatzoulis MA, et al. Treatment of sarcoidosis-associated pulmonary hypertension: a single centre retrospective experience using targeted therapies. Sarcoidosis Vasc Diffuse Lung Dis 2014;31(2):82–90.

88. Sadek MM, Yung D, Birnie DH, et al. Corticosteroid therapy for cardiac sarcoidosis: a systematic review. Can J Cardiol 2013;29(9):1034–41.

89. Osborne MT, Hulten EA, Singh A, et al. Reduction in ^{18}F-fluorodeoxyglucose uptake on serial cardiac positron emission tomography is associated with improved left ventricular ejection fraction in patients with cardiac sarcoidosis. J Nucl Cardiol 2014;21(1): 166–74.

90. Thachil A, Christopher J, Sastry BK, et al. Monomorphic ventricular tachycardia and mediastinal adenopathy due to granulomatous infiltration in patients with preserved ventricular function. J Am Coll Cardiol 2011;58(1):48–55.

91. Akashi H, Kato TS, Takayama H, et al. Outcome of patients with cardiac sarcoidosis undergoing cardiac transplantation—single-center retrospective analysis. J Cardiol 2012;60(5):407–10.

Consequences of Sarcoidosis

Marjolein Drent, MD, PhD[a,b,c,*], Bert Strookappe, MSc[c,d], Elske Hoitsma, MD, PhD[c,e], Jolanda De Vries, MSc, PhD[c,f,g]

KEYWORDS

- Cognitive impairment • Depressive symptoms • Exercise limitation • Fatigue • Pain • Rehabilitation
- Sarcoidosis • Small fiber neuropathy • Quality of life

KEY POINTS

- Consequences of sarcoidosis are wide ranging, and have a great impact on patients' lives.
- Sarcoidosis patients suffer not only from organ-related symptoms, but also from a wide spectrum of rather nonspecific disabling symptoms.
- Absence of evidence does not mean evidence of absence.
- Management of sarcoidosis requires a multidisciplinary personalized approach that focuses on somatic as well as psychosocial aspects of the disease.

INTRODUCTION

The clinical expression, natural history, and prognosis of sarcoidosis are highly variable and its course is often unpredictable.[1] Clinical manifestations vary with the organs involved.[1,2] The lungs are affected in approximately 90% of patients with sarcoidosis, and the disease frequently also involves the lymph nodes, skin, and eyes. Remission occurs in more than one-half of patients within 3 years of diagnosis, and within 10 years in two-thirds, with few or no remaining consequences.[2] Unfortunately, up to one-third of patients have persistent disease, leading to significant impairment of their quality of life (QoL).[3] Interpretation of the severity of the sarcoidosis can be complicated by its heterogeneity. Several major concerns of sarcoidosis patients include symptoms that cannot be explained by granulomatous involvement of a particular organ.[4] Apart from lung-related symptoms (eg, coughing, breathlessness, and dyspnea on exertion), patients may suffer from a wide range of rather nonspecific disabling symptoms.[2,5] These symptoms, such as fatigue, fever, anorexia, arthralgia, muscle pain, general weakness, muscle weakness, exercise limitation, and cognitive failure, often do not correspond with objective physical evidence of disease.[2,5–9] These issues are often troubling to pulmonologists and other sarcoidologists because they do not relate directly to a physiologic abnormality, are difficult to quantify and hence to monitor, and are challenging to treat.[4]

The authors have nothing to disclose.

[a] Department of Pharmacology and Toxicology, Faculty of Health, Medicine and Life Science, Maastricht University, PO Box 616, Maastricht 6200 MD, The Netherlands; [b] ILD Center of Excellence, St. Antonius Hospital, Koekoekslaan 1, Nieuwegein 3435 CM, The Netherlands; [c] ILD Care Foundation Research Team, PO Box 18, Bennekom 6720 AA, The Netherlands; [d] Department of Physical Therapy, Gelderse Vallei Hospital (ZGV), PO Box 9025, Ede 6710HN, The Netherlands; [e] Department of Neurology, Alrijne Hospital, PO Box 9650, Leiden 2300 RD, The Netherlands; [f] Department of Medical Psychology, St. Elisabeth Hospital Tilburg, Tilburg, The Netherlands; [g] Department of Medical and Clinical Psychology, Tilburg University, PO Box 90153, Tilburg 5000 LE, The Netherlands
* Corresponding author. ILD Care Foundation Research Team, PO Box 18, Bennekom 6720 AA, The Netherlands.
E-mail address: m.drent@maastrichtuniversity.nl

Symptoms such as fatigue can be nonspecific and difficult to objectify. Moreover, absence of evidence does not mean evidence of absence.[5,7] Sarcoidosis-related complaints, including fatigue, may become chronic and affect patients' QoL even after all other signs of disease activity have disappeared.[7,10,11] Hence, patients consult their physician not only with organ-specific symptoms—directly related to the organ(s) involved—but also with nonspecific health complaints, such as fatigue, cognitive failure, exercise intolerance, and muscle weakness.[12] These impairments in sarcoidosis are disabling, especially when they become chronic.[13,14] Sarcoidosis consists of several overlapping clinical syndromes ("the sarcoidosis"), each with its own specific pathogenesis. A complete evaluation of sarcoidosis could make use of a panel with 4 disease domains or dimensions: extent of disease, severity, activity, and impact.[15–17] Severity of sarcoidosis in each organ is defined as the degree of organ damage sustained from sarcoidosis. The interpretation of the severity of sarcoidosis can be complicated by its heterogeneity. The organ damage can be estimated subjectively by the intensity of symptoms, objectively as a percentage decline from normal capacity (eg, percentage of the predicted normal value on pulmonary function testing), or by critical location of lesions (eg, cardiac block). However, pulmonary function test results do not always represent changes in the severity of pulmonary sarcoidosis,[18] which illustrates that the demonstration of sarcoid activity remains an enigma. Assessment of inflammatory activity in sarcoidosis patients without deteriorating lung function or radiologic deterioration but with unexplained persistent disabling symptoms is an important and often problematic issue. Historically, evaluation of the various available tools for the assessment of inflammatory activity has been hampered by the lack of a gold standard. This article focuses on the impact of the broad range of sarcoidosis-related problems on patients' lives.

SYMPTOMS

In addition to symptoms related to the organs involved, patients may suffer from all kinds of less specific symptoms. These sarcoidosis-related disabling symptoms can significantly decrease a person's QoL, especially in chronic sarcoidosis.[19] All these symptoms may have major consequences and impact on the patients' lives and those of their relatives.

Fatigue

Fatigue is the most frequently described and devastating symptom in sarcoidosis, and is globally recognized as a disabling symptom. The reported prevalence varies from 60% to 90% of sarcoidosis patients,[5] and up to 25% of fatigued sarcoidosis patients report extreme fatigue. Physicians generally assess disease severity and progression in sarcoidosis on the basis of clinical tests, such as pulmonary function tests, chest radiographs, and serologic tests. However, these objective clinical parameters correlate poorly with the patients' subjective sense of well-being.[8,20] Sarcoidosis patients may suffer from substantial fatigue even in the absence of other symptoms or disease-related abnormalities. For example, fatigue and general weakness may persist even after routine clinical test results have returned to normal.[5] There is a positive association between symptoms of suspected small fiber neuropathy (SFN) and fatigue, as well as between dyspnea and fatigue.[13,21,22] So far, no organic substrate has been found for the symptoms of sarcoidosis-associated fatigue.

To date, no appropriate definition of fatigue exists. Fatigue can be seen and measured as a unidimensional or multidimensional concept. The multidimensional concept of fatigue can be divided into at least 2 categories: physical and mental or passive and active fatigue.[5,10]

Some sarcoidosis patients are debilitated by the symptoms of their disease and are unable to work; others are underemployed and incapable of achieving their full potential owing to their health issues.[23] Individuals affected by the disease frequently seem to be completely healthy, so their symptoms are often not taken seriously by family, friends, employers, and health care professionals. Consequently, some patients lose their desire and ability to socialize with others effectively, causing relationships and family dynamics to ultimately suffer. These combined factors impact on an individual's economic status, interpersonal relationships, and family dynamics, increase their stress levels, and induce depression in patients.

The etiology of this troublesome problem remains elusive and is usually multifactorial. Fatigue can be a consequence of the treatment itself, for instance, as a complication of corticosteroid therapy. The diagnosis of sarcoidosis-associated fatigue requires extensive evaluation to identify and treat potentially reversible causes.[5,6] Its etiology may involve granuloma formation and cytokine release. However, despite effective treatment of the sarcoidosis, many patients continue to experience fatigue.[5,24] Comorbidities associated with sarcoidosis, including depression, anxiety, hypothyroidism, and altered sleep patterns, may all contribute to fatigue.[23,25]

Despite an exhaustive search for treatable clinical causes of fatigue, most patients' complaints of fatigue are not correlated with clinical parameters of disease activity.[5,24]

Dyspnea

Dyspnea is, by definition, subjective, but a greater value should be given to its quantification by validated scales in the initial evaluation and follow-up of patients with sarcoidosis. The mechanism for dyspnea in sarcoidosis is multifactorial.[12,22,26] Research has found that the degree of dyspnea in sarcoidosis does not correlate with lung function tests.[27] Pulmonary function test results do not always reflect changes in the severity of pulmonary sarcoidosis. Moreover, several studies have reported that neither lung function test results nor chest radiographs correlate with nonspecific health complaints or with QoL.[19,28] In the follow-up, the level of dyspnea often, but not always, changes in the same direction as the forced vital capacity.[29] Spontaneous resolution of radiographic lesions is more common in asymptomatic patients.[17] The intensity of dyspnea at initial evaluation correlates with the need for long-term treatment.[30]

Small Fiber Neuropathy and Autonomic Dysfunction

In 2002, SFN was recognized as a symptom of sarcoidosis.[31] Unlike granulomatous large neuron involvement, SFN seems to be a common complication occurring in up to 40%[32] to 60% of patients with sarcoidosis.[33]

SFN is a peripheral nerve disorder that selectively affects thinly myelinated Aδ fibers and unmyelinated C fibers.[34] These fibers are associated with thermal and nociceptive sensations, and pathology of these nerves may lead to a "painful neuropathy." However, these nerves also affect the autonomic nervous system, and SFN may also lead to an "autonomic neuropathy" (**Box 1**).[35,36]

Symptoms of SFN are disabling for patients, have a high impact on QoL, and are often difficult to treat.[35] Damage to or loss of small somatic nerve fibers results in pain, burning, or tingling sensations, or numbness, typically affecting the limbs in a distal to proximal gradient. Symptoms can be very severe, are usually worse at night, and often affect sleep. People sometimes sleep with their feet uncovered because they cannot bear the touch of the sheets. Walking may be difficult owing to severe pain caused by the pressure on the floor. When autonomic fibers are affected, patients may experience dry eyes, dry mouth, orthostatic

---

> **Box 1**
> **Symptoms suggestive of small fiber neuropathy**
>
> *Sensory symptoms*
>
> Pain[a]
>
> Paresthesias
>
> Sheet intolerance
>
> Restless legs syndrome[b]
>
> *Symptoms of autonomic dysfunction*
>
> Hyperhidrosis or hyperhidrosis
>
> Diarrhea or constipation
>
> Urinary incontinence or urine retention
>
> Gastroparesis
>
> Sicca syndrome
>
> Blurry vision
>
> Facial flushing
>
> Orthostatic intolerance
>
> Sexual dysfunction
>
> [a] Pain in small fiber neuropathy often has a burning, tingling, shooting, or prickling character.
> [b] Restless legs syndrome is a disorder characterized by disagreeable leg sensations that usually occur before sleep onset and cause an almost irresistible urge to move.

---

dizziness, constipation, bladder incontinence, sexual dysfunction, trouble sweating, or red or white skin discolorations (see also **Box 1**).[34] Involvement of cardiac sympathetic nerves might play a role in the prognosis, because indices of autonomic cardiac dysfunction have been identified as strong predictors of cardiovascular morbidity and mortality.[34]

Because routine nerve conduction tests evaluate only large nerve fiber function, and quantitative techniques for the assessment of small nerve fibers are not routinely applied, the diagnosis of SFN can easily be missed.[35,37] This lack may lead to frustration for both physician and patient owing to the failure to diagnose a neuropathic pain syndrome. There is as yet no gold standard for the diagnosis of SFN. Diagnosis is usually established on the basis of clinical features, in combination with abnormal findings of specialized tests such as the assessment of intraepidermal nerve fiber density in skin biopsy, temperature sensation tests for sensory fibers, and sudomotor and cardiovagal testing for autonomic fibers.[32,33,38] The Small Fiber Neuropathy Screening List was developed in a sarcoidosis population as a first screening tool.[21]

PSYCHOLOGICAL BURDEN
Depressive Symptoms

Depressive symptoms in sarcoidosis are at least partly an expression of exhaustion owing to the ongoing disease. Depressive symptoms have been found to be associated negatively with and affect patients' fatigue scores.[10] In addition, the relationship between fatigue and depressive symptoms parallels the findings for other chronic illnesses, such as diabetes, chronic obstructive pulmonary disease, cardiac disease, and rheumatoid arthritis.[39] Moreover, the severity and nature of fatigue moderate anxiety and depressive symptoms in sarcoidosis. Fatigue and autonomic dysfunction are both dominant symptoms and risk factors for depression.[40] The symptoms may share several neurobiological abnormalities, for example, an increase in tumor necrosis factor-α.[40] The relationship between depressive symptoms and fatigue may also be based on a cytokine imbalance, initiated by an inflammatory immune response in sarcoidosis.[39,41] The cytokine balance of patients suffering from depression also seems to be disturbed.[42]

Not only fatigue, but also psychological symptoms such as depressive symptoms and anxiety, play an important role in sarcoidosis.[15,43–46] They have been reported in 17% to 66% of patients with sarcoidosis. Understanding the nature of the relationships between fatigue, depressive symptoms, and anxiety remains difficult however. The nature of fatigue moderates the relationships between fatigue and anxiety and between fatigue and depressive symptoms in sarcoidosis. In a study by De Kleijn and colleagues,[47] fatigue was often reported with concurrent depressive symptoms (34%–36%) and anxiety (43%–46%). About one-third of the patients (31%) reported high-trait anxiety as well as high levels of depressive symptoms at baseline. The study also suggested that the relationship between depressive symptoms and fatigue is bidirectional. Depressive symptoms may indirectly lead to more symptoms, because they are associated with poor self-care (diet, exercise, giving up smoking, and medication regimens) in patients with chronic diseases in general.[39] However, physical symptoms and the resulting functional impairments caused by complications of medical illness are also likely to impose a burden on the patient's life and to provoke depression.[39] Hence, not only fatigue but also depressive symptoms and anxiety should be an integral part of the multidisciplinary management of sarcoidosis patients.

Anxiety and Stress

Several studies have shown that the prevalence of anxiety in sarcoidosis patients is 33% to 36%.[47,48]

Studies also showed that anxiety was more common in sarcoidosis patients than in the general population and among healthy persons.[49,50] The percentages for anxiety disorders are obviously lower; for instance, 6.3% of sarcoidosis patients have a panic disorder.[51] In any case, anxiety is a major problem in sarcoidosis patients. Because fatigue is 1 symptom that is known to cooccur with anxiety, it is not surprising that anxiety in general and trait anxiety were found to be related to fatigue.[5,24,47] One study also found that trait anxiety predicted fatigue at follow-up.[47] Trait anxiety refers to the tendency of persons to react with anxiety in new situations. In contrast, state anxiety is defined as anxiety that is elicited in a particular situation and does not last long. In addition to fatigue, 1 study found that the severity of sarcoidosis symptoms was also related to anxiety.[52] Studies of the relation between anxiety and dyspnea reported inconsistent results.[49,53]

Studies examining stress in sarcoidosis are still scarce. One study found that the magnitude of stressful life events was higher in sarcoidosis patients than in healthy controls.[54] Patients also seemed to use inadequate coping strategies with regard to stress.[54] Another study reported a relation between increased life stress and impaired lung function.[55] Finally, 1 study focusing on perceived stress found it to be high and related to sarcoidosis symptoms.[23] Perceived/experienced stress is caused by interpreting a situation as threatening. This indicates that the same situation may be perceived as stressful by 1 person and as a challenge by another. Interpreting a situation as threatening may result in several reactions known as fight or flight, or freeze. In each of these, the person is scared, but this translates into different behavior: anger and aggressive behavior (fight), anxiety and escaping from the situation (flight), or no reaction at all (freeze). Fight and flight reactions require a physical reaction.

Anxiety consists of physical or hyperarousal symptoms, such as increased heart rate, perspiration, and dizziness, which are inherent to the reaction of the sympathetic nervous system.[56] In addition to a physical component, anxiety also has a cognitive component, that is, a thought (or chain of thoughts) that determines the emotion experienced. If someone is confronted with a situation and has thoughts such as, "I can do this" and "I want to test whether I can overcome this," the situation is regarded as a challenge, and the noted physical symptoms will not occur. If the same situation induces thoughts such as "I cannot handle this" and "I must do something, but I have no idea what," the situation is perceived as threatening and the physical symptoms related to anxiety occur. This relationship between stress and anxiety—and the 2 components of anxiety (cognitive and physical)—might explain the relationships found between symptoms and anxiety/stress.

Another aspect to take into consideration is the duration of stress or anxiety. A brief feeling of stress and anxiety is very common and is considered healthy, because the person uses the fight or flight reactions to cope with the situation. In this sense, a parallel can be drawn with pain and fatigue, which are both healthy responses to a stimulus that may harm the body or demand too much of the body, respectively. It becomes unhealthy when the stress and anxiety become persistent, because this will have negative effects on the immune system. In our modern society, physical reactions are often elicited by thoughts that do not require physical action. Think about (recurrent) negative thoughts, such as "I am a loser," "My illness makes me a burden to other people," "Symptoms will probably become worse," and "I will soon die from this disease."

From this perspective, various researchers have justly suggested that sarcoidosis patients may benefit from psychological interventions[47,51] focusing on coping and appraisal, such as stress reduction treatment.[23,55] In each case, the basis for the interventions should be a type of cognitive–behavioral therapy, including so-called third-generation cognitive-behavioral therapy–like mindfulness-based cognitive therapy, because this type of therapy has proved to be effective in patients with anxiety disorder. Finally, it is important to realize that anxiety (just like depressive symptoms/depression) is known to be among the factors prolonging chronic fatigue, and that

chronic fatigue can be successfully treated with cognitive–behavioral therapy.

Cognitive Impairment and Memory Loss

In addition to organ-specific symptoms and nonspecific health complaints such as fatigue and physical impairments, patients also have to deal with side effects of medical treatment. Patients with sarcoidosis often report everyday cognitive deficits.[6] There is growing interest in cognitive failure research in populations of patients with various chronic diseases.[57,58] Functional cognitive impairment, if present, may lead to increased fatigue and low compliance with medical treatment. Currently, however, no data are available on the extent of cognitive underperformance among sarcoidosis patients. Research in multiple sclerosis patients found that memory complaints were not associated with memory performance, but were associated with fatigue complaints.[58] It is tempting to speculate that this may also be the case in sarcoidosis patients. There is a special interest in sarcoidosis owing to the high prevalence of fatigue and everyday cognitive failure, together with the relatively young age of the patients.

Physical Impairment

Sarcoidosis obviously imposes a burden on patients' lives (**Fig. 1**).[12,59] Symptoms of fatigue and dyspnea induce exercise limitation, and fatigue also leads to physical inactivity, and the specific sarcoidosis symptoms, or the thought of living with a progressive, incurable condition, create anxiety and mood disturbance, and affect emotional well-being. Although less recognized

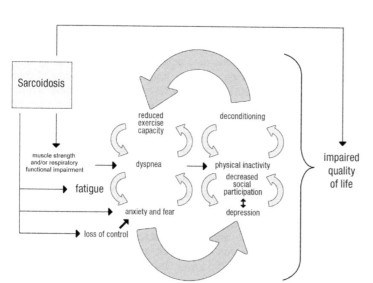

Fig. 1. Negative vicious circle of physical deconditioning: disabling symptoms in sarcoidosis can reduce daily physical activities, resulting in general deconditioning and a reduced quality of life. (*Adapted from* Swigris JJ, Brown KK, Make BJ, et al. Pulmonary rehabilitation in idiopathic pulmonary fibrosis: a call for continued investigation. Respir Med 2008;102(12):167580, and Marcellis RG, Lenssen AF, de Vries J, et al. Reduced muscle strength, exercise intolerance and disabling symptoms in sarcoidosis. Curr Opin Pulm Med 2013;19(5):528.)

than exertional dyspnea, lack of energy or exhaustion is a very common and frustrating physical symptom in patients with sarcoidosis. Patients with sarcoidosis (as well as other interstitial lung diseases) often have diminished exercise capacity and reduced muscle strength, as demonstrated by reduced oxygen uptake (measured during a maximal cardiopulmonary exercise test) or a shorter-than-predicted distance covered during a 6-minute walking test. Monitoring that takes muscle strength and exercise capacity into account has been found to improve the routine monitoring of sarcoidosis.[28,60,61] Like others, Marcellis and colleagues[28] found exercise intolerance and muscle weakness to be frequent problems in sarcoidosis, both in fatigued and nonfatigued patients.

Exercise intolerance in sarcoidosis is most often multifactorial, involving lung–mechanical, musculoskeletal, and gas exchange abnormalities.[12,28,62–64] Several studies have reported that neither lung function test results nor chest radiographs correlate with these nonspecific health complaints, nor with QoL.[11,23,44–46] Moreover, pulmonary function test results at rest seem to be poor predictors of exercise capacity. Changes in gas exchange upon exercise can be fairly accurately predicted by percent diffusing capacity of the lung for carbon monoxide,[65,66] but can be present even with normal diffusing capacity of the lung for carbon monoxide.[67] Fatigue that, as mentioned, is among the major problems in sarcoidosis, can reduce patients' day-to-day functioning.[5] Consequently, decreased physical activity can induce general deconditioning, which in turn contributes to increased perceived fatigue and a sense of dyspnea, as well as insufficient physical activity.[60,68] Assessment of the presence of physical impairments is recommended, because it provides additional information about the patient's functional status, disease severity, and progression.[28,60,62–64] Because the patients' ability to handle physical activity is clearly decreased, however, the activities should be adjusted, and rehabilitation programs should be designed carefully.[61,69,70]

Overall Impact on Patients' Lives: Quality of Life

The impact of any disease depends on the way the patient perceives the disease and modifies his or her activities of daily living. Living with a long-term disease like sarcoidosis significantly affects QoL, with negative consequences for general health and social and psychosocial well-being.[3,71–73] QoL is an important outcome measure of treatment, especially with regard to chronic diseases. It is a concept that concerns patients' evaluation of their functioning in a wide range of domains, but always including the physical, psychological, and social domains.[3] Assessment covering only these three domains is known as assessment of health-related QoL.[3,73]

QoL is often confused with health status, which concerns patients' physical, psychological, and social functioning.[3] Psychological factors such as burnout, emotional distress, and work-related social support influence levels of QoL.[72] A study among sarcoidosis patients found that the strongest predictor of all dimensions of QoL was the corresponding QoL at baseline.[13] This trend might be explained by the fact that sarcoidosis-related symptoms remain relatively stable over time.[13,47] Social support has been described as a buffer against pain and disability, and also as being associated with greater activity levels among individuals with pain.[72,74] Support from friends and family can also be related to the psychological dimensions of QoL.[75] A study among people with chronic pain found that a rich social network was related to higher perceived QoL.[76] Moreover, work-related social support is known to positively predict return to work, whereas lack of social support at work is a well-known risk factor for development of pain.[77] In sarcoidosis, there is poor agreement between physicians and patients with regard to the perceived symptoms attributable to the disease, with a particular failure of clinicians to recognize the impact of non–organ-specific features.[15,17] It has been proposed that assessment of the health status and QoL of sarcoidosis patients would help to bridge this gap, aiding communication and treatment, and complementing existing clinical assessments. Various aspects of sarcoidosis, such as the relatively young age at disease onset, the often unpredictable and chronic nature of the disease, the uncertainly about the cause and the broad range of frequently persistent symptoms may account for the aggravating influence on patients' lives as well as those of their families and friends, especially because a truly appropriate treatment of sarcoidosis is still lacking.

Fatigue, breathlessness, reduced exercise capacity, and arthralgia are the most frequently reported symptoms. It seems that these sarcoidosis-related symptoms are associated with a lower QoL.[8,13,44,47,53,78] Women have lower scores on the physical health, psychological health, social relationships, and environmental domains, and the general assessment of overall QoL. Research found that the use of corticosteroids predicted a lower QoL in all domains except spirituality. Having a partner was associated with the

QoL domains of psychological health and level of independence, whereas a low educational level predicted better scores for the social relationships domain, and arthralgia predicted poorer scores for this domain.[8] Fatigue had a negative effect on patients' QoL scores for the physical health, psychological health, and level of independence domains.

TREATMENT OPTIONS
Pharmacologic Treatment

There is a lack of standardized management strategies for sarcoidosis. Most sarcoidosis patients show spontaneous resolution of the disease and do not require systemic pharmacologic treatment.[2] Glucocorticoids are the cornerstone therapeutic agent, and have a favorable short-term effect on functional impairments, including respiratory impairment and symptoms. However, the long-term beneficial effect remains uncertain. In view of the limitations we are aware of presently, authorization would be doubtful if glucocorticoids were to be introduced at present. A subset of patients require more aggressive treatment. The published data on the different treatment options in sarcoidosis are limited and treatment therefore remains mostly empirical.[2] The decision on whether to start systemic immunosuppressive treatment or not should be based on the patients' symptomatology, including the impact on their QoL, as well as the extent of compromised organ function.

Recent studies have demonstrated the effectiveness of various neurostimulants, including methylphenidate, for the treatment of fatigue associated with sarcoidosis. These and other agents may be useful adjuncts for the treatment of this type of fatigue. There is obviously a need for studies evaluating the causes of, and new therapeutic options for, sarcoidosis-associated fatigue. Psychological interventions should also be examined. Standard sarcoidosis treatments such as those using corticosteroids and other immunosuppressive agents are often ineffective for SFN-related symptoms.[4] Symptomatic neuropathic pain treatment in sarcoidosis patients is not different from the treatment of neuropathic pain from other causes, and consists of antidepressants, anticonvulsants and prolonged-release opioids. However, in common with their effects in other neuropathic pain states, these agents provide limited pain relief in just 30% to 60% of patients, at the cost of considerable side effects. These data indicate that there is an urgent need for analgesic agents with high efficacy for neuropathic pain patients, causing no debilitating side effects. Case reports mention beneficial effects of intravenous immunoglobulin and anti–tumor necrosis factor-α therapy.[6,79,80] The precise potency of these drugs needs further study however.

Additional Alternatives to Pharmacologic Treatment

Developing the most appropriate therapeutic approach for sarcoidosis, including rehabilitation programs, requires careful consideration of the possible impact of pain, the SFN-related symptoms, the fatigue and coping strategies, as well as all other relevant aspects of this multisystem disease.[3,4,6,49,81] Various treatments are available for fatigue with a partly psychological cause, and patients with a clinical depression can be prescribed antidepressants. Some patients may require help to improve their coping and self-management skills, to improve their QoL. Cognitive therapy may be indicated to treat coping problems or stress perception. Sleeping problems should be treated appropriately.[25] In general, care providers have to raise supportive care issues and provide information about alternative care programs beside medication, which aim to reduce the symptoms and improve the well-being of sarcoidosis patients. Patients should be informed about the importance of exercise and they should be encouraged to stay active.

REHABILITATION

Patients should be instructed to lead an as active and involved a life as possible because exercise intolerance and muscle weakness are frequent problems in sarcoidosis influencing QoL (see Fig. 1).[28] Rehabilitation has many benefits for patients with sarcoidosis, including social participation, psychological well-being, maintaining levels of activity, learning to use breathing exercises and ways to adapt exercises for the home environment.[69,70,82,83] In the broader context of medical encounters, physical therapy or rehabilitation can help to avoid a negative vicious circle of deconditioning.[61,69] Research has found that fatigue in patients with sarcoidosis was reduced after a period of physical training.[69,70] Moreover, their psychological health and physical functioning also improved.[69] Sarcoidosis patients generally benefit from additional nonpharmacologic treatments, not only physical training but also nutritional supplements and counseling.[69,70,84,85] Patients should be counseled about their responsibilities in managing their own condition, about ways to engage different services when required, and about lifestyle, for example, the importance of regular exercise as well as pulmonary rehabilitation programs. Patients' self-perceived knowledge about the importance of exercise for their health (in addition to drug therapy) should be improved. Care providers should be able to refer patients to rehabilitation (including pulmonary rehabilitation) by physical therapists or other professionals with an awareness and knowledge of sarcoidosis, if they expect these patients to benefit, or if the patients ask for referral. Rehabilitation services or programs led by physical therapists should be available to patients at reasonable cost. Prospective studies should be designed to answer lingering questions about the value of exercise training for patients with sarcoidosis, including what benefits can be expected of maintenance programs and how long these benefits will last. Our own research found that patients reported fewer feelings of uncertainty and anxiety after a training program.[86] This finding has promising implications for clinical practice. Because sarcoidosis patients may suffer from various impairments, such as arthralgia, muscle pain, and fatigue, the intensity of the training should be personalized to avoid training aggravating these impairments, resulting in high dropout rates. This need also argues for a multidisciplinary approach to the routine management of sarcoidosis.

More research is needed to provide evidence for the relationship between physical therapy and recall. Such studies should assess whether awareness of the importance of physical activities in daily life and their consequences for sarcoidosis patients might affect adherence to treatment or medication regimens. The duration, frequency, and intensity of exercise programs are critical to achieve physical benefits.[82,86] In general "high-frequency, low-impact" exercise can be recommended. Future prospective studies are warranted to fine-tune the training parameters, duration, and frequency.

COMMUNICATION AND PATIENT PARTICIPATION

Providing information and communication can be hampered by the complexity of sarcoidosis and its heterogeneity. Moreover, management of patients with sarcoidosis requires more than prescribing drugs. It is important for physicians to listen to their patients; it is wise to take what the patient says seriously. Obviously, understanding and remembering medical information is crucial for every patient, because it is a prerequisite for coping with their disease and making informed treatment decisions. Most patients do remember their diagnosis, but have difficulty remembering information about things like treatment plans, recommendations, and side effects. Patients'

information recall may be enhanced by addressing emotions by means of affective communication. Extensive research has shown that physicians' affective communication (ie, being emotionally supportive and adopting a warm, empathic, and reassuring manner) may improve patients' outcomes, including decreased levels of anxiety and distress.[87,88] Physicians' affective communication not only tempers emotional arousal, but also enhances recall of medical information.[88] Research in various disorders has shown that such affective statements improved recall, especially with regard prognostic information and, to some extent, treatment information. Obviously, because sarcoidosis requires a multidisciplinary approach in view of its wide range of symptoms, communication among the various health care workers involved and between them and the patients is of great importance.[89] Although the effect of affective communication has not yet been studied in sarcoidosis, this may be expected to improve patient compliance. Patient participation is increasingly recognized as a key component in the design of health care processes and is also advocated as a means of improving patient compliance. The concept has been applied successfully to various areas of patient care, such as decision making and the management of chronic diseases. Patient participation in shared treatment decision making is hypothesized to improve treatment adherence and clinical outcomes. Although this has not yet been studied in sarcoidosis, other research findings reveal the significance of patient participation as a key factor in improving treatment adherence and clinical outcome. Quality improvement strategies for sarcoidosis management should, therefore, emphasize patient participation. Further research is essential to establish key determinants of the success of patient participation in improving efficacy of care for sarcoidosis patients.

Patient participation has promising implications for the multidisciplinary management of sarcoidosis. However, the effect of affective communication on recall should be established further because evidence is lacking, especially for extensive consultations. Other interesting topics for future studies include whether self-perceived medical knowledge about sarcoidosis and its related consequences, including treatment options, is sufficient to achieve beneficial effects.

SUMMARY

Sarcoidosis is a multisystem disorder of unknown cause(s) that imposes a burden on patient's lives. In addition to the specific organ-related symptoms, less specific disabling symptoms, including fatigue and physical impairments, may have a major influence on the daily activities and the social and professional lives of the patients, resulting in a reduced QoL. A multidisciplinary approach is recommended for these patients, one that focuses on somatic as well as psychosocial aspects of this erratic disorder. Patients self-perceived knowledge about the importance of exercise and lifestyle for their health (in addition to drugs) should be improved. Developing the most appropriate therapeutic approach for sarcoidosis, including rehabilitation programs, requires careful consideration of the possible impact of fatigue, SFN symptoms, pain, cognitive functioning, and coping strategies, as well as all other relevant aspects of this multisystem disease. Therefore, personalized medicine and appropriate communication are beneficial.

REFERENCES

1. Statement on sarcoidosis. Joint Statement of the American Thoracic Society (ATS), the European Respiratory Society (ERS) and the World Association of Sarcoidosis and Other Granulomatous Disorders (WASOG) adopted by the ATS Board of Directors and by the ERS Executive Committee, February 1999. Am J Respir Crit Care Med 1999; 160(2):736–55.

2. Valeyre D, Prasse A, Nunes H, et al. Sarcoidosis. Lancet 2014;383:1155–67.

3. De Vries J, Drent M. Quality of life and health status in sarcoidosis: a review of the literature. Clin Chest Med 2008;29(3):525–32.

4. Judson MA. Small fiber neuropathy in sarcoidosis: something beneath the surface. Respir Med 2011; 105(1):1–2.

5. Drent M, Lower EE, De Vries J. Sarcoidosis-associated fatigue. Eur Respir J 2012;40(1):255–63.

6. Elfferich MD, Nelemans PJ, Ponds RW, et al. Everyday cognitive failure in sarcoidosis: the prevalence and the effect of anti-TNF-alpha treatment. Respiration 2010;80(3):212–9.

7. Korenromp IH, Heijnen CJ, Vogels OJ, et al. Characterization of chronic fatigue in patients with sarcoidosis in clinical remission. Chest 2011;140(2):441–7.

8. Michielsen HJ, Peros-Golubicic T, Drent M, et al. Relationship between symptoms and quality of life in a sarcoidosis population. Respiration 2007; 74(4):401–5.

9. Baydur A, Alavy B, Nawathe A, et al. Fatigue and plasma cytokine concentrations at rest and during exercise in patients with sarcoidosis. Clin Respir J 2011;5(3):156–64.

10. De Kleijn WP, Drent M, Vermunt JK, et al. Types of fatigue in sarcoidosis patients. J Psychosom Res 2011;71(6):416–22.

11. Sharma OP. Fatigue and sarcoidosis. Eur Respir J 1999;13(4):713–4.

12. Marcellis RG, Lenssen AF, de Vries J, et al. Reduced muscle strength, exercise intolerance and disabling symptoms in sarcoidosis. Curr Opin Pulm Med 2013;19(5):524–30.

13. Drent M, Marcellis R, Lenssen A, et al. Association between physical functions and quality of life in sarcoidosis. Sarcoidosis Vasc Diffuse Lung Dis 2014;31(2):117–28.

14. Morgenthau AS, Iannuzzi MC. Recent advances in sarcoidosis. Chest 2011;139(1):174–82.

15. Cox CE, Donohue JF, Brown CD, et al. Health-related quality of life of persons with sarcoidosis. Chest 2004;125(3):997–1004.

16. Judson MA, Costabel U, Drent M, et al. The WASOG sarcoidosis organ assessment instrument: an update of a previous clinical tool. Sarcoidosis Vasc Diffuse Lung Dis 2014;31(1):19–27.

17. Pereira CA, Dornfeld MC, Baughman R, et al. Clinical phenotypes in sarcoidosis. Curr Opin Pulm Med 2014;20(5):496–502.

18. Baughman RP, Lower EE, Gibson K. Pulmonary manifestations of sarcoidosis. Presse Med 2012; 41(6 Pt 2):e289–302.

19. Michielsen HJ, Drent M, Peros-Golubicic T, et al. Fatigue is associated with quality of life in sarcoidosis patients. Chest 2006;130(4):989–94.

20. Wirnsberger RM, de Vries J, Breteler MH, et al. Evaluation of quality of life in sarcoidosis patients. Respir Med 1998;92(5):750–6.

21. Hoitsma E, De Vries J, Drent M. The small fiber neuropathy screening list: construction and cross-validation in sarcoidosis. Respir Med 2011;105(1): 95–100.

22. Hinz A, Fleischer M, Brahler E, et al. Fatigue in patients with sarcoidosis, compared with the general population. Gen Hosp Psychiatry 2011;33(5):462–8.

23. De Vries J, Drent M. Relationship between perceived stress and sarcoidosis in a Dutch patient population. Sarcoidosis Vasc Diffuse Lung Dis 2004; 21(1):57–63.

24. Korenromp IH, Grutters JC, van den Bosch JM, et al. Post-inflammatory fatigue in sarcoidosis: personality profiles, psychological symptoms and stress hormones. J Psychosom Res 2012;72(2):97–102.

25. Verbraecken J, Hoitsma E, van der Grinten CP, et al. Sleep disturbances associated with periodic leg movements in chronic sarcoidosis. Sarcoidosis Vasc Diffuse Lung Dis 2004;21(2):137–46.

26. Baughman RP, Sparkman BK, Lower EE. Six-minute walk test and health status assessment in sarcoidosis. Chest 2007;132(1):207–13.

27. Baughman RP, Teirstein AS, Judson MA, et al. Clinical characteristics of patients in a case control study of sarcoidosis. Am J Respir Crit Care Med 2001;164(10 Pt 1):1885–9.

28. Marcellis RG, Lenssen AF, Elfferich MD, et al. Exercise capacity, muscle strength and fatigue in sarcoidosis. Eur Respir J 2011;38(3):628–34.

29. Judson MA, Baughman RP, Thompson BW, et al. Two year prognosis of sarcoidosis: the ACCESS experience. Sarcoidosis Vasc Diffuse Lung Dis 2003;20(3):204–11.

30. Baughman RP, Judson MA, Teirstein A, et al. Presenting characteristics as predictors of duration of treatment in sarcoidosis. QJM 2006;99(5):307–15.

31. Hoitsma E, Marziniak M, Faber CG, et al. Small fibre neuropathy in sarcoidosis. Lancet 2002;359(9323): 2085–6.

32. Bakkers M, Merkies IS, Lauria G, et al. Intraepidermal nerve fiber density and its application in sarcoidosis. Neurology 2009;73(14):1142–8.

33. Hoitsma E, Drent M, Verstraete E, et al. Abnormal warm and cold sensation thresholds suggestive of small-fibre neuropathy in sarcoidosis. Clin Neurophysiol 2003;114(12):2326–33.

34. Hoitsma E, Reulen JP, de Baets M, et al. Small fiber neuropathy: a common and important clinical disorder. J Neurol Sci 2004;227(1):119–30.

35. Hoitsma E, Drent M, Sharma OP. A pragmatic approach to diagnosing and treating neurosarcoidosis in the 21st century. Curr Opin Pulm Med 2010; 16(5):472–9.

36. Tavee J, Zhou L. Small fiber neuropathy: a burning problem. Cleve Clin J Med 2009;76(5):297–305.

37. Hoitsma E, Faber CG, Drent M, et al. Neurosarcoidosis: a clinical dilemma. Lancet Neurol 2004;3(7):397–407.

38. Tavee J, Culver D. Sarcoidosis and small-fiber neuropathy. Curr Pain Headache Rep 2011;15(3):201–6.

39. Katon W, Lin EH, Kroenke K. The association of depression and anxiety with medical symptom burden in patients with chronic medical illness. Gen Hosp Psychiatry 2007;29(2):147–55.

40. Freeman R, Komaroff AL. Does the chronic fatigue syndrome involve the autonomic nervous system? Am J Med 1997;102(4):357–64.

41. Korenromp IH, Grutters JC, van den Bosch JM, et al. Reduced Th2 cytokine production by sarcoidosis patients in clinical remission with chronic fatigue. Brain Behav Immun 2011;25(7):1498–502.

42. Kim YK, Na KS, Shin KH, et al. Cytokine imbalance in the pathophysiology of major depressive disorder. Prog Neuropsychopharmacol Biol Psychiatry 2007; 31(5):1044–53.

43. Chang B, Steimel J, Moller DR, et al. Depression in sarcoidosis. Am J Respir Crit Care Med 2001; 163(2):329–34.

44. De Vries J, Rothkrantz-Kos S, van Dieijen-Visser MP, et al. The relationship between fatigue and clinical parameters in pulmonary sarcoidosis. Sarcoidosis Vasc Diffuse Lung Dis 2004;21(2):127–36.

45. Drent M, Wirnsberger RM, Breteler MH, et al. Quality of life and depressive symptoms in patients suffering from sarcoidosis. Sarcoidosis Vasc Diffuse Lung Dis 1998;15(1):59–66.

46. Elfferich MD, De Vries J, Drent M. Type D or 'distressed' personality in sarcoidosis and idiopathic pulmonary fibrosis. Sarcoidosis Vasc Diffuse Lung Dis 2011;28(1):65–71.

47. de Kleijn WP, Drent M, De Vries J. Nature of fatigue moderates depressive symptoms and anxiety in sarcoidosis. Br J Health Psychol 2013;18(2):439–52.

48. Ireland J, Wilsher M. Perceptions and beliefs in sarcoidosis. Sarcoidosis Vasc Diffuse Lung Dis 2010;27(1):36–42.

49. Hinz A, Brähler E, Möde R, et al. Anxiety and depression in sarcoidosis: the influence of age, gender, affected organs, concomitant diseases and dyspnea. Sarcoidosis Vasc Diffuse Lung Dis 2012;29:139–46.

50. Spruit MA, Janssen DJ, Franssen FM, et al. Rehabilitation and palliative care in lung fibrosis. Respirology 2009;14(6):781–7.

51. Goracci A, Fagiolini A, Martinucci M, et al. Quality of life, anxiety and depression in sarcoidosis. Gen Hosp Psychiatry 2008;30(5):441–5.

52. Holas P, Krejtz I, Urbankowski T, et al. Anxiety, its relation to symptoms severity and anxiety sensitivity in sarcoidosis. Sarcoidosis Vasc Diffuse Lung Dis 2013;30(4):282–8.

53. de Boer S, Kolbe J, Wilsher ML. The relationships among dyspnoea, health-related quality of life and psychological factors in sarcoidosis. Respirology 2014;19(7):1019–24.

54. Yamada Y, Tatsumi K, Yamaguchi T, et al. Influence of stressful life events on the onset of sarcoidosis. Respirology 2003;8(2):186–91.

55. Klonoff EA, Kleinhenz ME. Psychological factors in sarcoidosis: the relationship between life stress and pulmonary function. Sarcoidosis 1993;10(2):118–24.

56. Chaturvedi SK, Peter Maguire G, Somashekar BS. Somatization in cancer. Int Rev Psychiatry 2006; 18(1):49–54.

57. Shin SY, Katz P, Wallhagen M, et al. Cognitive impairment in persons with rheumatoid arthritis. Arthritis Care Res 2012;64(8):1144–50.

58. Jougleux-Vie C, Duhin E, Deken V, et al. Does fatigue complaint reflect memory impairment in multiple sclerosis? Mult Scler Int 2014;2014:692468.

59. Swigris JJ, Brown KK, Make BJ, et al. Pulmonary rehabilitation in idiopathic pulmonary fibrosis: a call for continued investigation. Respir Med 2008; 102(12):1675–80.

60. Marcellis RG, Lenssen AF, Kleynen S, et al. Exercise capacity, muscle strength, and fatigue in sarcoidosis: a follow-up study. Lung 2013;191(3):247–56.

61. Spruit MA, Thomeer MJ, Gosselink R, et al. Skeletal muscle weakness in patients with sarcoidosis and its relationship with exercise intolerance and reduced health status. Thorax 2005;60(1):32–8.

62. Baughman RP, Lower EE. Six-minute walk test in managing and monitoring sarcoidosis patients. Curr Opin Pulm Med 2007;13(5):439–44.

63. Wallaert B, Talleu C, Wemeau-Stervinou L, et al. Reduction of maximal oxygen uptake in sarcoidosis: relationship with disease severity. Respiration 2011; 82(6):501–8.

64. Wirnsberger RM, Drent M, Hekelaar N, et al. Relationship between respiratory muscle function and quality of life in sarcoidosis. Eur Respir J 1997; 10(7):1450–5.

65. Barros WG, Neder JA, Pereira CA, et al. Clinical, radiographic and functional predictors of pulmonary gas exchange impairment at moderate exercise in patients with sarcoidosis. Respiration 2004;71(4): 367–73.

66. Medinger AE, Khouri S, Rohatgi PK. Sarcoidosis: the value of exercise testing. Chest 2001;120(1): 93–101.

67. Marcellis RG, Lenssen AF, de Vries GJ, et al. Is there an added value of cardiopulmonary exercise testing in sarcoidosis patients? Lung 2013;191(1):43–52.

68. Braam AW, de Haan SN, Vorselaars AD, et al. Influence of repeated maximal exercise testing on biomarkers and fatigue in sarcoidosis. Brain Behav Immun 2013;33:57–64.

69. Marcellis RG, Veeke MAF, Mesters I, et al. Does physical training reduce fatigue in sarcoidosis? Sarcoidosis Vasc Diffuse Lung Dis 2015;32(1): 53–62.

70. Strookappe EW, Elfferich MDP, Swigris JJ, et al. Benefits of physical training in patients with idiopathic or end-stage sarcoidosis-related pulmonary fibrosis: a pilot study. Sarcoidosis Vasc Diffuse Lung Dis 2015;32(1):43–52.

71. De Vries J, Drent M. Quality of life and health status in sarcoidosis: a review. Semin Respir Crit Care Med 2007;28(1):121–7.

72. Thomten J, Soares JJ, Sundin O. The influence of psychosocial factors on quality of life among women with pain: a prospective study in Sweden. Qual Life Res 2011;20(8):1215–25.

73. Patel AS, Siegert RJ, Creamer D, et al. The development and validation of the King's sarcoidosis questionnaire for the assessment of health status. Thorax 2013;68(1):57–65.

74. Holtzman S, Newth S, Delongis A. The role of social support in coping with daily pain among patients with rheumatoid arthritis. J Health Psychol 2004; 9(5):677–95.

75. Goldberg GM, Kerns RD, Rosenberg R. Pain-relevant support as a buffer from depression among

chronic pain patients low in instrumental activity. Clin J Pain 1993;9(1):34–40.

76. Dysvik E, Lindstrom TC, Eikeland OJ, et al. Health-related quality of life and pain beliefs among people suffering from chronic pain. Pain Manag Nurs 2004; 5(2):66–74.

77. Marhold C, Linton SJ, Melin L. Identification of obstacles for chronic pain patients to return to work: evaluation of a questionnaire. J Occup Rehabil 2002;12(2):65–75.

78. De Vries J, Wirnsberger RM. Fatigue, quality of life and health status in sarcoidosis. Eur Respir Mon 2005;32:92–104.

79. Parambil JG, Tavee JO, Zhou L, et al. Efficacy of intravenous immunoglobulin for small fiber neuropathy associated with sarcoidosis. Respir Med 2011; 105(1):101–5.

80. Wijnen PA, Cremers JP, Nelemans PJ, et al. Association of the TNF-alpha G-308A polymorphism with TNF-inhibitor response in sarcoidosis. Eur Respir J 2014;43(6):1730–9.

81. Holland AE, Hill CJ, Conron M, et al. Short term improvement in exercise capacity and symptoms following exercise training in interstitial lung disease. Thorax 2008;63(6):549–54.

82. Spruit MA, Wouters EFM, Gosselink R. Rehabilitation programmes in sarcoidosis: a multidisciplinary approach. Eur Respir J 2005;32:316–26.

83. Swigris JJ, Fairclough DL, Morrison M, et al. Benefits of pulmonary rehabilitation in idiopathic pulmonary fibrosis. Respir Care 2011;56(6):783–9.

84. Boots AW, Drent M, de Boer VC, et al. Quercetin reduces markers of oxidative stress and inflammation in sarcoidosis. Clin Nutr 2011;30(4):506–12.

85. Boots AW, Drent M, Swennen EL, et al. Antioxidant status associated with inflammation in sarcoidosis: a potential role for antioxidants. Respir Med 2009; 103(3):364–72.

86. Strookappe B, Swigris J, De Vries J. Benefits of physical training in sarcoidosis. Lung 2015. [Epub ahead of print].

87. van Osch M, Sep M, van Vliet LM, et al. Reducing patients' anxiety and uncertainty, and improving recall in bad news consultations. Health Psychol 2014;33(11):1382–90.

88. Derksen F, Bensing J, Kuiper S, et al. Empathy: what does it mean for GPs? A qualitative study. Fam Pract 2015;32(1):94–100.

89. Drent M. Sarcoidosis: benefits of a multidisciplinary approach. Eur J Intern Med 2003;14(4):217–20.

Quality of Life Assessment in Sarcoidosis

Marc A. Judson, MD

KEYWORDS

- Sarcoidosis • Health-related quality of life • Patient-reported outcomes • Symptoms • Function

KEY POINTS

- Health-related quality of life (HRQL) is important in assessing sarcoidosis; quality of life issues are important in determining the need for treatment.
- HRQL can be assessed accurately using established patient-reported outcome measures (PROs).
- Recently, several sarcoidosis-specific PROs assessing HRQL have been developed for clinical use.

INTRODUCTION

Health-related quality of life (HRQL) has become an important aspect of patient evaluation. This may be especially true with sarcoidosis, because the disease is rarely fatal and the physiologic manifestations of the disease are often mild. Over the last few decades, the assessment of HRQL has become more rigorous, as patient-reported outcome measures (PROs) have been developed that have the capacity to quantify this patient assessment. In this article, we describe the importance, relevance, general methodology of construction, and application of PROs and HRQL assessment in sarcoidosis.

THE IMPORTANCE OF QUALITY OF LIFE ASSESSMENT IN SARCOIDOSIS

Sarcoidosis may involve any organ. The disease course is highly variable, ranging from an asymptomatic state to a progressive condition that may, occasionally, be life threatening. The pathologic hallmark of sarcoidosis is the granuloma that may resolve spontaneously or with antisarcoidosis therapy. Approximately 10% to 30% of sarcoidosis patients develop significant fibrosis that may result in permanent organ injury.[1]

Regardless of the clinical course, the decision to treat sarcoidosis is usually based on the presence of 1 or both of the following 2 conditions resulting from the disease: a situation of potential danger to the patient or a significant worsening of the patient's quality of life. Of these 2 treatment indications, sarcoidosis-induced significant worsening of quality of life is, far and away, the more common.

Despite the importance of the impact of sarcoidosis on quality of life, clinicians often fail to give this issue adequate importance and base treatment decisions on other factors. This situation is depicted in **Fig. 1** in relation to pulmonary sarcoidosis.[2] Sarcoidosis causes granulomatous inflammation. This granulomatous inflammation may not cause a significant physiologic derangement or result in a significant decrease in quality of life. Even when the granulomatous inflammation of pulmonary sarcoidosis does cause physiologic abnormalities, they are often minor[3,4] and do not always lead to appreciable symptoms.[4] In these situations, unless these minor physiologic derangements are associated with dangerous consequences, there is not an adequate indication for treatment. Nonetheless, clinicians often initiate antisarcoidosis treatment based on the presence of granulomatous inflammation (eg, increased

Disclosures: The author is a consultant for Mallinckrodt, Celgene, and Mitsubishi-Tanabe.
Division of Pulmonary and Critical Care Medicine, Department of Medicine, Albany Medical College, MC 91, 47 New Scotland Avenue, Albany, NY 12208, USA
E-mail address: judsonm@mail.amc.edu

chestmed.theclinics.com

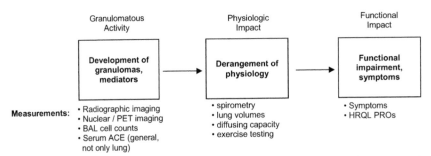

Fig. 1. Relationship of granulomatous inflammation, physiologic derangements, and HRQL impairment in pulmonary sarcoidosis. ACE, angiotensin-converting enzyme; BAL, bronchoalveolar lavage; HRQL, health-related quality of life; PRO, patient-reported outcome measure. (*Adapted from* Judson MA. The treatment of pulmonary sarcoidosis. Respir Med 2012;106(10):1353; with permission.)

serum angiotensin-converting enzyme levels, nodularity on chest imaging) or on the basis of physiologic change (eg, decrements in spirometry) when the patients quality of life is not affected appreciably. Previous studies have shown that sarcoidosis experts are relatively poor judges of the impact of the disease on the patient's quality of life.[5]

HRQL is a multidimensional construct composed of several domains, including physical, social, mental/emotional, cognitive, and spiritual, and refers to the extent to which 1 or several of these domains are affected by a medical condition and/or its treatment.[6] Serious consideration of HRQL results in a paradigm shift in patient care that has several significant consequences. First, attention to HRQL actively engages the patient in his or her health care, because patient input is required to make such assessments. Second, clinicians are obligated to focus on clinical information beyond objective laboratory data in considering HRQL. Such a process tends to redirect caregiver focus toward the real patient and away from the "iPatient," the virtual construct of the patient consisting of the patient's electronic medical record where patient assessment primarily involves interacting with a computer screen and not the real patient.[7] Third, giving major consideration to HRQL allows the clinician and the patient to work toward a common goal of maximizing the patient's sense of health as opposed to maximizing laboratory test results that, in the case of sarcoidosis, are very often discordant.[5]

THE ASSESSMENT OF HEALTH-RELATED QUALITY OF LIFE

The assessment of HRQL does not necessarily mandate the use of objective measures. Clinicians often use qualitative measures by asking the patient to describe his or her symptoms and inquiring about how those symptoms affect their ability to

function and their quality of life. Although such an approach is often reliable when therapy results in changes of great magnitude that lead to substantial improvements in HRQL, such an approach may be less reliable in detecting small but significant changes in HRQL. In the case of pulmonary sarcoidosis, the sarcoidosis-induced physiologic decrements are often relatively minor,[3,4] suggesting that a qualitative approach may be inadequate. Furthermore, in the case of assessing an intervention in a clinical trial, it is problematic to apply such qualitative assessments. Finally, as mentioned, clinical sarcoidosis experts only have a fair agreement with patients in the assessment of perceived sarcoidosis symptoms.[5]

HRQL can be quantitatively assessed using PROs. A PRO is any report coming directly from patients, without interpretation by physicians or others, about how they function or feel in relation to a health condition and its therapy.[8,9] PROs have been used to evaluate general HRQL as well as specific symptoms experienced by the patient. Furthermore, PROs may be scaled and validated so that PRO measures accurately quantify the patient's perception of a specific symptom or state. PROs have become a standard measure used in clinical trials, because some effects of a health condition and its therapy are known only to patients. Properly developed and evaluated PRO instruments have the potential to provide more accurate measurements of the effects of medical therapies, thereby increasing the efficiency of clinical trials that attempt to measure the meaningful treatment benefits.[9]

PROs have become a standard measure used in clinical trials to assess the impact of interventions on the patient's sense of well-being. The US Food and Drug Administration (FDA) has published the draft guidance for industry, "Patient-Reported Outcome Measures: Use in Medical Product Development to Support Labeling Claims," to inform sponsors, clinicians, and researchers of the FDA's current thinking on how best to develop and use PROs to support potential claims in product labeling.[8,9]

PROBLEMS IN THE ASSESSMENT OF HEALTH-RELATED QUALITY OF LIFE IN SARCOIDOSIS

Despite the aforementioned rationale for using PROs to assess HRQL in sarcoidosis, there is often resistance in performing such an assessment for many reasons. Some of these reasons relate to the general concept of using such PROs, whereas others specifically relate to PRO use for sarcoidosis.

General Resistance to the Use of Patient-Reported Outcome Measures to Assess Health-Related Quality Of Life

There are many causes of resistance to use PROs to assess HRQL that are not specific to sarcoidosis. First, the clinician often believes that PROs cannot be quantified accurately and that questioning patients concerning their symptoms and functional limitations will suffice. However, as demonstrated in a subsequent section, many aspects of HRQL can be quantified objectively and accurately. Furthermore, as mentioned, qualitative assessments of HRQL are unlikely to identify small but significant changes that are often observed with sarcoidosis. Second, the clinician is often concerned that his or her interventions have relatively less effect on change in the patient's HRQL than in objective physiologic measures. Third, the distinction between quality of life and HRQL is often blurred so that the patient's assessment of HRQL may involve the effects of non–health-related issues. This idea may lead to a concern on the part of the clinician that a patient's assessment of HRQL incorporates issues unrelated to health status. Fourth, even if a PRO accurately assesses the patient's HRQL, it is possible that this measurement is impacted by medical issues unrelated to sarcoidosis that are not under the control of the sarcoidosis doctor. Indeed, there is evidence that sarcoidosis patients may have a disproportional number of comorbidities and psychological disorders.[10,11] Furthermore, there is some evidence that increased health care use by sarcoidosis patients for comorbid illnesses is related to high corticosteroid use.[12] Finally, patients are not computers and often do not reliably quantify their sensations or assessments of functional impairment. However, well-designed PROs incorporate such potential errors by a variety of techniques, including transitional measurements where the patient compares sensations in the present to previously (eg, the Transitional Dyspnea

Index[13]), a reliance on distribution changes and effect size,[14] the use of some external anchor, such as patient judgments of change, that is used to compute a minimally important difference (MID) or clinically important difference,[14] using item response theory (IRT) to scale items that can be used to construct computer-adaptive testing (CAT) where patient inconsistencies can be detected.

Sarcoidosis-specific Resistance to the Use of Patient-Reported Outcome Measures to Assess Health-Related Quality of Life

There are also several sarcoidosis-specific issues that lead to clinician resistance to use PROs to assess HRQL. First, sarcoidosis has numerous clinical manifestations and may affect any organ in the body. Therefore, a general HRQL instrument may be inadequate to drill down to the HRQL effects of sarcoidosis specifically. As discussed in a subsequent section, several specific sarcoidosis instruments have been developed recently to address specific organ involvement so that the HRQL effects specifically attributable to sarcoidosis can be disentangled from the effects of other illnesses. Second, many of the PROs used to assess sarcoidosis are not disease specific in that they have not been validated in a sarcoidosis population. Although this is a potential limitation of these instruments, it is unlikely that symptoms such as dyspnea and fatigue are assessed differently in sarcoidosis patients than in patients with other disorders. Finally, although successful treatment of sarcoidosis may improve HRQL, the toxicity of therapy may also lead to worsening of HRQL.[5] Indeed, it has been shown recently that patients in a sarcoidosis clinic receiving a greater yearly total dose of corticosteroids had a worse HRQL compared with those receiving a lesser yearly total dose after adjustment for disease severity.[15] Therefore, a complete assessment of HRQL needs to incorporate both the positive and negative effects of antisarcoidosis therapy to make accurate treatment decisions. Recently, sarcoidosis-specific PROs have been developed that include "modules" that address both the positive and negative effects of antisarcoidosis therapy on HRQL.

CHARACTERISTICS OF PATIENT-REPORTED OUTCOME MEASURES

The development of appropriate PROs to measure HRQL is a complex process that is beyond the scope of this article and is well-outlined in the FDA guidance document concerning PROs.[8] The PRO should ideally measure traits that are unidimensional constructs, meaning that they can be measured on 1 scale from completely lacking the trait to having the trait in abundance (eg, dyspnea). The items used to construct the PRO should be based on expert opinion and rigorous patient input, usually involving patient focus groups and individual patient interviews.[8] Integral to the development of a PRO is the development of a "conceptual framework" that schematically articulates the expected relationships between the PRO items within each PRO domain and the larger instrument.[8] HRQL usually has multidimensional aspects that depend on several domains. The conceptual framework organizes the interrelationships between these domains so that the HRQL PRO can be constructed logically. An example of a conceptual framework in the development of a sarcoidosis HRQL PRO is depicted in **Fig. 2**.

Traditionally, PROs use "items" that are statements or questions that are posed to patients. In most PROs, the items may be answered by selecting one of several choices across a Likert scale, often with a range of severity (eg, "none," "minimal," "mild," "moderate," "moderately severe," and "severe") or of frequency (eg, "never," "seldom," "occasionally," "commonly," "most of the time," and "all of the time.")

Validation of an instrument is the process of assessing whether the instrument credibly measures what it is intended to measure.[16] PROs are required to be validated in 3 general dimensions: (a) content validity, which examines if the PRO items are sensible and reflect the trait of interest,

(b) criterion validity, which considers if the PRO reflects "external criteria," usually previously established measures for the trait, and (c) construct validity, which examines whether the PRO behaves according to the conceptual framework.[16] To give some examples of PROs that fail to meet these dimensions of validation, a pulmonary symptom PRO would fail to meet content validity if it failed to measure symptoms of cough. A pulmonary symptom PRO would fail to meet criterion validity if PRO measure moved in the opposite direction to the Saint George Respiratory Questionnaire (SGRQ), an established pulmonary symptom PRO.[17] A pulmonary symptom PRO would fail to meet construct validity if the PRO assessed patients as having less cough or wheeze during asthma exacerbations then when they were free of exacerbations.

An additional feature of a PRO measure is its reliability, which refers to the consistency of a measurement. One form of reliability is repeatability or test–retest reliability, which examines the variation in a PRO measure administered repeatedly under the same conditions. A special form of reliability is the internal consistency of the PRO, which can be assessed if HRQL measure involves summing up the scores of individual items to a single total score. The internal consistency examines if the individual items are consistent with each other in terms of them moving in the same direction.

Another characteristic of a PRO is whether it is "disease specific." Most PROs were developed and validated in certain populations and that may

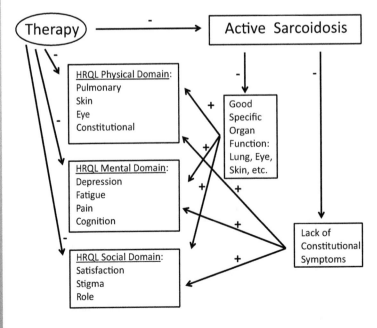

Fig. 2. A sample conceptual framework depicting the interrelationships between domains related to a proposed sarcoidosis HRQL patient-reported outcome measure. Effective therapy lowers the activity of sarcoidosis. Active sarcoidosis worsens organ function and constitutional symptoms. HRQL is composed of several domains (physical, mental, and social are depicted in this conceptual framework), that may each be adversely affected by therapy (eg, corticosteroids). Each of the boxes in the figure could be expanded to drill down further on these factors. A rational patient-reported outcome measure should comply with the proposed conceptual framework. HRQL, health-related quality of life; +, improves; −, worsens; each arrow relates only the 2 factors between them.

not reflect the individual or cohort to which the PRO is administered. In the case of sarcoidosis, most but not all of the HRQL PROs that have been used were not constructed using sarcoidosis patients. This circumstance does not invalidate the use of these PROs in sarcoidosis patients, provided there is no plausible rationale that sarcoidosis patients would assess the trait being measured in a different way than the cohort in which the PRO was validated. Although the debate regarding the use of generic versus disease-specific measures persists, generic measures are most useful for cross-illness comparisons of treatments and illnesses whereas disease-specific measures may be more sensitive to changes in patient functional capacity.[18]

Another important characteristic of an HRQL PRO is the MID, otherwise known as the clinically important difference. The MID has been defined as the smallest difference that patients perceive and that would mandate a change in clinical management.[19] A PRO may identify a statistically significant difference in HRQL in 2 groups. However, that difference would need to exceed the MID of the PRO to be clinically significant. Calculation of the MID is beyond the scope of this article, but involves examining changes in the PRO over time and correlating the PRO change against other accepted clinically meaningful outcomes, called anchor variables.

Ideally, an HRQL PRO could be used not only to assess the response of cohorts of subjects in clinical trials, but to monitor specific individuals over time, using these PROs to notify clinicians in "real time" regarding symptom fluctuations or worsening.[20] Unfortunately, the multidimensional natures of most current PROs are too crude for individual patient assessment in the clinical setting.[20–22]

IRT is a relatively new measurement approach with the potential to provide precise assessments at the individual level.[20,22,23] The traditional PRO incorporates items that have associated point scores that, when summed, yield a total score that is supposed to reflect that state of a certain trait. This is similar to most tests that students undergo to assess their mastery of a subject. With IRT, it is the item that determines the state of a certain trait. To continue the student test analogy, an IRT test would give the student increasingly difficult problems to determine the level of student mastery of a subject. The level of student mastery would not be determined by the percentage of correct questions answered, but rather by the most difficult question that the student answered correctly.

IRT involves constructing questionnaire items along a continuum of an underlying trait (eg, fatigue, dyspnea; **Fig. 3**). These items, called "an item bank," are calibrated mathematically, using information from experts in the disease and from patients, to identify their specific position along the trait continuum. Through calibration of this item bank, IRT enables the approximation of an individual's location along a hierarchically ordered (eg, mild, moderate, and severe) trait that is being measured (see **Fig. 3**).[24] A well-constructed item bank can be used to construct a short form PRO, where a small subgroup of items from the entire item bank can provide superior precision when compared with non-IRT PROs, and nearly equivalent accuracy when compared with the entire item bank (**Fig. 4**).[20] In addition, using a well-calibrated item bank, researchers may create short forms to uniquely individualize and tailor the questions to a particular target population or study aim (**Fig. 5**). Finally, IRT allows for the application of CAT. With CAT, items are selected from the item bank iteratively, based on the subject's previous responses, so that the most informative item is used to estimate the subject's location along the continuum of the trait (**Fig. 6**A). One advantage of CAT is that a relatively small number of items need to be answered to obtain a precise estimate. In addition, a CAT test that "fails to converge" with iterative items suggests that the subject may be giving inconsistent responses, and implies that the PRO measure may be unreliable (see **Fig. 6**B). Without CAT, it would be problematic to detect such a deficiency in a PRO.

There are additional pragmatic issues that must be addressed for a PRO to be reliable. The PRO forms/computer display must be legible and clear for the patient to read. In addition, some individual or computer must check the accuracy of the patient responses in real time in front of the patient so that they may be corrected, if needed. This is because patients may inadvertently skip an item, or mistakenly give 2 different responses to the same item. If these mistakes are not identified and corrected, it may invalidate the PRO assessment, although some PROs have developed algorithms for dealing with both skipped items and item response duplication.[25]

Because language is not devoid of cultural and social aspects, the translation of a PRO into another language requires a rigorous methodology.[26,27] The aspects of this approach are beyond the scope of this article. Suffice it to say that a PRO translated from 1 another language unless it undergoes a detailed validation process.

Several pragmatic issues must be addressed before a PRO can be reliably administered. The items should be clearly readable. Care should be taken that "copies of copies" of forms are not

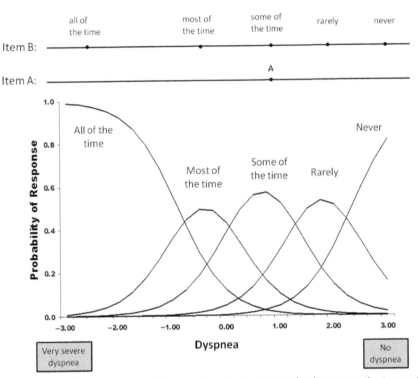

Fig. 3. The scaling of 1 item by item response theory in the development of a dyspnea patient-reported outcome measure (PRO). This PRO uses a 5-point Likert scale ("all of the time," "most of the time," "some of the time," "rarely," "never"). With scaling, the 5 responses are not equidistant from each other. The actual scaling involves field testing in patients and is truly represented by probability curves depicted in the figure. Because these probability curves are problematic to depict in subsequent figures, each item is depicted as a single point in **Figs. 4** and **5** (example, item *A* in this figure) and as a mean of each of the 5 possible responses in **Fig. 6**A and B (example, item *B* in this figure).

administered that are problematic to read. The subject should have the PRO administered in a comfortable and quiet environment. The subject should be encouraged to answer the items independently, without supervision or guidance from friends or relatives. If the patient is illiterate, it is acceptable to read the questions to the subject. It is recommended that this be done by someone other than a friend or relative if possible. Although there is a concern for patient confidentiality, efforts

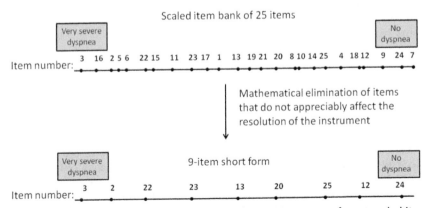

Fig. 4. Construction of a short form dyspnea patient-reported outcome measure from a scaled item back developed through item response theory. Using mathematical techniques, the 9-item short form has nearly the same power of resolution as the complete 25-item item bank. See **Fig. 3**, item *A* for what each dot represents.

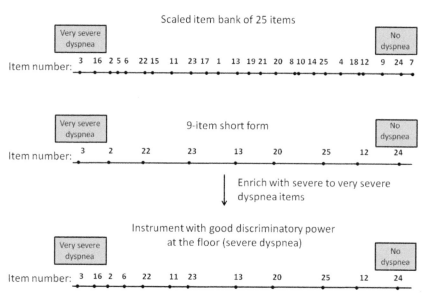

Fig. 5. Development of an item response theory-derived patient-reported outcome measure examining a cohort with severe dyspnea (eg, New York Heart Association Class 3 and 4 pulmonary hypertension, end-stage pulmonary sarcoidosis). Items focusing on severe dyspnea were added to the short form to increase resolution at the more severe end of the dyspnea trait because fewer questions in this range may not adequately identify an improvement with an intervention ("floor effect"). As with all of these patient-reported outcome measures, they would need to be validated to be used clinically. See **Fig. 3**, item A for what each dot represents.

should be made to review the subject's responses in real time, because the subject may have forgotten to answer 1 item, or, alternatively, given 2 responses to the same item. As previously mentioned for most PROs, failure to correct these errors invalidates the evaluation. Some PROs, such as the SGRQ, do have calculators to correct for such error, although most do not. PROs may be administered in hard copy form or on a computer. Hard copy forms are, obviously, less expensive. Computer administration does have the potential advantages of easily and confidentially tracking subject errors in item responses (absent or multiple responses). Furthermore, computer administration of a PRO can be formatted to construct CAT.

SPECIFIC HEALTH-RELATED QUALITY OF LIFE MEASURES USED IN SARCOIDOSIS

Table 1 shows some common HRQL PROs that have been used in sarcoidosis trials. General HRQL measures that are not specific for sarcoidosis have been studied in sarcoidosis patients, including the Short Form-36 (SF-36),[28–31] World Health Organization – Quality of Life 100 (WHO-QOL-100),[32–34] and WHOQOL-BREF.[35] The SF-36, although a general HRQL measure, has been shown to have a good correlation with sarcoidosis-specific PROs.[36–38] Sarcoidosis-

specific general HRQL measures include the Sarcoidosis Health Questionnaire (SHQ),[36] Kings Sarcoidosis Questionnaire (KCQ),[37] and Sarcoidosis Assessment Tool (SAT).[39,40] MIDs have not been determined for the SHQ and the KCQ, so that their clinical application is somewhat limited. Both the KCQ and SAT have specific modules/domains for organ-specific manifestations of sarcoidosis so that impact of specific organ involvement can be assessed by the patient. In addition, both the KCQ and SAT have a module focusing on the patient assessment of medication effects that is a major concern for sarcoidosis patients.

The SGRQ is a general, pulmonary-oriented HRQL PRO that has been used in several sarcoidosis studies.[41–46] Although the SGRQ is not sarcoidosis specific, it has been shown to correlate well with sarcoidosis-specific PROs.[36–38] The Medical Research Council (MRC) general dyspnea scale that also has been shown to correlate with sarcoidosis-specific PROs.[36,37] Although the Baseline Dyspnea Index (BDI)/Transitional Dyspnea Index (TDI) has also been used in a pulmonary sarcoidosis trial,[28] this measure has never been correlated to a sarcoidosis-specific PRO.

Fatigue is a common complaint of sarcoidosis patients, with 60% to 81% reporting significant fatigue.[35,47,48] The cause of fatigue in sarcoidosis is multifactorial and may be caused from inflammatory mediators associated with granulomatous

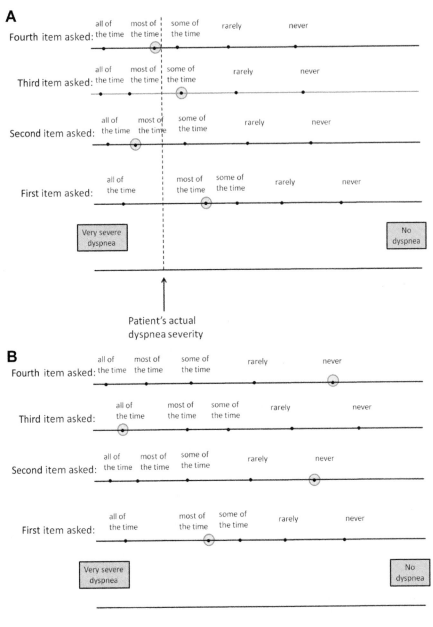

Fig. 6. (*A*) Computer-adaptive testing of a dyspnea patient-reported outcome measure developed using item response theory logic. The gray circles show the patient's responses to each item. The computer selects an initial dyspnea item from the item bank. The patient's response to the first item results in the computer selecting a second item that strategically maximizes the likelihood of localizing the exact level of dyspnea of the patient. The computer continues with this approach, which often results in an accurate assessment of the patient's trait (dyspnea, in this case) after posing very few questions. See **Fig. 3**, item *B* for what the dots represent. (*B*) Because people are not always logical or consistent in their assessment of their symptoms, computer-adaptive testing allows for patient inconsistency to be detected. The gray circles show the patient's responses to each item. In this example, the patient's responses suggest great inconsistency in the patients assessment of dyspnea on different items (eg, a patient who is never short of breath walking 1 mile but always short of breath walking 100 feet). In this case, computer-adaptive testing concludes that this patient's dyspnea cannot be assessed reliably by this patient-reported outcome measure. This would be problematic to detect without using computer-adaptive testing. See **Fig. 3**, item *B* for what the dots represent.

Table 1
Selected quality of life measures used in sarcoidosis trials

Measure	Domains/Symptoms Assessed	Sarcoidosis Specific	MID Determined	Number of Items	Approximate Time to Complete PRO (min)	Sarcoidosis Studies Using Measure
SF-36	General HRQL • Physical composite with 4 subscales • Mental composite with 4 subscales	−	+	36	3–10	—
WHOQOL-100	General HRQL • Physical health • Psychological independence • Social relationships • Environment • Spirituality	−	+[a]	100	Literate 30; semiliterate 40–90	—
WHOQOL-BREF	General HRQL • Physical health • Psychological social relationships • Environment	−	−	26	5–15	—
SHQ	General HRQL • Daily functioning • Physical functioning • Emotional functioning	+	−	29	5–15	—
KCQ	General HRQL • General health • Lung • Eye • Skin • Medications	+	−	29[c]	5–15	—
SAT	General HRQL • Physical functioning • Satisfaction • Pain • Sleep • Fatigue • Lung • Skin • Skin stigma	+	+	51[c]	10–20	—
SGRQ	General respiratory HRQL	−	+	50	10–20	—
MRC	Dyspnea	−	−	1	1	—
BDI/TDI	Dyspnea • Functional impairment • Magnitude of task • Magnitude of effort	−	−	24	1–3	—
FAS	Fatigue	+	+	10	1–5	—
FACIT-F	Fatigue	−	+[b]	13	3–10	—
PROMIS fatigue scale	Fatigue	+	+	10	1–5	—

(continued on next page)

Table 1
(continued)

Measure	Domains/Symptoms Assessed	Sarcoidosis Specific	MID Determined	Number of Items	Approximate Time to Complete PRO (min)	Sarcoidosis Studies Using Measure
SAT fatigue subscale	Fatigue	+	+	5	1–3	—
Beck Depression Inventory	Depression	—	—	21	5–10	—
CES-D	Depression	—	—	20	5–10	—

Abbreviations: BDI/TDI, Baseline Dyspnea Index/Transitional Dyspnea Index; CES-D, Center for Epidemiologic Studies-Depression Scale; FACIT-F, Functional Assessment of Chronic Illness Therapy Fatigue; FAS, fatigue assessment scale; HRQOL, health-related quality of life; KCQ, Kings College Questionnaire; MRC, Medical Research Council (MRC) general dyspnea scale; PROMIS, Patient Reported Outcomes Measurement Information Systems; SAT, Sarcoidosis Assessment Tool; SF-36, Short form–36; SGRQ, Saint George Respiratory Questionnaire; SHQ, Sarcoidosis Health Questionnaire; WHOQOL-100, World Health Organization – Quality of Life 100; WHOQOL-BREF, short (brief) version of the WHOQOL-100.

[a] In breast cancer patients.[30]
[b] In rheumatoid arthritis, chemotherapy, and anemia patients[54]; +, yes; −, no.
[c] Fewer items are needed to measure specific organs and/or domains.

inflammation,[49] corticosteroid and other antisarcoidosis therapy, adrenal insufficiency from withdrawal of chronic corticosteroid therapy, organ dysfunction caused by sarcoidosis, depression[11] and other psychological factors from coping with a chronic disease, and factors indirectly related to sarcoidosis, such as obesity and obstructive sleep apnea from chronic corticosteroid use.[50,51] Several medications have been suggested to be of benefit for sarcoidosis-associated fatigue.[49,52] Therefore, it is important identify fatigue in sarcoidosis patients, as well as determine its cause, monitor it, and consider therapy for fatigue.

Several fatigue PROs have been evaluated in sarcoidosis patients. The Fatigue Assessment Scale (FAS) is a sarcoidosis-specific fatigue measure that has been used in several sarcoidosis studies.[48,53–55] In addition, an MID has been established for the FAS.[56] One concern with the FAS is that because 2 of the 10 items in the measure ask fatigue questions with a Likert scale in the opposite direction from the 8 other items, the internal consistency of this PRO is poor compared with other fatigue measures and was in the "questionable range" in a female sarcoidosis subgroup.[57] Three other fatigue PROs that have been used in sarcoidosis patients are the Functional Assessment of Chronic Illness Therapy Fatigue (FACIT-F), and the Patient Reported Outcomes Measurement Information Systems (PROMIS) Fatigue Instrument (PFI), and the SAT fatigue subscale. The FACIT-F was developed for oncology trials[58] and has been used in drug intervention studies in sarcoidosis,[49] although it is not

sarcoidosis specific. The PFI is an IRT-based PRO, has been shown to have an excellent internal consistency, and has been used in sarcoidosis[57] The SAT fatigue subscale is IRT based,[39,40] has been used in a clinical sarcoidosis trial,[38] and a minimal clinically important difference has been established for this measure.[38]

Depression is common in sarcoidosis, having been reported in 60% of patients in 1 series.[11] Depression may be described as fatigue by some patients; therefore, a psychological evaluation should be considered in all sarcoidosis patients with unexplained fatigue. Although no PRO is sarcoidosis specific, both the Beck Depression Inventory and Center for Epidemiologic Studies-Depression Scale have been used in sarcoidosis cohorts.[11,49,51]

SUMMARY

HRQL is important to sarcoidosis patients. Ideally, most indications for the treatment of sarcoidosis relate to disease-associated HRQL. However, clinicians often focus on objective clinical and laboratory tests that often do not reflect HRQL well. PROs have been constructed that can reliably quantify HRQL. Many of these PROs are disease specific and have had minimally important clinical differences established that allows for a determination of clinically relevant changes in these measures. These PROs are clearly useful in sarcoidosis intervention trials involving cohorts of sarcoidosis patients. Properly scaled PROs, including those based on IRT, may be useful to follow HRQL measures in individual patients over time.

REFERENCES

1. Lynch JP 3rd, Ma YL, Koss MN, et al. Pulmonary sarcoidosis. Semin Respir Crit Care Med 2007; 28(1):53–74.

2. Judson MA. The treatment of pulmonary sarcoidosis. Respir Med 2012;106(10):1351–61.

3. Judson MA, Boan AD, Lackland DT. The clinical course of sarcoidosis: presentation, diagnosis, and treatment in a large white and black cohort in the United States. Sarcoidosis Vasc Diffuse Lung Dis 2012;29(2):119–27.

4. Baydur A, Alsalek M, Louie SG, et al. Respiratory muscle strength, lung function, and dyspnea in patients with sarcoidosis. Chest 2001;120(1):102–8.

5. Cox CE, Donohue JF, Brown CD, et al. Health-related quality of life of persons with sarcoidosis. Chest 2004;125(3):997–1004.

6. Cella DF, Bonomi AE. Measuring quality of life: 1995 update. Oncology (Williston Park) 1995;9(Suppl 11): 47–60.

7. Verghese A. Culture shock–patient as icon, icon as patient. N Engl J Med 2008;359(26):2748–51.

8. U.S. Department of Health and Human Services FDA Center for Drug Evaluation and Research, U.S. Department of Health and Human Services FDA Center for Biologics Evaluation and Research, U.S. Department of Health and Human Services FDA Center for Devices and Radiological Health. Guidance for industry: patient-reported outcome measures: use in medical product development to support labeling claims: draft guidance. Health Qual Life Outcomes 2006;4:79.

9. Patrick DL, Burke LB, Powers JH, et al. Patient-reported outcomes to support medical product labeling claims: FDA perspective. Value Health 2007; 10(Suppl 2):S125–37.

10. Reynolds HY. Sarcoidosis: impact of other illnesses on the presentation and management of multi-organ disease. Lung 2002;180(5):281–99.

11. Chang B, Steimel J, Moller DR, et al. Depression in sarcoidosis. Am J Respir Crit Care Med 2001; 163(2):329–34.

12. Ligon CB, Judson MA. Impact of systemic corticosteroids on healthcare utilization in patients with sarcoidosis. Am J Med Sci 2011;341(3):196–201.

13. Mahler DA, Weinberg DH, Wells CK, et al. The measurement of dyspnea. Contents, interobserver agreement, and physiologic correlates of two new clinical indexes. Chest 1984;85(6):751–8.

14. Norman GR, Sridhar FG, Guyatt GH, et al. Relation of distribution- and anchor-based approaches in interpretation of changes in health-related quality of life. Med Care 2001;39(10):1039–47.

15. Judson MA, Chaudhry H, Louis A, et al. The effect of corticosteroids on quality of life in a sarcoidosis clinic: the results of a propensity analysis. Respir Med 2015;109(4):526–31.

16. Fayers P, Machin D. Quality of life: the assessment, analysis, and interpretation of patient-reported outcomes. 2nd edition. West Sussex (Untied Kingdom): John Wiley and Sons, LTD; 2007.

17. Jones PW, Quirk FH, Baveystock CM, et al. A self-complete measure of health status for chronic airflow limitation. The St. George's respiratory questionnaire. Am Rev Respir Dis 1992;145(6):1321–7.

18. Beaser RS, Garbus SB, Jacobson AM. Diabetes mellitus. In: Spilker B, editor. Quality of life and pharmacoeconomics in clinical trials. 2nd edition. Philadelphia: Lippincott-Raven; 1996. p. 983–91.

19. Jaeschke R, Singer J, Guyatt GH. Measurement of health status. Ascertaining the minimal clinically important difference. Control Clin Trials 1989;10(4):407–15.

20. Victorson DE, Cella D, Judson MA. Quality of life evaluation in sarcoidosis: current status and future directions. Curr Opin Pulm Med 2008;14(5):470–7.

21. Cella D, Nowinski CJ. Measuring quality of life in chronic illness: the functional assessment of chronic illness therapy measurement system. Arch Phys Med Rehabil 2002;83(12 Suppl 2):S10–7.

22. Ware JE Jr, Bjorner JB, Kosinski M. Practical implications of item response theory and computerized adaptive testing: a brief summary of ongoing studies of widely used headache impact scales. Med Care 2000;38(Suppl 9):II73–82.

23. Cella D, Chang CH. A discussion of item response theory and its applications in health status assessment. Med Care 2000;38(Suppl 9):II66–72.

24. Stansfeld SA, Roberts R, Foot SP. Assessing the validity of the SF-36 general health survey. Qual Life Res 1997;6(3):217–24.

25. Basagana X, Barrera-Gomez J, Benet M, et al. A framework for multiple imputation in cluster analysis. Am J Epidemiol 2013;177(7):718–25.

26. Hagell P, Hedin PJ, Meads DM, et al. Effects of method of translation of patient-reported health outcome questionnaires: a randomized study of the translation of the Rheumatoid Arthritis Quality of Life (RAQoL) Instrument for Sweden. Value Health 2010;13(4):424–30.

27. Eremenco SL, Cella D, Arnold BJ. A comprehensive method for the translation and cross-cultural validation of health status questionnaires. Eval Health Prof 2005;28(2):212–32.

28. Judson MA, Silvestri J, Hartung C, et al. The effect of thalidomide on corticosteroid-dependent pulmonary sarcoidosis. Sarcoidosis Vasc Diffuse Lung Dis 2006;23(1):51–7.

29. Jastrzebski D, Ziora D, Lubecki M, et al. Fatigue in sarcoidosis and Exercise Tolerance, dyspnea, and quality of life. Adv Exp Med Biol 2015;833:31–6.

30. Bourbonnais JM, Malaisamy S, Dalal BD, et al. Distance saturation product predicts health-related quality of life among sarcoidosis patients. Health Qual Life Outcomes 2012;10:67.

31. Heij L, Niesters M, Swartjes M, et al. Safety and efficacy of ARA 290 in sarcoidosis patients with symptoms of small fiber neuropathy: a randomized, double-blind pilot study. Mol Med 2012;18:1430–6.

32. Hoitsma E, De Vries J, van Santen-Hoeufft M, et al. Impact of pain in a Dutch sarcoidosis patient population. Sarcoidosis Vasc Diffuse Lung Dis 2003; 20(1):33–9.

33. Wirnsberger RM, De Vries J, Jansen TL, et al. Impairment of quality of life: rheumatoid arthritis versus sarcoidosis. Neth J Med 1999;54(3):86–95.

34. Den Oudsten BL, Zijlstra WP, De Vries J. The minimal clinical important difference in the World Health Organization Quality of Life instrument–100. Support Care Cancer 2013;21(5):1295–301.

35. Marcellis RG, Lenssen AF, Elfferich MD, et al. Exercise capacity, muscle strength and fatigue in sarcoidosis. Eur Respir J 2011;38(3):628–34.

36. Cox CE, Donohue JF, Brown CD, et al. The Sarcoidosis health questionnaire: a new measure of health-related quality of life. Am J Respir Crit Care Med 2003;168(3):323–9.

37. Patel AS, Siegert RJ, Creamer D, et al. The development and validation of the King's Sarcoidosis Questionnaire for the assessment of health status. Thorax 2013;68(1):57–65.

38. Judson MA, Mack M, Beaumont JL, et al. Differences for the sarcoidosis assessment tool. A new patient-reported outcome measure. Am J Respir Crit Care Med 2015;191(7):786–95.

39. Victorson DE, Cella D, Grund H, et al. A conceptual model of health-related quality of life in sarcoidosis. Qual Life Res 2013;23(1):89–101.

40. Victorson DE, Choi S, Judson MA, et al. Development and testing of item response theory-based item banks and short forms for eye, skin and lung problems in sarcoidosis. Qual Life Res 2014;23(4): 1301–13.

41. Judson MA, Highland KB, Kwon S, et al. Ambrisentan for sarcoidosis associated pulmonary hypertension. Sarcoidosis Vasc Diffuse Lung Dis 2011; 28(2):139–45.

42. Baughman RP, Judson MA, Lower EE, et al. Inhaled iloprost for sarcoidosis associated pulmonary hypertension. Sarcoidosis Vasc Diffuse Lung Dis 2009; 26(2):110–20.

43. Gvozdenovic BS, Mihailovic-Vucinic V, Ilic-Dudvarski A, et al. Differences in symptom severity and health status impairment between patients with pulmonary and pulmonary plus extrapulmonary sarcoidosis. Respir Med 2008;102(11):1636–42.

44. Baughman RP, Sparkman BK, Lower EE. Six-minute walk test and health status assessment in sarcoidosis. Chest 2007;132(1):207–13.

45. Antoniou KM, Tzanakis N, Tzouvelekis A, et al. Quality of life in patients with active sarcoidosis in Greece. Eur J Intern Med 2006;17(6):421–6.

46. de Boer S, Kolbe J, Wilsher ML. The relationships among dyspnoea, health-related quality of life and psychological factors in sarcoidosis. Respirology 2014;19(7):1019–24.

47. Michielsen HJ, Drent M, Peros-Golubicic T, et al. Fatigue is associated with quality of life in sarcoidosis patients. Chest 2006;130(4):989–94.

48. De Vries J, Michielsen H, Van Heck GL, et al. Measuring fatigue in sarcoidosis: the fatigue assessment scale (FAS). Br J Health Psychol 2004;9(Pt 3): 279–91.

49. Lower EE, Harman S, Baughman RP. Double-blind, randomized trial of dexmethylphenidate hydrochloride for the treatment of sarcoidosis-associated fatigue. Chest 2008;133(5):1189–95.

50. Drent M, Verbraecken J, van der Grinten C, et al. Fatigue associated with obstructive sleep apnea in a patient with sarcoidosis. Respiration 2000;67(3):337–40.

51. Turner GA, Lower EE, Corser BC, et al. Sleep apnea in sarcoidosis. Sarcoidosis Vasc Diffuse Lung Dis 1997;14(1):61–4.

52. Wagner MT, Marion SD, Judson MA. The effects of fatigue and treatment with methylphenidate on sustained attention in sarcoidosis. Sarcoidosis Vasc Diffuse Lung Dis 2005;22(3):235.

53. De Vries J, Rothkrantz-Kos S, van Dieijen-Visser MP, et al. The relationship between fatigue and clinical parameters in pulmonary sarcoidosis. Sarcoidosis Vasc Diffuse Lung Dis 2004;21(2):127–36.

54. Hinz A, Fleischer M, Brahler E, et al. Fatigue in patients with sarcoidosis, compared with the general population. Gen Hosp Psychiatry 2011;33(5):462–8.

55. de Kleijn WP, Elfferich MD, De Vries J, et al. Fatigue in sarcoidosis: American versus Dutch patients. Sarcoidosis Vasc Diffuse Lung Dis 2009;26(2):92–7.

56. de Kleijn WP, De Vries J, Wijnen PA, et al. Minimal (clinically) important differences for the fatigue assessment scale in sarcoidosis. Respir Med 2011;105(9):1388–95.

57. Kalkanis A, Yucel RM, Judson MA. The internal consistency of PRO fatigue instruments in sarcoidosis: superiority of the PFI over the FAS. Sarcoidosis Vasc Diffuse Lung Dis 2013;30(1):60–4.

58. Cella D, Eton DT, Lai JS, et al. Combining anchor and distribution-based methods to derive minimal clinically important differences on the Functional Assessment of Cancer Therapy (FACT) anemia and fatigue scales. J Pain Symptom Manage 2002; 24(6):547–61.

Treatment of Sarcoidosis

Marlies S. Wijsenbeek, MD, PhD[a], Daniel A. Culver, DO[b,c],*

KEYWORDS

- Sarcoidosis • Treatment • Corticosteroids • Steroid sparing • TNF antagonists • Prognosis
- Patient preferences

KEY POINTS

- The treatment of sarcoidosis can be divided into the key questions of "whom to treat" and "how to treat".
- The decision to treat depends on the degree of organ impairment; threat to organ function; impact of symptoms on quality of life; and the extent, activity, and chronicity of disease.
- The patient's preferences and input are central in the process of deciding when and how to treat.
- Noninflammatory manifestations of sarcoidosis are commonly the salient feature, and treatment of them is usually not with immunosuppressive medications.
- The dosing, duration, and choices of steroids and nonsteroid medications should be adjusted empirically to the individual patient.

INTRODUCTION

Sarcoidosis is a multisystem granulomatous disease with large variability in presentation, disease behavior, and outcome. The cause of sarcoidosis and explanation for its wide phenotypic differences are not yet fully understood. Interaction between a presumed trigger and a genetically susceptible host is considered the mainstay of sarcoidosis pathogenesis. Genetic factors may play an important role in modifying the risk for the disease, its phenotype, and the outcome. As a result of the disease heterogeneity, treatment varies from none to a range of medications, including corticosteroids, cytotoxic agents, and biologic agents.[1–3] Despite important advances in the understanding of the disease, there is a paucity of evidence-based treatment protocols and data supporting a beneficial treatment effect on long-term outcomes.[4,5] Furthermore, despite more available therapies, some data suggest an increasing mortality trend over the past 2 decades.[6] Treatment of sarcoidosis should be tailored to the individual patient's needs; it encompasses balancing natural prognosis, severity, and impact of disease; likelihood of response to therapy; and potential side effects, leading to the central questions: whom to treat and how to treat?

WHOM TO TREAT

A decision to initiate treatment often implies that treatment will be necessary over the long term.[7,8] Thus, careful delineation of the goals of treatment is necessary. Some variables that should be considered include the expected prognosis; extent of disease; severity (impact on organ function and symptoms); whether it is active; and, most importantly, the opinion of the patient.

Prognosis

In many patients with sarcoidosis the disease resolves spontaneously. Even if the disease persists, it may not cause sufficient problems to require therapy. For example, in a survey of 500 patients

Disclosures: Dr D.A. Culver has received consulting fees from Mallinkrodt Pharmaceuticals.
[a] Department of Pulmonary Medicine, Erasmus Medical Center, University Medical Center Rotterdam, Gravendijkwal 230, 3015 CE Rotterdam, The Netherlands; [b] Department of Pulmonary Medicine, Respiratory Institute, Cleveland Clinic, 9500 Euclid Avenue, Cleveland, OH 44195, USA; [c] Department of Pathobiology, Lerner Research Institute, Cleveland Clinic, 9500 Euclid Avenue, Cleveland, OH 44195, USA
* Corresponding author. 9500 Euclid Avenue, Desk A90, Cleveland, OH 44195.
E-mail address: culverd@ccf.org

Clin Chest Med 36 (2015) 751–767
http://dx.doi.org/10.1016/j.ccm.2015.08.015
0272-5231/15/$ – see front matter © 2015 Elsevier Inc. All rights reserved.

from 10 tertiary centers around the world, only 43% of patients who were still being seen at the centers were still using any therapy 5 years after diagnosis, similar to the proportion with persistent but untreated disease in those centers, which are also skewed to include the most severe case mix.[9] However, a substantial minority has chronic or progressive disease with concomitant morbidity, and a small proportion of these patients might even die from the disease. Having insight regarding the prognosis influences treatment decisions; if the risk of a poor outcome is high, there is a greater incentive to commence therapy. When instituting therapy, it is important to realize that not only the disease itself but also its treatments might (negatively) affect morbidity and mortality.

Reported mortalities in sarcoidosis vary from 1% to 7 % depending on the setting and population studied.[6,10–13] Swigris and colleagues[6] reported an increase in age-adjusted, sarcoidosis-related mortality of 50.5% in women and 30.1% in men over 2 decades. In the United Kingdom a 2-fold increased risk for death in sarcoidosis was reported, which was also greater in women.[14] A population-based cohort study in the United States uncovered a 2-fold increase in sarcoidosis-related hospitalizations in a decade.[15] However, it is debatable whether these numbers also reflect a possible better recognition of disease, an increase of severity, and/or an aging sarcoidosis population. In Europe and the United States deaths are primarily a result of progressive pulmonary fibrosis with subsequent respiratory failure.[16] Other causes are severe neurologic or cardiac involvement. In Japan, death is mostly attributed to cardiac involvement.[17,18]

Scadding's[19] landmark study from 1961 about the prognosis of sarcoidosis followed 136 patients with sarcoidosis for 5 years after their diagnosis. At the end of this study 97% of the patients with stage I disease and 58% with stage II were asymptomatic, whereas only 25% of the patients with stage III were asymptomatic.[19] These trends have subsequently been confirmed in other studies.[20–22] A commonly adopted clinical approach is the concept of 3 broad, partially overlapping groups: acute disease, which often resolves within 2 to 5 years of diagnosis; chronic disease, which persists beyond 5 years after diagnosis; and refractory disease, which progresses despite adequate therapy and is typically also chronic in duration.[23,24]

It is generally appreciated that patients with acute-onset disease have a good chance of spontaneous remission.[16,20,25,26] Löfgren syndrome, with its acute onset consisting of bilateral hilar lymphadenopathy, erythema nodosum, and polyarthritis, usually resolves spontaneously and generally does not require treatment.[22,27] Apart from Löfgren syndrome, the definition of acute sarcoidosis has varied considerably in the literature. In the past, disease resolution within 2 years was used as definition of the acute form.[23,25,28] However, several studies reported a substantial rate of resolution of disease between 2 and 5 years from diagnosis, which has led to the redefinition of chronic as that disease persisting after 5 years.[24,26,29,30] Nevertheless, persistence of active inflammation more than 2 years from diagnosis reduces the chances of resolution substantially.[24]

Studying the natural history of sarcoidosis is limited by differences in case identification, dissimilarities in racial background, differences in techniques for assessing organ involvement, and the confounding effects of variable treatment.[8,19,27,28,31,32] In the past decade, several approaches have been proposed to phenotype patients with sarcoidosis in relation to clinical outcome.[9,33–37] Recently, Walsh and colleagues[37] showed that a combination of a composite physiologic index and high-resolution chest computed tomography findings of fibrosis and pulmonary artery/aorta size ratio predicted mortality. A disadvantage of this approach is that the model focuses primarily on advanced disease, and therefore does not have clear-cut relevance for predicting the likelihood of a poor outcome at the time of sarcoidosis onset.

Until now, no study has comprehensively established which features most strongly determine the chance of spontaneous resolution or of serious organ involvement. Besides ascertainment bias related to referral patterns and evolving technologies, there have been few attempts to systematically assess manifestations and then to follow patients for an adequate length of time to conclusively define which features independently carry the most weight for long-term prognosis. As an example, several studies have suggested that African Americans have a worse prognosis than white Americans in the United States.[27,38,39] However, multivariable analysis in a large US study suggested that the worse prognosis in African Americans may relate primarily to their greater frequency of extrapulmonary organ involvement, rather than to race itself.[7] Some of the features that have most commonly been associated with a worse prognosis are listed in **Table 1**.

Effect of Treatment on Natural History

Granuloma formation in sarcoidosis is thought to result from interaction of an environmental antigen and a genetically susceptible host. This interplay

Table 1
Selected prognostic features at the time of diagnosis

Features	References
Age>40 y	20,40
African American race	27,39
Requirement for therapy	7,8
Extrapulmonary Involvement	
Cardiac	25,41
Neurologic (except isolated CN palsy)	42–44
Lupus pernio/cutaneous sarcoidosis	19,25
Splenomegaly	20,25
Hypercalcemia/ nephrocalcinosis	25,45
Osseous disease	32,46
Pulmonary Features	
Stage 3–4 chest radiograph	19,20,25,30,47,48
Pulmonary hypertension	49
Significant lung function impairment	47,50
Moderate to severe dyspnea	7,51
BAL neutrophilia at presentation	52,53

Abbreviations: BAL, bronchoalveolar lavage; CN, cranial nerve.

between particular combinations of triggers and host responses would also explain the differences found in hypotheses on the pathogenesis of disease.[54] However, it may be that the primary cause of sarcoidosis is more an intrinsic abnormal immunologic response than an environmental antigen per se.[4,54] It has been speculated that in sarcoidosis the granulomatous reaction is needed to clear the antigen.[3] In this theory, suppressing the granulomatous inflammation by effective therapy for sarcoidosis may lead to failure of clearance of the assumed antigen, which could lead to relapse of disease when treatment is stopped.[3,55] Evidence supporting this theory is the observation that relapse of disease may be more common in patients previously treated with corticosteroids or in patients who received a higher dose of corticosteroids.[8,56] In a Swedish patient cohort presenting with Löfgren syndrome, 80% of the patients who were HLA-DRB1*03 negative and treated with corticosteroids had persisting disease at 2 years versus 37% of the nontreated patients.[57] Several other studies have failed to show improved rates of normalization of chest radiography at long-term follow-up when instituting early treatment in sarcoidosis.[58–62]

Although these studies have shown that routine institution of therapy for the purpose of improving long-term outcome in sarcoidosis might even have the opposite effect, there are also some studies suggesting some long-term benefits with therapy. A study conducted by the British Thoracic Society evaluated the effect of 18 months of corticosteroids in patients with stage II and III sarcoidosis on 5-year outcome, compared with observation only.[57,63] Before treatment allocation, all patients were observed for 6 months to exclude patients with rapidly progressive disease or resolution. In the follow-up period only 6 of 31 patients in the observation arm needed treatment because of deterioration of disease. At the end of the study at 5 years, the patients treated with corticosteroids showed a lower incidence of any radiographic fibrosis (26% vs 42%), a lower incidence of reporting any dyspnea (15% vs 39%), and greater improvement in forced vital capacity (FVC; +10.6% vs +2.65%) compared with the observation group. In a trial in 189 Finnish patients, patients were double-blind randomized to either placebo or oral prednisone for 3 months followed by inhaled budesonide for 15 months. At 5 years, the prednisone-treated group showed more resolution of radiographic changes (74% vs 62%) and also less relapse and better pulmonary function than the untreated group for the patients with radiographic stage II and III, but not for stage I.[64] However, effect size in these trials was of unclear clinical benefit and baseline imbalances between treated groups were present. Overall, these data have led to a general appreciation that there is no clear-cut long-term benefit of routine treatment in all patients with acute pulmonary sarcoidosis.[23,65]

Approach to Treatment Decisions

Systematic assessment of extent, severity, and activity of disease and the impact on the patient's life helps to guide treatment decisions. These decisions should always be weighed against the chances for spontaneous resolution, possible treatment toxicities, and the patient's wishes and expectations (**Fig. 1**).

Extent of disease

After the diagnosis of sarcoidosis has been established, additional work-up is recommended to evaluate the extent of disease.[16] In the ACCESS study (A Case Control Etiologic Study of Sarcoidosis), 23% of patients developed new organ involvement during 2-years' follow-up, suggesting that reassessment needs to be performed.[27] Recently a new tool, the World Association of Sarcoidosis and Other Granulomatous Disorders (WASOG) Sarcoidosis Organ Assessment Instrument, was developed to systematically assess

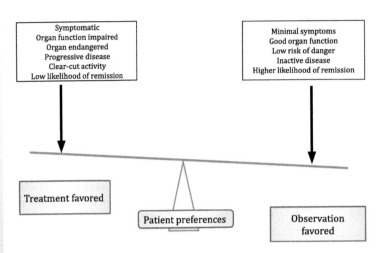

Fig. 1. The major factors influencing the decision to start immunosuppressive therapy for sarcoidosis. Symptoms and organ impairment refer to those from active granulomatous inflammation, not those from consequences of the disease (eg, fibrosis). The patient's input occupies a central position.

organ involvement in sarcoidosis.[66] PET and MRI can also play a role, when clinically indicated, to detect occult sites of sarcoidosis.[67,68]

Severity of disease

Severity of organ involvement can be measured objectively as percentage decline from normal capacity (eg, pulmonary function, cardiac ejection fraction, renal clearance) or subjectively by the intensity of symptoms.[33] In sarcoidosis, a considerable burden of disease is also caused by less organ-specific but often very troublesome symptoms, termed the sarcoidosis penumbra by Lazar and Culver.[24] One of these most common problems is fatigue, which has been reported in 50% to 70% of patients with sarcoidosis.[69–71] Even when sarcoidosis is clinically in remission, fatigue may remain present and become a chronic problem causing impaired quality of life and reduced socioeconomic participation.[72] Until now, the exact mechanism for chronic fatigue in sarcoidosis remains unknown, but it is most likely multifactorial.[73] Both the disease and its comorbidities, such as deconditioning, depression, stress, sleep pattern disturbance, thyroid problems, anemia, medication, and weight gain, could contribute to fatigue.[72,74] Depression is encountered in 46% to 66% of patients, depending on the method used to screen.[75–77] Also, the prevalence of perceived stress is higher in patients with sarcoidosis.[78,79] Sleep apnea is another potential cause for fatigue and depression, and is reported to be more prevalent in patients with sarcoidosis.[73,80] Sleep apnea is typically treatable, whereas most other causes for fatigue in sarcoidosis are therapy resistant. Another frequently encountered, therapy-resistant, and disabling symptom is pain.[81] Small-fiber neuropathy may be a cause of pain, but more fibromyalgialike pain is also reported.[82]

Both fatigue and pain can be extremely problematic for the patient and frustrating to the treating clinician because the symptoms are difficult to quantify objectively and therapeutic options are largely unrecognized or nonexistent. When attempting to alleviate symptoms in these situations careful discussion about expectations and potential side effects are crucial.[83]

Besides these less organ-specific symptoms, with a more relative treatment indication, there are also several situations that in general necessitate treatment to prevent organ damage with poor outcome.[1,2] The most common are listed in **Box 1**. Treatment of any of these indications should be initiated when there is a high suspicion of active granulomatous inflammation using clinical, serologic, or imaging data.

Activity of disease

Unlike most other diseases, active disease in sarcoidosis does not mean that therapy is necessary. In contrast, severe organ damage can be present in advanced disease despite the absence of ongoing inflammation, in which case immunosuppressive therapy may also not be warranted. Activity can be measured by showing active granulomatous inflammation or by observing organ function deterioration. Multiple tests have been studied to assess active inflammation. Proposed markers of disease activity are serum angiotensin-converting enzyme, serum soluble interleukin (IL)-2 receptor, and serum human chitotriosidase; however, the clinical value of these markers in staging disease or predicting or detecting change is debated.[84,85] Testing for chitotriosidase is also not widely available yet.

Pulmonary PET activity in sarcoidosis probably represents active disease,[86] but is expensive and exposes patients to a radiation burden and is therefore not suitable for standard management of sarcoidosis. In patients with persistent symptoms

---

Box 1
Indications for immunosuppressive therapy

Respiratory

Symptomatic pulmonary disease with infiltrates

Progressive deterioration of pulmonary function tests

Significant upper respiratory tract sarcoidosis

Ocular

Posterior or intermediate uveitis

Anterior uveitis refractory to topical therapy or with toxicities from topical therapy

Cutaneous

Disfiguring lesions (patient choice)

Hepatic

Impaired synthetic function

Hyperbilirubinemia

Progressive increase of transaminase levels

Portal hypertension

Splenic

Pain or early satiety caused by enlargement

Cytopenias caused by hypersplenism

Cardiac[a]

Second-degree or third-degree conduction block

Ventricular dysrhythmias

Cardiomyopathy

Neurologic[b]

Any brain or spinal cord involvement

Granulomatous peripheral nerve disease

Symptomatic myositis

Bone marrow

Cytopenia

Endocrine

Significant hypercalcemia/hypercalciuria

Nephrolithiasis

Pituitary sarcoidosis

[a] Treatment of diastolic heart failure and supraventricular dysrhythmias is unclear.
[b] Possible exceptions include isolated cranial nerve 7 palsy, and mild acute aseptic meningitis.

---

high-resolution computed tomography suggests fibrosis.[68] Other signs of disease activity are hypercalciuria and hypercalcemia.[87,88] Hypercalciuria is reported to be present in 40% to 62% of patients with sarcoidosis; hypercalcemia is far less common, with a prevalence of approximately 5% to 8%.[88,89]

Impact of disease on patients' lives

Having sarcoidosis may greatly affect quality of life and it has been shown that physicians' perception of disease severity frequently does not correspond with the impact patients experience.[75] Quality of life is impaired in most patients with sarcoidosis because of symptoms such as dyspnea, persistent cough, peripheral pain, fatigue, and cognitive dysfunction, which might result in a downward spiral of limitations in activities, social isolation, stress, and depression.[90–92] Also, sarcoidosis treatments might negatively affect quality of life.[75,93] Established physiologic measures such as pulmonary function and radiography do not capture the impact that sarcoidosis may have on a patient's life and are found to correlate poorly with questionnaires measuring health-related quality of life.[75,94,95] Recently, progress has been made in developing patient-reported outcome measures (PROMs) specific for sarcoidosis.[95–97] Both Judson[96] and Patel[95] have developed questionnaires with organ-specific modules, reflecting the systemic nature of sarcoidosis. No comparisons between these 2 questionnaires have been done so far. In testing, optimizing, and developing PROMs, collaboration between patients, doctors, and researchers is crucial.[98]

Patient Involvement

When treating patients with sarcoidosis, clinicians should always bear in mind that treatment is not only about improving physiologic parameters but also about restoring quality of life. Adequate information enables patients to make more balanced decisions and set realistic goals. However, giving information is a unidirectional way of communication in which patients are thought to have values and doctors to have knowledge. Ideally, medical experts should also learn from the experience experts and collaborate in optimizing treatment decisions and care. Also, on a larger scale than the individual contact in the consultancy room, patient involvement can change priorities in care improvement.[99]

HOW TO TREAT

and radiological signs of fibrosis PET scanning seems a helpful technique to guide treatment decisions, because some patients with PET activity show reversibility of abnormalities even when the

Similar to the decision to treat, the strategy for treatment should also be tailored to each individual patient. Decisions include the choice of which medications to use, the dose, and the duration of treatment. Although systemic corticosteroids have long been advocated as the first-line therapy for treatment-requiring sarcoidosis, clinical practice has evolved in the past several years toward earlier and broader use of steroid-sparing therapies. There has also been new recognition that the minimum dose of corticosteroids necessary to control sarcoidosis may be lower than traditionally advocated. In contrast, there are few empiric data to guide decision making about the dose of cytotoxic steroid-sparing medications and very few data about the optimal duration of treatment in general.

Corticosteroids

The benefits of corticosteroids in sarcoidosis have been known since 1948. Compared with many other approaches, corticosteroids are inexpensive, widely available, rapidly effective, very reliable, easily titrated, and clinical experience with them is vast. They also have the theoretic advantage of downregulating multiple arms of the immune response. However, the toxicities of corticosteroids for management of sarcoidosis have not been carefully enumerated. In 2 controlled trials of corticosteroids versus placebo, the median weight gain in the treated group was 3.6 and 11 kg, respectively.[63,100] Other toxicities have not been comprehensively assessed in large populations of patients with sarcoidosis, but one analysis suggested that health-related quality of life is significantly lower in those treated with corticosteroids, even after adjustment for disease severity.[75] In addition, the risk from corticosteroids may be based on a threshold dose for some toxicities (eg, obesity, ocular complications) but for others may be linear regardless of the use of lower doses (eg, fluid retention, insomnia).[101] Given these considerations, a decision to use corticosteroids as monotherapy, or as a mainstay of therapy, should be individualized for each patient and alternatives should be discussed. In patients with a high risk for toxic effects of steroids (diabetes, psychiatric disorders, osteoporosis), other agents may be more appropriate for first-line therapy (**Fig. 2**).

For pulmonary sarcoidosis, most treatment guidelines suggest initial doses between 20 and 40 mg daily.[1,24,28,102] However, there have been no dose-ranging studies to define the optimal dose. A retrospective study at one institution found that a median dose of 19 mg daily was sufficient to treat acutely decompensated pulmonary sarcoidosis, although the doses used ranged from 10 to 40 mg daily.[103] Several early prospective trials with positive results used doses as low as 10 to 20 mg daily.[104–106] Therefore, it is not evident that higher doses of corticosteroids offer additional benefit for pulmonary sarcoidosis. In practice, the dose is usually titrated according to the response. The optimal tapering schedule is not known, but carefully monitoring of effect and tailored tapering might reduce the cumulative dose of corticosteroids and their side effects. The bulk of the response in pulmonary sarcoidosis is typically evident in 3 to 4 weeks' time.[103,107] After gauging response, the dose is typically tapered to a maintenance level in stepwise increments every 3 to 4 weeks. Most experts consider a taper to 10 mg or less of prednisone to be successful,[102,108] although, as mentioned earlier, the goal maintenance dose must be individualized for each patient.

The optimal duration of therapy for pulmonary sarcoidosis is unknown, but is typically at least 6 months for sarcoidosis of recent onset (<5 years). If treatment with corticosteroids is required, the chances of relapse after stopping therapy have been reported to range from 14% to 74% for acute disease,[8,31,104] and to be 75% for those with chronic sarcoidosis.[109] In one observational series, most relapses were observed 2 to 6 months after stopping therapy, but occurred after more than 12 months in 20% of the cohort, and after 24 months in 10%.[8] When relapses do occur, repeat treatment with previously adequate doses is generally adequate to regain control of the inflammatory process.[31]

Management of sarcoidosis with corticosteroids mandates attention to prevention of common complications of corticosteroids, including

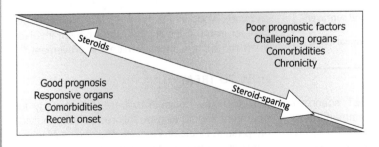

Good prognosis
Responsive organs
Comorbidities
Recent onset

Steroids

Poor prognostic factors
Challenging organs
Comorbidities
Chronicity

Steroid-sparing

Fig. 2. The main therapy used for the long-term control of sarcoidosis should be tailored to the situation and patient. Situations with briefer expected treatment courses, with a good possibility of control with lower doses, may favor corticosteroid monotherapy; when a protracted or refractory course is more likely, early initiation of steroid-sparing agents should be considered.

infection and bone fragility. The intention to use corticosteroids for a limited time at the initiation of therapy commonly leads to neglect of their associated health maintenance requirements. Because a high proportion of patients require ongoing therapy (discussed earlier), consideration of vaccination status, need for antibiotic prophylaxis against *Pneumocystis jiroveci*, and osteoporosis prophylaxis should be addressed at the initiation of therapy. The optimal strategy for preserving bone health is unknown, because supplemental calcium and/or vitamin D may lead to hypercalciuria or hypercalcemia. However, it has also been suggested that low vitamin D level is related more to disease activity in sarcoidosis and that supplementing vitamin D and calcium can be done safely, if monitored carefully.[88] In some patients, prophylactic bisphosphonates alone may be sufficient to maintain bone density.[110] If supplemental calcium or vitamin D is prescribed, measurement of 1,25-dihydroxyvitamin D, serum calcium, and urine calcium levels should be performed. Measurement of 25-hydroxyvitamin D alone is insufficient to monitor the risks of vitamin D toxicity, because bioconversion to the active dihydroxy form is not linked to calcium levels in active sarcoidosis.[111]

Inhaled corticosteroids and other topical therapy

Inhaled corticosteroids are most useful for treatment of cough or airways hyperreactivity in sarcoidosis. Budesonide is the best studied inhaled steroid. Finnish patients who received budesonide for 15 months, after a 3-month run-in period with prednisolone, showed modestly improved lung function and fewer relapses compared with placebo.[112] Other studies in pulmonary disease have yielded conflicting results.[113–116] In contrast, there are few data to support fluticasone.[108,117] Topical therapy may also be helpful in mild to moderately severe ocular, upper respiratory, and cutaneous sarcoidosis.

Cytotoxic Medications

Commonly described agents in this group include methotrexate (MTX), azathioprine, leflunomide, and mycophenolate mofetil. Although they are often called cytotoxic agents, their mechanisms of action are diverse, and are not entirely caused by destruction of immune cells or inhibition of their growth.[118] There are limited data comparing the effectiveness of the cytotoxic medications, so the choice of use often depends on clinician familiarity with the medications, patient preferences, comorbidities, and availability. A single study retrospectively compared the effectiveness of MTX (155 Dutch patients) and azathioprine (45 Belgian patients) when used as second-line therapy for pulmonary sarcoidosis.[119] Both medications resulted in similar improvements in pulmonary function tests and reductions of steroid dose. Azathioprine was associated with more apparent infections (35% vs 18%), but the putative difference was likely caused, at least in part, by differences in classification of antibiotic use episodes between the two study centers. Besides this single study, any conclusions regarding the relative efficacy of the cytotoxic agents are based on comparisons of reported outcomes from separate studies, and are therefore tenuous.

Methotrexate

MTX is the most widely studied and widely used cytotoxic medication for sarcoidosis. In a Delphi study of primarily US sarcoidosis experts, MTX was chosen by 80% as the first choice for steroid-sparing therapy in sarcoidosis.[102] It is the only cytotoxic agent tested in a randomized, placebo-controlled trial in a sarcoidosis population, in which it exerted a moderate steroid-sparing effect when used for a 12-month period.[100] Subsequent case series showed improvements in chronic pulmonary, cutaneous, hepatic, ocular, neurologic, and cardiac sarcoidosis with MTX.[120–123]

For sarcoidosis the typical dose is 10 to 20 mg orally or by transdermal injection once a week.[121,124] In a rheumatoid arthritis population, switching from oral to parenteral dosing has been shown to be effective for a subset of patients, presumably by achieving higher and more predictable levels of the drug.[125] In our experience, a subset of patients switching from oral to parenteral MTX experience abatement of side effects and/or substantial clinical responses. It is said that the benefits of MTX require up to 6 months to manifest,[126] so tapering of steroids should be delayed for at least several months after initiating MTX. It seems that MTX is safe and well tolerated even when used for prolonged treatment.[127]

MTX can cause several toxicities, including liver injury, bone marrow suppression, and pneumonitis. A guideline for use of MTX in sarcoidosis has been developed, which suggests monitoring of transaminase levels and complete blood count every 4 to 6 weeks, until a stable dose is reached, whereupon the monitoring interval can be extended to every 3 months.[127] The dose should be reduced, or the MTX stopped altogether, depending on the severity of monitored toxicity. Common side effects include nausea and fatigue; rash and headache may also occur occasionally.

Most of the side effects occur around the day of medication administration, and generally resolve within 2 to 3 days. The risk for most of these side effects can be mitigated by supplementation with folic acid of 1 to 2 mg/d, or 5 mg once or twice weekly. In most studies of folic acid supplementation in patients with rheumatoid arthritis, its use led to reduced toxicity, fewer medication discontinuations, and no loss of clinical effectiveness.[128,129]

Azathioprine

Azathioprine inhibits lymphocytes by blocking purine synthesis. The data for the use of azathioprine are limited primarily to case series. The largest of these was the Belgian cohort (described earlier), which described pulmonary responses and steroid-sparing effects in 45 patients. In a small, nonrandomized study of patients with disease refractory to steroids, 7 of 10 had improvement of symptoms and chest radiograph, but no change in pulmonary function tests after 6 months of azathioprine therapy.[130] Standard doses for azathioprine are typically 1.5 to 2.5 mg/kg ideal body weight per day, in divided doses. Similar to MTX, the effect of azathioprine may require months of treatment.

Bone marrow suppression, especially of granulocytes, is the most serious toxicity from azathioprine. Some centers routinely measure thiopurine methyltransferase (TPMT) level before initiation of therapy, because deficiency leads to accumulation of azathioprine metabolites and higher chances of severe neutropenia. Low TPMT levels occur in 11% of the population, and the enzyme is absent in 0.3%.[131] An alternate strategy is to check blood counts more frequently during initiation of therapy. Once a stable dose has been reached, the monitoring interval can be extended to every 3 months. Although liver function abnormalities are not typically as severe as for MTX, they should be monitored as well with the same frequency as the blood count. The risk for malignancy in patients who use azathioprine for the long term remains controversial. A retrospective cohort study among 4734 US patients treated with azathioprine for ulcerative colitis found an adjusted hazard ratio for development of lymphoma of 4.2 (95% confidence interval, 2.5–6.8) compared with other patients with ulcerative colitis.[132] However, some of the risk may relate to greater disease severity in the treated group.

Leflunomide

Another antilymphocyte agent, leflunomide, has been evaluated in 2 retrospective series involving a total of 108 patients.[133,134] Those 2 series used a dose of 20 mg daily for most patients. The rate of complete response, as assessed by the treating physician, for target organ involvement was approximately 50% for both series, and most of the remaining patients had at least partial responses. For pulmonary disease, the series reported by Sahoo and colleagues[133] described improvements in the rate of change of FVC, which had declined by 0.1 ± 0.3 L during the 6-month period before initiation of leflunomide, but improved by 0.09 ± 0.3 L in the 6-month period after starting therapy, despite reduction of the median prednisone dose from 10 mg daily to 0 mg daily. Leflunomide seems to be most effective when used in combination with MTX.[133]

The most common side effects from leflunomide include diarrhea, abdominal discomfort, nausea, and fatigue.[133] Hepatic toxicity may occur, with a higher incidence in those using concomitant MTX or those with preexisting liver dysfunction.[135] In clinical trials for rheumatoid arthritis, increases of alanine aminotransferase level greater than 3 times the upper limits of normal were observed in 2% to 4% of patients.[136–138] Most hepatic toxicity occurs within 6 months of initiating therapy, but can at times lead to liver failure, so the US Food and Drug Administration (FDA) now recommends monthly transaminase measurement for the first 6 months of therapy. Peripheral neuropathy has also been reported in case series,[139–141] and patients should be counseled to be vigilant for its onset. In patients with preexisting uncontrolled diabetes who have diabetic neuropathy, it may be prudent to treat with other agents preferentially. If toxicity does occur, because of the long circulating half-life of leflunomide metabolites, it should be actively removed using cholestyramine 8 g 3 times a day for 2 days.

Mycophenolate mofetil

The mechanism of the antiinflammatory activity of mycophenolate is unclear but it may be secondary to inhibition of purine synthesis by lymphocytes. In a small retrospective series, mycophenolate improved visual acuity and ocular inflammation from sarcoid uveitis in all 7 patients reviewed after a median time of only 6.7 weeks.[142] The largest series to date included 37 patients who were started on mycophenolate for pulmonary sarcoidosis.[143] There was no statistically significant improvement in the rate of change of FVC or carbon monoxide diffusion in the lung, although the mean daily prednisone dose was successfully tapered from 14 mg to 9 mg. A series of 10 patients with pulmonary disease described improvements in spirometry and reduction of prednisone doses in most of them.[144] Other series reporting beneficial effects from mycophenolate are confounded by concomitant initiation of other agents.[145–147] A possible exception to the limited evidence of efficacy for mycophenolate may be renal sarcoidosis, which is appealing, because dose adjustment is unnecessary except in severe renal failure.[148,149]

Biologic Tumor Necrosis Factor Antagonists

Tumor necrosis factor (TNF) is a key mediator of granulomatous inflammation. Anti-TNF monoclonal antibodies are now widely used for management of sarcoidosis, but the soluble receptor construct that also antagonizes TNF, etanercept, is not effective. Infliximab is the most studied and widely used TNF antagonist in the sarcoidosis population. A recent WASOG publication provides practical advice and evidence for the use of TNF antagonists for sarcoidosis.[150] In general, the TNF antagonists are commonly used as third-line medications when other agents fail,[1,24] but there are certain situations in which they seem to be most effective, and may be used earlier in the treatment algorithm; examples include moderate to severe neurosarcoidosis, and lupus pernio.[151,152] A retrospective analysis from a randomized trial of infliximab for pulmonary sarcoidosis suggested that there may be little additional benefit from TNF antagonists in patients receiving baseline prednisone doses greater than 15 mg/d.[153] However, it is unlikely that this threshold applies equally to all patients and organs.

Opportunistic infections are the major complication of the TNF inhibitors, including tuberculosis and fungal infections.[154–156] Screening for latent tuberculosis infection is required before initiating TNF-alpha inhibitors and untreated latent tuberculosis (TB) infection is considered a relative contraindication. Reactivation of tuberculosis may be atypical and disseminated, leading to delayed diagnosis and increased mortality. Although skin testing and/or interferon gamma release assays should be checked, they may be unreliable because peripheral cellular anergy is common in sarcoidosis. Therefore, a very careful exposure history and a low threshold for presumptive treatment of latent TB before starting these medications are advisable.

The FDA has mandated a black box warning against the use of TNF antagonists in patients with cardiomyopathy, because increased mortality from worsened heart failure and de novo heart failure have been reported.[157] However, it is unclear whether these concerns apply to sarcoidosis cardiomyopathy; 2 case reports have described patients with refractory cardiac sarcoidosis who were successfully treated with infliximab.[158,159]

Antibodies to infliximab, and less commonly adalimumab, can develop in some patients and lead to allergic reactions and loss of efficacy.[160] This phenomenon may be at least partially mitigated by pretreatment with steroids before infusions.[154] In nonsarcoidosis populations, the use of concomitant MTX or leflunomide improves response rates, possibly by reducing the rate of formation of antichimeric antibodies.[161–163] The optimal duration of therapy for TNF-alpha inhibitors remains unclear, but it seems that most patients relapse within 3 to 12 months after treatment is stopped.[164]

Infliximab

Infliximab is a chimeric murine-human TNF antagonist that binds to both soluble and membrane TNF, blocking bioactivity and inducing apoptosis of TNF-expressing leukocytes. It has been the subject of 2 double-blind, randomized, placebo-controlled trials for pulmonary sarcoidosis, and has also been shown to be effective in numerous case series. As a result of the accumulated data, infliximab is now a community-accepted standard of care therapy for refractory or severe sarcoidosis.

In a randomized double-blind trial comparing infliximab with placebo in 138 patients with moderate to severe chronic pulmonary sarcoidosis, treated patients experienced a statistically significant FVC improvement of 3.4% at week 24.[165] Subgroup analysis revealed that patients with more severe impairment or a longer duration of disease were more likely to respond.[165] In addition, there was a statistically significant improvement in the extrapulmonary manifestations of sarcoidosis in the patients receiving infliximab compared with placebo.[166] Case series have shown that infliximab can also be effective for neurologic, ocular, cutaneous, and bone sarcoidosis.[146,151,166–169]

Adalimumab and other anti–tumor necrosis factor biologics

Adalimumab is a fully humanized monoclonal TNF antagonist with the advantage of subcutaneous administration and lower rates of immunogenicity.[160] There have been fewer studies of adalimumab than infliximab for sarcoidosis, and no placebo-controlled trials. Adalimumab seems to be effective in sarcoidosis in uncontrolled series.[170–172] In a prospective observational study of 10 patients, treatment with adalimumab 40 mg subcutaneously every other week resulted in approximately 50% reduction in fluorodeoxyglucose uptake on PET scan after 24 weeks.[172] For cutaneous sarcoidosis, a small double-blind, randomized, placebo-controlled trial in 16 patients showed improvements in lesion area after 12 weeks of therapy.[173]

The dosing regimen for adalimumab in sarcoidosis has not been studied carefully, so the optimal approach is unclear. In the Crohn population, loading doses of 160 mg at week 0, and 80 mg at week 2, followed by 40 mg weekly, have been shown to be more effective and generate a quicker response than the standard rheumatology approach of 40 mg every other week.[174] A loading dose has been used in several of the reported sarcoidosis experiences.[171,173] Compared with infliximab, it seems that the time to response is slower for adalimumab.

A third anti-TNF biologic medication, golimumab, was evaluated in 173 patients with pulmonary or cutaneous disease, who were randomized to 28 weeks of golimumab, ustekinumab (an IL-12/IL-23 antagonist), or placebo.[175] The trial was negative, perhaps because of the dosing regimen, patient population, study design, or the pharmacokinetics of the subcutaneous medication. Etanercept, a soluble receptor construct that blocks TNF bioavailability, is also ineffective for sarcoidosis.[176,177]

Antimalarial Medications

Chloroquine and hydroxychloroquine reduce inflammation through several mechanisms, including inhibition of lysosome acidification necessary for antigen presentation, and toll-like receptor activation.[178] Chloroquine is more potent than hydroxychloroquine but also more toxic; as a result, hydroxychloroquine is more widely used. The antimalarial medications are mostly used for cutaneous sarcoidosis and hypercalcemia.[179–181] Chloroquine has also been evaluated for chronic pulmonary sarcoidosis in a small study, in which patients treated with and maintained on chloroquine had sustained improvements in lung function decline compared with placebo.[182] Ophthalmic screening every 6 to 12 months is recommended during treatment with these agents, because toxicity can usually be discerned before substantial irreversible vision loss. Other important toxicities of the antimalarial agents include nausea and myopathy.

Adrenocorticotropic Hormone Gel

Pituitary extracts containing primarily adrenocorticotropic hormone (ACTH) exert antiinflammatory effects through stimulation of cortisol production in the adrenal glands but also by activation of the melanocortin receptor (MCR) family.[183,184] The 5 MCRs are expressed on various immune cells, including myeloid and lymphoid cell lineages.[183] Experimental data suggest that the effects of ACTH are mediated by both glucocorticoid receptor–dependent pathways and mechanisms independent of glucocorticoid receptor activation,

Table 2
Rarely used antisarcoidosis medications

Medication	Main Target Organ[a]	Major Toxicity
Cyclophosphamide	Neurologic[188] Renal[189]	Bone marrow suppression Opportunistic infection Hematologic or uroepithelial malignancy Hemorrhagic cystitis
Chlorambucil	Multiple[190]	Bone marrow suppression Hematologic malignancy
Thalidomide	Cutaneous[191,192] Pulmonary[193]	Peripheral neuropathy Hypersomnolence Venous thrombosis Teratogenicity
Minocycline	Cutaneous[194]	GI upset
Pentoxifylline	Pulmonary[195,196] GLUS	GI upset
Rituximab	Pulmonary[197] Ocular[198,199]	Opportunistic infections Infusion reactions
Apremilast	Cutaneous[200]	GI upset
Progenitor cell infusion	Pulmonary[201]	Unknown

Abbreviation: GI, gastrointestinal.
  [a] May refer to the organ that has been the subject of investigation; most have not been evaluated carefully in multiple organs.

supporting a role for the steroid-independent anti-inflammatory mechanisms of ACTH.[184]

The effectiveness of ACTH for treatment of sarcoidosis was first recognized in the early 1950s,[185,186] leading to FDA approval for symptomatic pulmonary sarcoidosis. However, the efficacy, low cost, and wide availability of corticosteroids have relegated ACTH therapy to a third-line or fourth-line option at present. ACTH gel requires parenteral administration, typically twice weekly. Clinical trials with this agent will be helpful to define its position in the therapeutic armamentarium, and the degree to which its side effect profile overlaps that of glucocorticoids.

Other Agents

Other agents have been used historically, or in selected situations. These other agents may broadly be categorized into (largely) effective therapies that have been nearly abandoned because of toxicity, weaker agents that are sometimes useful for adjunctive treatment, and new medications with an as-yet unsettled role. Cyclophosphamide, chlorambucil, and thalidomide are examples of medications with waning use. Minocycline and pentoxifylline may be useful adjunctive therapies, but are weaker agents. An unusual use for pentoxifylline may be for treatment of a rare sarcoidosis mimic: the granulomatous lesions of uncertain significance (GLUS) syndrome.[187] Several newer approaches include the anti–B cell antibody rituximab; apremilast, a phosphodiesterase-4 inhibitor; and cell-based therapy, which was recently shown to be tolerated well and feasible in a small study of 3 patients. These agents are listed in **Table 2**.

SUMMARY

Treatment of sarcoidosis can roughly be considered in 2 steps: when to treat and how to treat. The decision about initiation of treatment may in part be influenced by the options for how to treat. At each step, the active participation of the patient should be solicited, and in general treatment planning should be formulated with a view to a long-term strategy. Two major indications for treatment are substantial impairment of organ function, especially if there is a high likelihood of irreversible damage, and significant impairment of the patient's quality of life. Other variables that influence the decision to treat the disease include its chronicity, prognosis, extent, severity, and the evidence for disease activity. Several noninflammatory consequences of sarcoidosis, such as pulmonary hypertension and fatigue, may require alternate (nonimmunosuppressive) therapeutic strategies. The number of immunosuppressive options for treating sarcoidosis continues to expand, diminishing the role for corticosteroids in many patients. In some patients, the optimal maintenance corticosteroid dose may be nil, depending on comorbidities and tolerance. Periodic attempts to de-escalate immunosuppressive therapy should be part of the management strategy.

REFERENCES

1. Baughman RP, Lower EE. Medical therapy of sarcoidosis. Semin Respir Crit Care Med 2014; 35(3):391–406.
2. Culver DA. Sarcoidosis. Immunol Allergy Clin North Am 2012;32(4):487–511.
3. Judson MA. Advances in the diagnosis and treatment of sarcoidosis. F1000Prime Rep 2014;6:89.
4. Spagnolo P. Sarcoidosis: a critical review of history and milestones. Clin Rev Allergy Immunol 2015; 49(1):1–5.
5. Fischer A, Grunewald J, Spagnolo P, et al. Genetics of sarcoidosis. Semin Respir Crit Care Med 2014;35(3):296–306.
6. Swigris JJ, Olson AL, Huie TJ, et al. Sarcoidosis-related mortality in the United States from 1988 to 2007. Am J Respir Crit Care Med 2011;183(11): 1524–30.
7. Baughman RP, Judson MA, Teirstein A, et al. Presenting characteristics as predictors of duration of treatment in sarcoidosis. QJM 2006;99(5):307–15.
8. Gottlieb JE, Israel HL, Steiner RM, et al. Outcome in sarcoidosis. The relationship of relapse to corticosteroid therapy. Chest 1997;111(3):623–31.
9. Baughman RP, Nagai S, Balter M, et al. Defining the clinical outcome status (COS) in sarcoidosis: results of the WASOG task force. Sarcoidosis Vasc Diffuse Lung Dis 2011;28(1):56–64.
10. Gribbin J, Hubbard RB, Le Jeune I, et al. Incidence and mortality of idiopathic pulmonary fibrosis and sarcoidosis in the UK. Thorax 2006;61(11):980–5.
11. Reich JM. Mortality of intrathoracic sarcoidosis in referral vs population-based settings: influence of stage, ethnicity, and corticosteroid therapy. Chest 2002;121(1):32–9.
12. Nicholson TT, Plant BJ, Henry MT, et al. Sarcoidosis in Ireland: regional differences in prevalence and mortality from 1996-2005. Sarcoidosis Vasc Diffuse Lung Dis 2010;27(2):111–20.
13. Tukey MH, Berman JS, Boggs Et Al DA. Mortality among African American women with sarcoidosis: data from the Black Women's Health Study. Sarcoidosis Vasc Diffuse Lung Dis 2013;30(2): 128–33.
14. Hanley A, Hubbard RB, Navaratnam V. Mortality trends in asbestosis, extrinsic allergic alveolitis and sarcoidosis in England and Wales. Respir Med 2011;105(9):1373–9.

15. Gerke AK. Morbidity and mortality in sarcoidosis. Curr Opin Pulm Med 2014;20(5):472–8.

16. Statement on sarcoidosis. Joint statement of the American Thoracic Society (ATS), the European Respiratory Society (ERS) and the World Association of Sarcoidosis and Other Granulomatous Disorders (WASOG) adopted by the ATS Board of Directors and by the ERS Executive Committee, February 1999. Am J Respir Crit Care Med 1999; 160(2):736–55.

17. Morimoto T, Azuma A, Abe S, et al. Epidemiology of sarcoidosis in Japan. Eur Respir J 2008;31(2): 372–9.

18. Sekiguchi M, Yazaki Y, Isobe M, et al. Cardiac sarcoidosis: diagnostic, prognostic, and therapeutic considerations. Cardiovasc Drugs Ther 1996; 10(5):495–510.

19. Scadding JG. Prognosis of intrathoracic sarcoidosis in England. A review of 136 cases after five years' observation. Br Med J 1961;2(5261): 1165–72.

20. Mana J, Salazar A, Manresa F. Clinical factors predicting persistence of activity in sarcoidosis: a multivariate analysis of 193 cases. Respiration 1994;61(4):219–25.

21. Baughman RP, Lower EE. Features of sarcoidosis associated with chronic disease. Sarcoidosis Vasc Diffuse Lung Dis 2015;31(4):275–81.

22. Grunewald J. HLA associations and Lofgren's syndrome. Expert Rev Clin Immunol 2012;8(1): 55–62.

23. Baughman RP, Costabel U, du Bois RM. Treatment of sarcoidosis. Clin Chest Med 2008;29(3):533–48.

24. Lazar CA, Culver DA. Treatment of sarcoidosis. Semin Respir Crit Care Med 2010;31(4):501–18.

25. Neville E, Walker AN, James DG. Prognostic factors predicting the outcome of sarcoidosis: an analysis of 818 patients. Q J Med 1983;52(208): 525–33.

26. Nagai S, Shigematsu M, Hamada K, et al. Clinical courses and prognoses of pulmonary sarcoidosis. Curr Opin Pulm Med 1999;5(5):293–8.

27. Judson MA, Baughman RP, Thompson BW, et al. Two year prognosis of sarcoidosis: the ACCESS experience. Sarcoidosis Vasc Diffuse Lung Dis 2003;20(3):204–11.

28. Hunninghake GW, Costabel U, Ando M, et al. ATS/ERS/WASOG statement on sarcoidosis. American Thoracic Society/European Respiratory Society/World Association of Sarcoidosis and other Granulomatous Disorders. Sarcoidosis Vasc Diffuse Lung Dis 1999;16(2):149–73.

29. Pietinalho A, Ohmichi M, Löfroos AB, et al. The prognosis of pulmonary sarcoidosis in Finland and Hokkaido, Japan. A comparative five-year study of biopsy-proven cases. Sarcoidosis Vasc Diffuse Lung Dis 2000;17(2):158–66.

30. Hillerdal G, Nöu E, Osterman K, et al. Sarcoidosis: epidemiology and prognosis. A 15-year European study. Am Rev Respir Dis 1984;130(1):29–32.

31. Hunninghake GW, Gilbert S, Pueringer R, et al. Outcome of the treatment for sarcoidosis. Am J Respir Crit Care Med 1994;149(4 Pt 1):893–8.

32. Siltzbach LE, James DG, Neville E, et al. Course and prognosis of sarcoidosis around the world. Am J Med 1974;57(6):847–52.

33. Pereira CA, Dornfeld MC, Baughman R, et al. Clinical phenotypes in sarcoidosis. Curr Opin Pulm Med 2014;20(5):496–502.

34. Wasfi YS, Rose CS, Murphy JR, et al. A new tool to assess sarcoidosis severity. Chest 2006;129(5): 1234–45.

35. Prasse A, Katic C, Germann M, et al. Phenotyping sarcoidosis from a pulmonary perspective. Am J Respir Crit Care Med 2008;177(3):330–6.

36. Rodrigues SC, Rocha NA, Lima MS, et al. Factor analysis of sarcoidosis phenotypes at two referral centers in Brazil. Sarcoidosis Vasc Diffuse Lung Dis 2011;28(1):34–43.

37. Walsh SL, Wells AU, Sverzellati N, et al. An integrated clinicoradiological staging system for pulmonary sarcoidosis: a case-cohort study. Lancet Respir Med 2014;2(2):123–30.

38. Sones M, Israel HL. Course and prognosis of sarcoidosis. Am J Med 1960;29:84–93.

39. Israel HL, Karlin P, Menduke H, et al. Factors affecting outcome of sarcoidosis. Influence of race, extrathoracic involvement, and initial radiologic lung lesions. Ann N Y Acad Sci 1986;465: 609–18.

40. Takada K, Ina Y, Noda M, et al. The clinical course and prognosis of patients with severe, moderate or mild sarcoidosis. J Clin Epidemiol 1993;46(4): 359–66.

41. Chapelon-Abric C, de Zuttere D, Duhaut P, et al. Cardiac sarcoidosis: a retrospective study of 41 cases. Medicine (Baltimore) 2004;83(6):315–34.

42. Chapelon C, Ziza JM, Piette JC, et al. Neurosarcoidosis: signs, course and treatment in 35 confirmed cases. Medicine (Baltimore) 1990;69(5):261–76.

43. Scott TF. Neurosarcoidosis: progress and clinical aspects. Neurology 1993;43(1):8–12.

44. Sohn M, Culver DA, Judson MA, et al. Spinal cord neurosarcoidosis. Am J Med Sci 2014; 347(3):195–8.

45. Rizzato G, Fraioli P, Montemurro L. Nephrolithiasis as a presenting feature of chronic sarcoidosis. Thorax 1995;50(5):555–9.

46. Neville E, Carstairs LS, James DG. Sarcoidosis of bone. Q J Med 1977;46(182):215–27.

47. Viskum K, Vestbo J. Vital prognosis in intrathoracic sarcoidosis with special reference to pulmonary function and radiological stage. Eur Respir J 1993;6(3):349–53.

48. Milman N, Selroos O. Pulmonary sarcoidosis in the Nordic countries 1950-1982. II. Course and prognosis. Sarcoidosis 1990;7(2):113–8.

49. Baughman RP, Engel PJ, Taylor L, et al. Survival in sarcoidosis-associated pulmonary hypertension: the importance of hemodynamic evaluation. Chest 2010;138(5):1078–85.

50. Baughman RP, Winget DB, Bowen EH, et al. Predicting respiratory failure in sarcoidosis patients. Sarcoidosis Vasc Diffuse Lung Dis 1997;14(2): 154–8.

51. Vestbo J, Viskum K. Respiratory symptoms at presentation and long-term vital prognosis in patients with pulmonary sarcoidosis. Sarcoidosis 1994; 11(2):123–5.

52. Ziegenhagen MW, Rothe ME, Schlaak M, et al. Bronchoalveolar and serological parameters reflecting the severity of sarcoidosis. Eur Respir J 2003;21(3):407–13.

53. Drent M, Jacobs JA, de Vries J, et al. Does the cellular bronchoalveolar lavage fluid profile reflect the severity of sarcoidosis? Eur Respir J 1999; 13(6):1338–44.

54. Chen ES, Moller DR. Etiologies of sarcoidosis. Clin Rev Allergy Immunol 2015;49(1):6–18.

55. Panselinas E, Judson MA. Acute pulmonary exacerbations of sarcoidosis. Chest 2012;142(4): 827–36.

56. Rizzato G, Montemurro L, Colombo P. The late follow-up of chronic sarcoid patients previously treated with corticosteroids. Sarcoidosis Vasc Diffuse Lung Dis 1998;15(1):52–8.

57. Grunewald J, Eklund A. Lofgren's syndrome: human leukocyte antigen strongly influences the disease course. Am J Respir Crit Care Med 2009; 179(4):307–12.

58. Eule H, Weinecke A, Roth I, et al. The possible influence of corticosteroid therapy on the natural course of pulmonary sarcoidosis. Late results of a continuing clinical study. Ann N Y Acad Sci 1986; 465:695–701.

59. Zaki MH, Lyons HA, Leilop L, et al. Corticosteroid therapy in sarcoidosis. A five-year, controlled follow-up study. N Y State J Med 1987;87(9):496–9.

60. Paramothayan NS, Lasserson TJ, Jones PW. Corticosteroids for pulmonary sarcoidosis. Cochrane Database Syst Rev 2005;(2):CD001114.

61. Paramothayan S, Lasserson T. Treatments for pulmonary sarcoidosis. Respir Med 2008;102(1):1–9.

62. Paramothayan S, Lasserson TJ, Walters EH. Immunosuppressive and cytotoxic therapy for pulmonary sarcoidosis. Cochrane Database Syst Rev 2006;(3):CD003536.

63. Gibson GJ, Prescott RJ, Muers MF, et al. British Thoracic Society Sarcoidosis study: effects of long term corticosteroid treatment. Thorax 1996; 51(3):238–47.

64. Pietinalho A, Tukiainen P, Haahtela T, et al. Early treatment of stage II sarcoidosis improves 5-year pulmonary function. Chest 2002;121(1):24–31.

65. Judson MA. An approach to the treatment of pulmonary sarcoidosis with corticosteroids: the six phases of treatment. Chest 1999;115(4): 1158–65.

66. Judson MA, Costabel U, Drent M, et al. The WASOG Sarcoidosis Organ Assessment Instrument: an update of a previous clinical tool. Sarcoidosis Vasc Diffuse Lung Dis 2014;31(1):19–27.

67. Hostettler KE, Bratu VA, Fischmann A, et al. Whole-body magnetic resonance imaging in extrathoracic sarcoidosis. Eur Respir J 2014;43(6):1812–5.

68. Mostard RL, van Kroonenburgh MJ, Drent M. The role of the PET scan in the management of sarcoidosis. Curr Opin Pulm Med 2013;19(5):538–44.

69. de Kleijn WP, De Vries J, Lower EE, et al. Fatigue in sarcoidosis: a systematic review. Curr Opin Pulm Med 2009;15(5):499–506.

70. Drent M, Lower EE, De Vries J. Sarcoidosis-associated fatigue. Eur Respir J 2012;40(1):255–63.

71. Sharma OP. Fatigue and sarcoidosis. Eur Respir J 1999;13(4):713–4.

72. Korenromp IH, Heijnen CJ, Vogels OJ, et al. Characterization of chronic fatigue in patients with sarcoidosis in clinical remission. Chest 2011; 140(2):441–7.

73. Fleischer M, Hinz A, Brähler E, et al. Factors associated with fatigue in sarcoidosis. Respir Care 2014;59(7):1086–94.

74. Drent M, Wirnsberger RM, de Vries J, et al. Association of fatigue with an acute phase response in sarcoidosis. Eur Respir J 1999;13(4):718–22.

75. Cox CE, Donohue JF, Brown CD, et al. Health-related quality of life of persons with sarcoidosis. Chest 2004;125(3):997–1004.

76. Yeager H, Rossman MD, Baughman RP, et al. Pulmonary and psychosocial findings at enrollment in the ACCESS study. Sarcoidosis Vasc Diffuse Lung Dis 2005;22(2):147–53.

77. Chang B, Steimel J, Moller DR, et al. Depression in sarcoidosis. Am J Respir Crit Care Med 2001; 163(2):329–34.

78. De Vries J, Drent M. Relationship between perceived stress and sarcoidosis in a Dutch patient population. Sarcoidosis Vasc Diffuse Lung Dis 2004;21(1):57–63.

79. Wilsher ML. Psychological stress in sarcoidosis. Curr Opin Pulm Med 2012;18(5):524–7.

80. Lower EE, Malhotra A, Sudurlescu V, et al. Sarcoidosis, fatigue, and sleep apnea. Chest 2013;144(6): 1976–7.

81. Hoitsma E, De Vries J, van Santen-Hoeufft M, et al. Impact of pain in a Dutch sarcoidosis patient population. Sarcoidosis Vasc Diffuse Lung Dis 2003; 20(1):33–9.

82. Tavee J, Culver D. Sarcoidosis and small-fiber neuropathy. Curr Pain Headache Rep 2011;15(3):201–6.

83. Eklund A, du Bois RM. Approaches to the treatment of some of the troublesome manifestations of sarcoidosis. J Intern Med 2014;275(4):335–49.

84. Keir G, Wells AU. Assessing pulmonary disease and response to therapy: which test? Semin Respir Crit Care Med 2010;31(4):409–18.

85. Vorselaars AD, van Moorsel CH, Zanen P, et al. ACE and sIL-2R correlate with lung function improvement in sarcoidosis during methotrexate therapy. Respir Med 2015;109(2):279–85.

86. Mostard RL, Verschakelen JA, van Kroonenburgh MJ, et al. Severity of pulmonary involvement and (18)F-FDG PET activity in sarcoidosis. Respir Med 2013;107(3):439–47.

87. Meyrier A, Valeyre D, Bouillon R, et al. Different mechanisms of hypercalciuria in sarcoidosis. Correlations with disease extension and activity. Ann N Y Acad Sci 1986;465:575–86.

88. Kamphuis LS, Bonte-Mineur F, van Laar JA, et al. Calcium and vitamin D in sarcoidosis: is supplementation safe? J Bone Miner Res 2014;29(11):2498–503.

89. Conron M, Young C, Beynon HL. Calcium metabolism in sarcoidosis and its clinical implications. Rheumatology (Oxford) 2000;39(7):707–13.

90. Victorson DE, Cella D, Grund H, et al. A conceptual model of health-related quality of life in sarcoidosis. Qual Life Res 2014;23(1):89–101.

91. Valeyre D, Prasse A, Nunes H, et al. Sarcoidosis. Lancet 2014;383(9923):1155–67.

92. Drent M, Wirnsberger RM, Breteler MH, et al. Quality of life and depressive symptoms in patients suffering from sarcoidosis. Sarcoidosis Vasc Diffuse Lung Dis 1998;15(1):59–66.

93. Judson MA, Chaudhry H, Louis A, et al. The effect of corticosteroids on quality of life in a sarcoidosis clinic: the results of a propensity analysis. Respir Med 2015;109(4):526–31.

94. Korenromp IH, van de Laar MA. Health-related quality of life in sarcoidosis. Curr Opin Pulm Med 2014;20(5):503–7.

95. Patel AS, Siegert RJ, Creamer D, et al. The development and validation of the King's Sarcoidosis Questionnaire for the assessment of health status. Thorax 2013;68(1):57–65.

96. Judson MA, Mack M, Beaumont JL, et al. Validation and important differences for the sarcoidosis assessment tool. A new patient-reported outcome measure. Am J Respir Crit Care Med 2015;191(7):786–95.

97. Cox CE, Donohue JF, Brown CD, et al. The Sarcoidosis Health Questionnaire: a new measure of health-related quality of life. Am J Respir Crit Care Med 2003;168(3):323–9.

98. Victorson DE, Choi S, Judson MA, et al. Development and testing of item response theory-based item banks and short forms for eye, skin and lung problems in sarcoidosis. Qual Life Res 2014;23(4):1301–13.

99. Boivin A, Lehoux P, Lacombe R, et al. Involving patients in setting priorities for healthcare improvement: a cluster randomized trial. Implement Sci 2014;9:24.

100. Baughman RP, Winget DB, Lower EE. Methotrexate is steroid sparing in acute sarcoidosis: results of a double blind, randomized trial. Sarcoidosis Vasc Diffuse Lung Dis 2000;17(1):60–6.

101. Huscher D, Thiele K, Gromnica-Ihle E, et al. Dose-related patterns of glucocorticoid-induced side effects. Ann Rheum Dis 2009;68(7):1119–24.

102. Schutt AC, Bullington WM, Judson MA. Pharmacotherapy for pulmonary sarcoidosis: a Delphi consensus study. Respir Med 2010;104(5):717–23.

103. McKinzie BP, Bullington WM, Mazur JE, et al. Efficacy of short-course, low-dose corticosteroid therapy for acute pulmonary sarcoidosis exacerbations. Am J Med Sci 2010;339(1):1–4.

104. Israel HL, Fouts DW, Beggs RA. A controlled trial of prednisone treatment of sarcoidosis. Am Rev Respir Dis 1973;107(4):609–14.

105. Sharma OP, Colp C, Williams MH Jr. Course of pulmonary sarcoidosis with and without corticosteroid therapy as determined by pulmonary function studies. Am J Med 1966;41(4):541–51.

106. James DG, Carstairs LS, Trowell J, et al. Treatment of sarcoidosis. Report of a controlled therapeutic trial. Lancet 1967;2(7515):526–8.

107. Goldstein DS, Williams MH. Rate of improvement of pulmonary function in sarcoidosis during treatment with corticosteroids. Thorax 1986;41(6):473–4.

108. Baughman RP, Iannuzzi MC, Lower EE, et al. Use of fluticasone in acute symptomatic pulmonary sarcoidosis. Sarcoidosis Vasc Diffuse Lung Dis 2002;19(3):198–204.

109. Johns CJ, Schonfeld SA, Scott PP, et al. Longitudinal study of chronic sarcoidosis with low-dose maintenance corticosteroid therapy. Outcome and complications. Ann N Y Acad Sci 1986;465:702–12.

110. Gonnelli S, Rottoli P, Cepollaro C, et al. Prevention of corticosteroid-induced osteoporosis with alendronate in sarcoid patients. Calcif Tissue Int 1997;61(5):382–5.

111. Stern PH, De Olazabal J, Bell NH. Evidence for abnormal regulation of circulating 1 alpha,25-dihydroxyvitamin D in patients with sarcoidosis and normal calcium metabolism. J Clin Invest 1980;66(4):852–5.

112. Pietinalho A, Tukiainen P, Haahtela T, et al. Oral prednisolone followed by inhaled budesonide in newly diagnosed pulmonary sarcoidosis: a

double-blind, placebo-controlled multicenter study. Finnish Pulmonary Sarcoidosis study group. Chest 1999;116(2):424–31.

113. Alberts C, van der Mark TW, Jansen HM. Inhaled budesonide in pulmonary sarcoidosis: a double-blind, placebo-controlled study. Dutch study group on pulmonary sarcoidosis. Eur Respir J 1995;8(5): 682–8.

114. Erkkila S, Fröseth B, Hellström PE, et al. Inhaled budesonide influences cellular and biochemical abnormalities in pulmonary sarcoidosis. Sarcoidosis 1988;5(2):106–10.

115. Milman N, Graudal N, Grode G, et al. No effect of high-dose inhaled steroids in pulmonary sarcoidosis: a double-blind, placebo-controlled study. J Intern Med 1994;236(3):285–90.

116. Zych D, Pawlicka L, Zielinski J. Inhaled budesonide vs prednisone in the maintenance treatment of pulmonary sarcoidosis. Sarcoidosis 1993;10(1): 56–61.

117. du Bois RM, Greenhalgh PM, Southcott AM, et al. Randomized trial of inhaled fluticasone propionate in chronic stable pulmonary sarcoidosis: a pilot study. Eur Respir J 1999;13(6):1345–50.

118. Chan ES, Cronstein BN. Molecular action of methotrexate in inflammatory diseases. Arthritis Res 2002;4(4):266–73.

119. Vorselaars AD, Wuyts WA, Vorselaars VM, et al. Methotrexate versus azathioprine in second line therapy of sarcoidosis. Chest 2013;144(3):805–12.

120. Baughman RP, Lower EE. Alternatives to corticosteroids in the treatment of sarcoidosis. Sarcoidosis Vasc Diffuse Lung Dis 1997;14(2):121–30.

121. Lower EE, Baughman RP. Prolonged use of methotrexate for sarcoidosis. Arch Intern Med 1995; 155(8):846–51.

122. Veien NK, Brodthagen H. Cutaneous sarcoidosis treated with methotrexate. Br J Dermatol 1977; 97(2):213–6.

123. Dev S, McCallum RM, Jaffe GJ. Methotrexate treatment for sarcoid-associated panuveitis. Ophthalmology 1999;106(1):111–8.

124. Webster GF, Razsi LK, Sanchez M, et al. Weekly low-dose methotrexate therapy for cutaneous sarcoidosis. J Am Acad Dermatol 1991;24(3):451–4.

125. Jundt JW, Browne BA, Fiocco GP, et al. A comparison of low dose methotrexate bioavailability: oral solution, oral tablet, subcutaneous and intramuscular dosing. J Rheumatol 1993; 20(11):1845–9.

126. Baughman RP, Lower EE. A clinical approach to the use of methotrexate for sarcoidosis. Thorax 1999;54(8):742–6.

127. Cremers JP, Drent M, Bast A, et al. Multinational evidence-based World Association of Sarcoidosis and Other Granulomatous Disorders recommendations for the use of methotrexate in sarcoidosis: integrating systematic literature research and expert opinion of sarcoidologists worldwide. Curr Opin Pulm Med 2013;19(5):545–61.

128. van Ede AE, Laan RF, Rood MJ, et al. Effect of folic or folinic acid supplementation on the toxicity and efficacy of methotrexate in rheumatoid arthritis: a forty-eight week, multicenter, randomized, double-blind, placebo-controlled study. Arthritis Rheum 2001;44(7):1515–24.

129. Morgan SL, Baggott JE, Vaughn WH, et al. Supplementation with folic acid during methotrexate therapy for rheumatoid arthritis. A double-blind, placebo-controlled trial. Ann Intern Med 1994; 121(11):833–41.

130. Pacheco Y, Marechal C, Marechal F, et al. Azathioprine treatment of chronic pulmonary sarcoidosis. Sarcoidosis 1985;2(2):107–13.

131. Lennard L, Van Loon JA, Weinshilboum RM. Pharmacogenetics of acute azathioprine toxicity: relationship to thiopurine methyltransferase genetic polymorphism. Clin Pharmacol Ther 1989;46(2): 149–54.

132. Khan N, Abbas AM, Lichtenstein GR, et al. Risk of lymphoma in patients with ulcerative colitis treated with thiopurines: a nationwide retrospective cohort study. Gastroenterology 2013;145(5): 1007–15.e3.

133. Sahoo DH, Bandyopadhyay D, Xu M, et al. Effectiveness and safety of leflunomide for pulmonary and extrapulmonary sarcoidosis. Eur Respir J 2011;38(5):1145–50.

134. Baughman RP, Lower EE. Leflunomide for chronic sarcoidosis. Sarcoidosis Vasc Diffuse Lung Dis 2004;21(1):43–8.

135. Food and Drug Administration. Labeling information: leflunomide. 2005. Available at: http://www.ncbi.nlm.nih.gov/pubmed/. Accessed September 29, 2015.

136. Emery P, Breedveld FC, Lemmel EM, et al. A comparison of the efficacy and safety of leflunomide and methotrexate for the treatment of rheumatoid arthritis. Rheumatology (Oxford) 2000; 39(6):655–65.

137. Smolen JS, Kalden JR, Scott DL, et al. Efficacy and safety of leflunomide compared with placebo and sulphasalazine in active rheumatoid arthritis: a double-blind, randomised, multicentre trial. European Leflunomide Study Group. Lancet 1999; 353(9149):259–66.

138. Strand V, Cohen S, Schiff M, et al. Treatment of active rheumatoid arthritis with leflunomide compared with placebo and methotrexate. Leflunomide Rheumatoid Arthritis Investigators Group. Arch Intern Med 1999;159(21):2542–50.

139. Bharadwaj A, Haroon N. Peripheral neuropathy in patients on leflunomide. Rheumatology (Oxford) 2004;43(7):934.

140. Carulli MT, Davies UM. Peripheral neuropathy: an unwanted effect of leflunomide? Rheumatology (Oxford) 2002;41(8):952–3.

141. Bonnel RA, Graham DJ. Peripheral neuropathy in patients treated with leflunomide. Clin Pharmacol Ther 2004;75(6):580–5.

142. Bhat P, Cervantes-Castañeda RA, Doctor PP, et al. Mycophenolate mofetil therapy for sarcoidosis-associated uveitis. Ocul Immunol Inflamm 2009; 17(3):185–90.

143. Hamzeh N, Voelker A, Forssén A, et al. Efficacy of mycophenolate mofetil in sarcoidosis. Respir Med 2014;108(11):1663–9.

144. Brill AK, Ott SR, Geiser T. Effect and safety of mycophenolate mofetil in chronic pulmonary sarcoidosis: a retrospective study. Respiration 2012; 86(5):376–83.

145. Androdias G, Khan TA, Shetty AK, et al. Mycophenolate mofetil may be effective in CNS sarcoidosis but not in sarcoid myopathy. Neurology 2011; 76(13):1168–72.

146. Moravan M, Segal BM. Treatment of CNS sarcoidosis with infliximab and mycophenolate mofetil. Neurology 2009;72(4):337–40.

147. Corbett J. Treating CNS sarcoidosis with infliximab and mycophenolate mofetil. Curr Neurol Neurosci Rep 2009;9(5):339–40.

148. Moudgil A, Przygodzki RM, Kher KK. Successful steroid-sparing treatment of renal limited sarcoidosis with mycophenolate mofetil. Pediatr Nephrol 2006;21(2):281–5.

149. MacPhee IA, Spreafico S, Bewick M, et al. Pharmacokinetics of mycophenolate mofetil in patients with end-stage renal failure. Kidney Int 2000;57(3): 1164–8.

150. Drent M, Cremers JP, Jansen TL, et al. Practical eminence and experience-based recommendations for use of TNF-alpha inhibitors in sarcoidosis. Sarcoidosis Vasc Diffuse Lung Dis 2014;31(2):91–107.

151. Sodhi M, Pearson K, White ES, et al. Infliximab therapy rescues cyclophosphamide failure in severe central nervous system sarcoidosis. Respir Med 2009;103(2):268–73.

152. Stagaki E, Mountford WK, Lackland DT, et al. The treatment of lupus pernio: the results of 116 treatment courses in 54 patients. Chest 2008;135(2): 468–76.

153. Judson MA, Baughman RP, Costabel U, et al. The potential additional benefit of infliximab in patients with chronic pulmonary sarcoidosis already receiving corticosteroids: a retrospective analysis from a randomized clinical trial. Respir Med 2014; 108(1):189–94.

154. Baughman RP, Lower EE, Drent M. Inhibitors of tumor necrosis factor (TNF) in sarcoidosis: who, what, and how to use them. Sarcoidosis Vasc Diffuse Lung Dis 2008;25(2):76–89.

155. Keane J, Gershon S, Wise RP, et al. Tuberculosis associated with infliximab, a tumor necrosis factor alpha-neutralizing agent. N Engl J Med 2001; 345(15):1098–104.

156. Wallis RS, Broder M, Wong J, et al. Granulomatous infections due to tumor necrosis factor blockade: correction. Clin Infect Dis 2004;39(8):1254–5.

157. Chung ES, Packer M, Lo KH, et al. Randomized, double-blind, placebo-controlled, pilot trial of infliximab, a chimeric monoclonal antibody to tumor necrosis factor-alpha, in patients with moderate-to-severe heart failure: results of the anti-TNF Therapy Against Congestive Heart Failure (ATTACH) trial. Circulation 2003;107(25):3133–40.

158. Uthman I, Touma Z, Khoury M. Cardiac sarcoidosis responding to monotherapy with infliximab. Clin Rheumatol 2007;26(11):2001–3.

159. Barnabe C, McMeekin J, Howarth A, et al. Successful treatment of cardiac sarcoidosis with infliximab. J Rheumatol 2008;35(8):1686–7.

160. Atzeni F, Talotta R, Salaffi F, et al. Immunogenicity and autoimmunity during anti-TNF therapy. Autoimmun Rev 2013;12(7):703–8.

161. Sandborn WJ. Optimizing anti-tumor necrosis factor strategies in inflammatory bowel disease. Curr Gastroenterol Rep 2003;5(6):501–5.

162. Rutgeerts P, Van Assche G, Vermeire S. Optimizing anti-TNF treatment in inflammatory bowel disease. Gastroenterology 2004;126(6):1593–610.

163. Finckh A, Dehler S, Gabay C, et al. The effectiveness of leflunomide as a co-therapy of tumour necrosis factor inhibitors in rheumatoid arthritis: a population-based study. Ann Rheum Dis 2009; 68(1):33–9.

164. Panselinas E, Rodgers JK, Judson MA. Clinical outcomes in sarcoidosis after cessation of infliximab treatment. Respirology 2009;14(4):522–8.

165. Baughman RP, Drent M, Kavuru M, et al. Infliximab therapy in patients with chronic sarcoidosis and pulmonary involvement. Am J Respir Crit Care Med 2006;174(7):795–802.

166. Judson MA, Baughman RP, Costabel U, et al. Efficacy of infliximab in extrapulmonary sarcoidosis: results from a randomised trial. Eur Respir J 2008;31(6):1189–96.

167. Carter JD, Valeriano J, Vasey FB, et al. Refractory neurosarcoidosis: a dramatic response to infliximab. Am J Med 2004;117(4):277–9.

168. Doty JD, Mazur JE, Judson MA. Treatment of sarcoidosis with infliximab. Chest 2005;127(3):1064–71.

169. Saleh S, Ghodsian S, Yakimova V, et al. Effectiveness of infliximab in treating selected patients with sarcoidosis. Respir Med 2006;100(11):2053–9.

170. Erckens RJ, Mostard RL, Wijnen PA, et al. Adalimumab successful in sarcoidosis patients with refractory chronic non-infectious uveitis. Graefes Arch Clin Exp Ophthalmol 2012;250(5):713–20.

171. Kamphuis LS, Lam-Tse WK, Dik WA, et al. Efficacy of adalimumab in chronically active and symptomatic patients with sarcoidosis. Am J Respir Crit Care Med 2011;184(10):1214–6.

172. Milman N, Graudal N, Loft A, et al. Effect of the TNF-alpha inhibitor adalimumab in patients with recalcitrant sarcoidosis: a prospective observational study using FDG-PET. Clin Respir J 2012; 6(4):238–47.

173. Pariser RJ, Paul J, Hirano S, et al. A double-blind, randomized, placebo-controlled trial of adalimumab in the treatment of cutaneous sarcoidosis. J Am Acad Dermatol 2013;68(5):765–73.

174. Sandborn WJ, Hanauer SB, Rutgeerts P, et al. Adalimumab for maintenance treatment of Crohn's disease: results of the CLASSIC II trial. Gut 2007; 56(9):1232–9.

175. Judson MA, Baughman RP, Costabel U, et al. Safety and efficacy of ustekinumab or golimumab in patients with chronic sarcoidosis. Eur Respir J 2014;44(5):1296–307.

176. Utz JP, Limper AH, Kalra S, et al. Etanercept for the treatment of stage II and III progressive pulmonary sarcoidosis. Chest 2003;124(1):177–85.

177. Baughman RP, Lower EE, Bradley DA, et al. Etanercept for refractory ocular sarcoidosis: results of a double-blind randomized trial. Chest 2005;128(2): 1062–147.

178. Wallace DJ, Gudsoorkar VS, Weisman MH, et al. New insights into mechanisms of therapeutic effects of antimalarial agents in SLE. Nat Rev Rheumatol 2012;8(9):522–33.

179. Adams JS, Diz MM, Sharma OP. Effective reduction in the serum 1,25-dihydroxyvitamin D and calcium concentration in sarcoidosis-associated hypercalcemia with short-course chloroquine therapy. Ann Intern Med 1989;111(5):437–8.

180. Siltzbach LE, Teirstein AS. Chloroquine therapy in 43 patients with intrathoracic and cutaneous sarcoidosis. Acta Med Scand Suppl 1964;425:302–8.

181. Zic JA, Horowitz DH, Arzubiaga C, et al. Treatment of cutaneous sarcoidosis with chloroquine. Review of the literature. Arch Dermatol 1991;127(7):1034–40.

182. Baltzan M, Mehta S, Kirkham TH, et al. Randomized trial of prolonged chloroquine therapy in advanced pulmonary sarcoidosis. Am J Respir Crit Care Med 1999;160(1):192–7.

183. Berkovich R, Agius MA. Mechanisms of action of ACTH in the management of relapsing forms of multiple sclerosis. Ther Adv Neurol Disord 2014; 7(2):83–96.

184. Catania A, Lonati C, Sordi A, et al. The melanocortin system in control of inflammation. ScientificWorldJournal 2010;10:1840–53.

185. Olson JA, Steffensen EH, Margulis RR, et al. Effect of ACTH on certain inflammatory diseases of the eye. JAMA 1950;45(3):274–300.

186. Miller MM, Bass HE. Effect of ACTHAR-C (ACTH) in sarcoidosis. Ann Intern Med 1952; 37(4):776–84.

187. Brincker H. Granulomatous lesions of unknown significance: the GLUS syndrome. In: James D, editor. Sarcoidosis and other granulomatous disorders. New York: Marcel Dekker; 1994. p. 69–76.

188. Doty JD, Mazur JE, Judson MA. Treatment of corticosteroid-resistant neurosarcoidosis with a short-course cyclophosphamide regimen. Chest 2003;124(5):2023–6.

189. Goldszer RC, Galvanek EG, Lazarus JM. Glomerulonephritis in a patient with sarcoidosis. Report of a case and review of the literature. Arch Pathol Lab Med 1981;105(9):478–81.

190. Kataria YP. Chlorambucil in sarcoidosis. Chest 1980;78(1):36–43.

191. Baughman RP, Judson MA, Teirstein AS, et al. Thalidomide for chronic sarcoidosis. Chest 2002; 122(1):227–32.

192. Droitcourt C, Rybojad M, Porcher R, et al. A randomized, investigator-masked, double-blind, placebo-controlled trial on thalidomide in severe cutaneous sarcoidosis. Chest 2014; 146(4):1046–54.

193. Fazzi P, Manni E, Cristofani R, et al. Thalidomide for improving cutaneous and pulmonary sarcoidosis in patients resistant or with contraindications to corticosteroids. Biomed Pharmacother 2012; 66(4):300–7.

194. Bachelez H, Senet P, Cadranel J, et al. The use of tetracyclines for the treatment of sarcoidosis. Arch Dermatol 2001;137(1):69–73.

195. Park MK, Fontana Jr, Babaali H, et al. Steroid-sparing effects of pentoxifylline in pulmonary sarcoidosis. Sarcoidosis Vasc Diffuse Lung Dis 2009;26(2):121–31.

196. Zabel P, Entzian P, Dalhoff K, et al. Pentoxifylline in treatment of sarcoidosis. Am J Respir Crit Care Med 1997;155(5):1665–9.

197. Sweiss NJ, Lower EE, Mirsaeidi M, et al. Rituximab in the treatment of refractory pulmonary sarcoidosis. Eur Respir J 2014;43(5):1525–8.

198. Lower EE, Baughman RP, Kaufman AH. Rituximab for refractory granulomatous eye disease. Clin Ophthalmol 2012;6:1613–8.

199. Beccastrini E, Vannozzi L, Bacherini D, et al. Successful treatment of ocular sarcoidosis with rituximab. Ocul Immunol Inflamm 2013;21(3):244–6.

200. Baughman RP, Judson MA, Ingledue R, et al. Efficacy and safety of apremilast in chronic cutaneous sarcoidosis. Arch Dermatol 2012;148(2):262–4.

201. Baughman RP, Culver DA, Jankovi V, et al. Placenta-derived mesenchymal-like cells (PDA-001) as therapy for chronic pulmonary sarcoidosis: a phase 1 study. Sarcoidosis Vasc Diffuse Lung Dis 2015;32(2):106–14.

Index

Note: Page numbers of article titles are in **boldface** type.

A

ACTH gel. See Adrenocorticotropic hormone (ACTH) gel
Adalimumab
  in sarcoidosis management, 759–760
Adaptive immune system
  in sarcoidosis immunopathogenesis, 551–554
    alveolar macrophages, 551–552
    APCs, 551
    T cells, 552–554 (See also T cells)
Admixture mapping studies
  in genetic epidemiology of sarcoidosis, 571
Adrenocorticotropic hormone (ACTH) gel
  in sarcoidosis management, 760–761
Air trapping
  in sarcoidosis diagnosis, 608
Alveolar macrophages
  in sarcoidosis immunopathogenesis, 551–552
Alveolar sarcoidosis
  large parenchymal nodules and, 606
Angiolupoid sarcoidosis, 690
Annexin A11
  in sarcoidosis, 578–579
Antigen(s)
  infectious
    in sarcoidosis pathogenesis, **561–568**
Antigen-presenting cells (APCs)
  in sarcoidosis immunopathogenesis, 551
Antimalarial agents
  in sarcoidosis management, 760
Antimicrobial agents
  in sarcoidosis
    clinical trials of, 565–566
Anxiety
  sarcoidosis and, 730–731
APCs. See Antigen-presenting cells (APCs)
Arrhythmia(s)
  atrial
    cardiac sarcoidosis and
      management of, 665
  ventricular
    cardiac sarcoidosis and
      management of, 663–664
Atrial arrhythmias
  cardiac sarcoidosis and
    management of, 665
Atrophic sarcoidosis, 690
Autonomic dysfunction
  sarcoidosis and, 729

B

Azathioprine
  in sarcoidosis management, 758

BAL. See Bronchoalveolar lavage (BAL)
Bioaerosol(s)
  microbial
    in sarcoidosis pathogenesis, 561
Biologic agents
  in sarcoid uveitis management, 677–678
Biomarker(s)
  in sarcoidosis
    genome-based approaches in identifying, **621–630** (See also Sarcoidosis, biomarkers in)
Blood
  gene signatures in
    in sarcoidosis diagnosis, 624–625
Blood gene expression profiling
  in sarcoidosis vs. TB, 625–626
Bronchoalveolar lavage (BAL)
  in pulmonary sarcoidosis, 635–636
BTNL2. See Butyrophilinlike 2 (BTNL2)
Butyrophilinlike 2 (BTNL2)
  in sarcoidosis, 576

C

Candidate gene studies
  in genetic epidemiology of sarcoidosis, 570–571
Cardiac magnetic resonance (CMR)
  in cardiac sarcoidosis diagnosis, 665
Cardiac sarcoidosis, **657–668**
  atrial arrhythmias in
    management of, 665
  clinical management of, 660–661
  clinical manifestations of, 657
  conduction abnormalities in
    management of, 662–663
  diagnosis of, 657–659
    CMR in, 665
  epidemiology of, 657
  future directions in, 665–666
  left ventricular dysfunction in
    management of, 661
  prognosis of, 659–660
  sudden cardiac death related to
    risk stratification for, 664–665

Clin Chest Med 36 (2015) 769–776
http://dx.doi.org/10.1016/S0272-5231(15)00129-X
0272-5231/15/$ – see front matter © 2015 Elsevier Inc. All rights reserved

United States Postal Service

Statement of Ownership, Management, and Circulation
(All Periodicals Publications Except Requestor Publications)

1. Publication Title: Clinics in Chest Medicine

2. Publication Number: 0 0 0 - 7 0 6

3. Filing Date: 9/18/15

4. Issue Frequency: Mar, Jun, Sep, Dec

5. Number of Issues Published Annually: 4

6. Annual Subscription Price: $345.00

7. Complete Mailing Address of Known Office of Publication (Not printer) (Street, city, county, state, and ZIP+4®):
Elsevier Inc.
360 Park Avenue South
New York, NY 10010-1710

Contact Person: Stephen R. Bushing

Telephone (Include area code): 215-239-3688

8. Complete Mailing Address of Headquarters or General Business Office of Publisher (Not printer):
Elsevier Inc., 360 Park Avenue South, New York, NY 10010-1710

9. Full Names and Complete Mailing Addresses of Publisher, Editor, and Managing Editor (Do not leave blank)

Publisher (Name and complete mailing address):
Linda Belfus, Elsevier Inc., 1600 John F. Kennedy Blvd., Suite 1800, Philadelphia, PA 19103

Editor (Name and complete mailing address):
Patrick Manley, Elsevier Inc., 1600 John F. Kennedy Blvd., Suite 1800, Philadelphia, PA 19103-2899

Managing Editor (Name and complete mailing address):
Adrianne Brigido, Elsevier Inc., 1600 John F. Kennedy Blvd., Suite 1800, Philadelphia, PA 19103-2899

10. Owner (Do not leave blank. If the publication is owned by a corporation, give the name and address of the corporation immediately followed by the names and addresses of all stockholders owning or holding 1 percent or more of the total amount of stock. If not owned by a corporation, give the names and addresses of the individual owners. If owned by a partnership or other unincorporated firm, give its name and address as well as those of each individual owner. If the publication is published by a nonprofit organization, give its name and address.)

Full Name	Complete Mailing Address
Wholly owned subsidiary of	1600 John F. Kennedy Blvd, Ste. 1800
Reed/Elsevier, US holdings	Philadelphia, PA 19103-2899

11. Known Bondholders, Mortgagees, and Other Security Holders Owning or Holding 1 Percent or More of Total Amount of Bonds, Mortgages, or Other Securities. If none, check box. ☐ None

Full Name	Complete Mailing Address
N/A	

12. Tax Status (For completion by nonprofit organizations authorized to mail at nonprofit rates) (Check one)
The purpose, function, and nonprofit status of this organization and the exempt status for federal income tax purposes:
☐ Has Not Changed During Preceding 12 Months
☐ Has Changed During Preceding 12 Months (Publisher must submit explanation of change with this statement)

13. Publication Title: Clinics in Chest Medicine

14. Issue Date for Circulation Data Below: September 2015

15. Extent and Nature of Circulation	Average No. Copies Each Issue During Preceding 12 Months	No. Copies of Single Issue Published Nearest to Filing Date
a. Total Number of Copies (Net press run)	1019	865
b. Legitimate Paid and/Or Requested Distribution (By Mail and Outside the Mail) (1) Mailed Outside-County Paid/Requested Mail Subscriptions stated on PS Form 3541. (Include paid distribution above nominal rate, advertiser's proof copies and exchange copies)	532	404
(2) Mailed In-County Paid/Requested Mail Subscriptions stated on PS Form 3541. (Include paid distribution above nominal rate, advertiser's proof copies and exchange copies)		
(3) Paid Distribution Outside the Mails Including Sales Through Dealers And Carriers, Street Vendors, Counter Sales, and Other Paid Distribution Outside USPS®	204	231
(4) Paid Distribution by Other Classes of Mail Through the USPS (e.g. First-Class Mail®)		
c. Total Paid and/or Requested Circulation (Sum of 15b (1), (2), (3), and (4))	736	635
d. Free or Nominal Rate Distribution (By Mail and Outside the Mail) (1) Free or Nominal Rate Outside-County Copies included on PS Form 3541	65	63
(2) Free or Nominal Rate In-County Copies included on PS Form 3541		
(3) Free or Nominal Rate Copies mailed at Other classes Through the USPS (e.g. First-Class Mail)		
(4) Free or Nominal Rate Distribution Outside the Mail (Carriers or Other means)		
e. Total Nonrequested Distribution (Sum of 15d (1), (2), (3) and (4))	65	63
f. Total Distribution (Sum of 15c and 15e)	801	698
g. Copies not Distributed (See instructions to publishers #4 (page #3))	218	167
h. Total (Sum of 15f and g)	1019	865
i. Percent Paid and/or Requested Circulation (15c divided by 15f times 100)	91.89%	90.97%

If you are claiming electronic copies go to line 16 on page 3. If you are not claiming Electronic copies, skip to line 17 on page 3.

16. Electronic Copy Circulation	Average No. Copies Each Issue During Preceding 12 Months	No. Copies of Single Issue Published Nearest to Filing Date
a. Paid Electronic Copies		
b. Total paid Print Copies (Line 15c) + Paid Electronic copies (Line 16a)		
c. Total Print Distribution (Line 15f) + Paid Electronic Copies (Line 16a)		
d. Percent Paid (Both Print & Electronic copies) (16b divided by 16c X 100)		

☐ **I certify that 50% of all my distributed copies (electronic and print) are paid above a nominal price.**

17. Publication of Statement of Ownership
If the publication is a general publication, publication of this statement is required. Will be printed in the **December 2015** issue of this publication.

18. Signature and Title of Editor, Publisher, Business Manager, or Owner

Stephen R. Bushing

Stephen R. Bushing – Inventory Distribution Coordinator

Date: September 18, 2015

I certify that all information furnished on this form is true and complete. I understand that anyone who furnishes false or misleading information on this form or who omits material or information requested on the form may be subject to criminal sanctions (including fines and imprisonment) and/or civil sanctions (including civil penalties).

PS Form 3526, July 2014 (Page 3 of 3) PSN 7530-01-000-9931 **PRIVACY NOTICE:** See our Privacy policy in www.usps.com.

PS Form 3526, July 2014 (Page 1 of 3) (Instructions Page 3))

Moving?

Make sure your subscription moves with you!

To notify us of your new address, find your **Clinics Account Number** (located on your mailing label above your name), and contact customer service at:

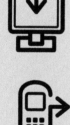

Email: journalscustomerservice-usa@elsevier.com

800-654-2452 (subscribers in the U.S. & Canada)
314-447-8871 (subscribers outside of the U.S. & Canada)

Fax number: 314-447-8029

Elsevier Health Sciences Division
Subscription Customer Service
3251 Riverport Lane
Maryland Heights, MO 63043

*To ensure uninterrupted delivery of your subscription, please notify us at least 4 weeks in advance of move.

ELSEVIER

Printed and bound by CPI Group (UK) Ltd, Croydon, CR0 4YY

03/10/2024

01040379-0001